PROGRESS IN CLINICAL AND BIOLOGICAL RESEARCH

RECENT TITLES

Please contact the publisher for information about previous titles in this series.

SKIN CARCINOGENESIS
Mechanisms and
Human Relevance

SKIN CARCINOGENESIS
Mechanisms and
Human Relevance

Proceedings of the Symposium Dermal Carcinogenesis: Research Directions for
Human Relevance, Held in Austin, Texas, December 1–4, 1987

Editors

Thomas J. Slaga
Department of Carcinogenesis
University of Texas
M.D. Anderson Cancer Center
Science Park—Research Division
Smithville, Texas

Andre J.P. Klein-Szanto
Department of Pathology
Fox Chase Cancer Center
Philadelphia, Pennsylvania

R.K. Boutwell
Department of Oncology
University of
Wisconsin Medical School
McArdle Laboratory for
Cancer Research
Madison, Wisconsin

Donald E. Stevenson
Shell Oil Company
Houston, Texas

Hugh L. Spitzer
American Petroleum Institute
Washington, D.C.

Bob D'Motto
Proctor and Gamble
Cincinnati, Ohio

ALAN R. LISS, INC. • NEW YORK

Address all Inquiries to the Publisher
Alan R. Liss, Inc., 41 East 11th Street, New York, NY 10003

While the authors, editors, and publisher believe that drug selection and dosage and the specifications and usage of equipment and devices, as set forth in this book, are in accord with current recommendations and practice at the time of publication, they accept no legal responsibility for any errors or omissions, and make no warranty, express or implied, with respect to material contained herein. In view of ongoing research, equipment modifications, changes in governmental regulations and the constant flow of information relating to drug therapy, drug reactions and the use of equipment and devices, the reader is urged to review and evaluate the information provided in the package insert or instructions for each drug, piece of equipment or device for, among other things, any changes in the instructions or indications of dosage or usage and for added warnings and precautions.

Library of Congress Cataloging-in-Publication Data

Skin carcinogenesis.

(Progress in clinical and biological research ;
v. 298)
    Includes index.
    1. Skin—Cancer—Etiology—Congresses.   2. Carcino-
genesis—Congresses.   I. Slaga, Thomas J.   II. Series.
[DNLM: 1. Skin Neoplasms—etiology—congresses.
WR 500 S62815 1987]
RC280.S5S585   1989   616.99′477071   89-2497
ISBN 0-8451-5148-7

Contents

Contributors

Thomas S. Argyris, Department of Pathology, State University of New York, Health Sciences Center, Syracuse, NY 13210 **[63]**

B. Bailleul, Beatson Institute for Cancer Research, Glasgow, Scotland G61 1BD, and U.124 INSERM, Institute de Recherches sur le Cancer, 59045 Lille Cedex, France **[137]**

James K. Baldwin, Department of Carcinogenesis, Science Park, The University of Texas M.D. Anderson Cancer Center, Smithville, TX 78957 **[249]**

Allan Balmain, Beatson Institute for Cancer Research, Glasgow, Scotland G61 1BD **[137]**

Martha A. Belury, Department of Carcinogenesis, Science Park, The University of Texas M.D. Anderson Cancer Center, Smithville, TX 78957 **[249]**

Peter M. Blumberg, Molecular Mechanisms of Tumor Promotion Section, Laboratory of Cellular Carcinogenesis and Tumor Promotion, National Cancer Institute, Bethesda, MD 20892 **[201]**

Keith Bonham, Department of Radiation Ocology, University of Arizona Health Sciences Center, Tucson, AZ 85724 **[147]**

R.K. Boutwell, Department of Oncology, University of Wisconsin Medical School, McArdle Laboratory for Cancer Research, Madison, WI 53706 **[xv,xix,3]**

G. Tim Bowden, Department of Radiation Oncology, University of Arizona Health Sciences Center, Tucson, AZ 85724 **[147]**

K. Brown, Beatson Institute for Cancer Research, Glasgow, Scotland G61 1BD **[137]**

Fredric J. Burns, Institute of Environmental Medicine, New York University Medical Center, New York, NY 10016 **[81]**

Gregory S. Cameron, Department of Carcinogenesis, Science Park, The University of Texas M.D. Anderson Cancer Center, Smithville, TX 78957 **[249]**

Peter H. Craig, Department of Environmental Health and Safety, Mobil Oil Corporation, Princeton, NJ 08540 **[381]**

The numbers in brackets are the opening page numbers of the contributors' articles.

Marie L. Dell'Aquila, Molecular Mechanisms of Tumor Promotion Section, Laboratory of Cellular Carcinogenesis and Tumor Promotion, National Cancer Institute, Bethesda, MD 20892 **[201]**

David J. de Vries, Molecular Mechanisms of Tumor Promotion Section, Laboratory of Cellular Carcinogenesis and Tumor Promotion, National Cancer Institute, Bethesda, MD 20892 **[201]**

John DiGiovanni, Department of Carcinogenesis, Science Park, The University of Texas M.D. Anderson Cancer Center, Smithville, TX 78957 **[167]**

Andrzej A. Dlugosz, Department of Dermatology, Hospital of the University of Pennsylvania, Philadelphia, PA 19104 **[213]**

Bob D'Motto, Proctor and Gamble, Cincinnati, OH 55247 **[xv,xix]**

Leonard Dzubow, Department of Dermatology, Hospital of the University of Pennsylvania, Philadelphia, PA 19104 **[213]**

William C. Eastin, Jr., Carcinogenesis and Toxicology Evaluation Branch, National Institute of Environmental Health Sciences, Research Triangle Park, NC 27709 **[295]**

Gerard F. Egan, Department of Toxicology, Exxon Biomedical Sciences, Inc., East Millstone, NJ 08875 **[363]**

Patricia A. Egner, Department of Environmental Health Sciences, Division of Biological Sciences, Johns Hopkins School of Hygiene and Public Health, Baltimore, MD 21205 **[233]**

Anthony J. Faras, Institute of Human Genetics and Department of Microbiology, University of Minnesota Medical School, Minneapolis, MN 55455 **[35]**

F. Fee, Beatson Institute for Cancer Research, Glasgow, Scotland G61 1BD **[137]**

Susan M. Fischer, Department of Carcinogenesis, Science Park, The University of Texas M.D. Anderson Cancer Center, Smithville, TX 78957 **[249]**

Hirota Fujiki, Cancer Prevention Division, National Cancer Center Research Institute, Tokyo 104, Japan **[281]**

Susan K. Gilmour, Wistar Institute, Philadelphia, PA 19104 **[213]**

Paul Grasso, Department of Experimental Pathology, Robens Institute, University of Surrey, Guildford, Surrey, England CR2 4AV **[17]**

Stephen S. Hecht, Division of Chemical Carcinogenesis, Naylor Dana Institute for Disease Prevention, American Health Foundation, Valhalla, NY 10595 **[331]**

Henry Hennings, Laboratory of Cellular Carcinogenesis and Tumor Promotion, National Cancer Institute, Bethesda, MD 20892 **[95,127]**

Oili Hietala, Wistar Institute, Philadelphia, PA 19104; present address: Department of Biochemistry, University of Oulu, Oulu, Finland **[213]**

Mitsuru Hirota, Cancer Prevention Division, National Cancer Center Research Institute, Tokyo 104, Japan **[281]**

Dietrich Hoffmann, Division of Environmental Carcinogenesis, Naylor Dana Institute for Disease Prevention, American Health Foundation, Valhalla, NY 10595 **[331]**

Deborah Jaffe, Department of Radiation Oncology, University of Chicago Medical School, Chicago, IL 60637 **[147]**

Susan Jaken, Alton Jones Cell Science Center, Lake Placid, NY 12946 **[127]**

Daniel W. Jasheway, Department of Carcinogenesis, Science Park, The University of Texas M.D. Anderson Cancer Center, Smithville, TX 78957 **[249]**

Ann R. Kennedy, Department of Radiation Oncology, University of Pennsylvania School of Medicine, Philadelphia, PA 19104 **[103]**

Thomas W. Kensler, Department of Environmental Health Sciences, Division of Toxicological Sciences, Johns Hopkins School of Hygiene and Public Health, Baltimore, MD 21205 **[233]**

Anne E. Kilkenny, Laboratory of Cellular Carcinogenesis and Tumor Promotion, National Cancer Institute, Bethesda, MD 20892 **[127]**

Andre J.P. Klein-Szanto, Department of Pathology, Fox Chase Cancer Center, Philadelphia, PA 19111 **[xv,xix,45]**

Kenneth H. Kraemer, Laboratory of Molecular Carcinogenesis, National Cancer Institute, Bethesda, MD 20892 **[25]**

Peter Krieg, Institute for Virus Research, German Cancer Research Center, 6900 Heidelberg, Federal Republic of Germany **[147]**

Stephen C. Lewis, Department of Toxicology, Exxon Biomedical Sciences, Inc., East Millstone, NJ 08875 **[363]**

Richard H. McKee, Department of Toxicology, Exxon Biomedical Sciences, Inc., East Millstone, NJ 08875 **[363]**

Assieh A. Melikian, Division of Environmental Carcinogenesis, Naylor Dana Institute for Disease Prevention, American Health Foundation, Valhalla, NY 10595 **[331]**

Hideki Nakakuma, Molecular Mechanisms of Tumor Promotion Section, Laboratory of Cellular Carcinogenesis and Tumor Promotion, National Cancer Institute, Bethesda, MD 20892 **[201]**

Stephen Nesnow, Carcinogenesis and Metabolism Branch, Health Effects Research Laboratory, U.S. Environmental Protection Agency, Research Triangle Park, NC 27711 **[347]**

Thomas G. O'Brien, Wistar Institute, Philadelphia, PA 19104 **[213]**

Kevin O'Donnell, Wistar Institute, Philadelphia, PA 19104 **[213]**

Ronald S. Ostrow, Institute of Human Genetics and Department of Microbiology, University of Minnesota Medical School, Minneapolis, MN 55455 **[35]**

Larry Ostrowski, Department of Radiation Oncology, University of Arizona Health Science Center, Tucson, AZ 85724 **[147]**

Kelly E. Patrick, Department of Carcinogenesis, Science Park, The University of Texas M.D. Anderson Cancer Center, Smithville, TX 78957 **[249]**

George R. Pettit, Cancer Research Institute and Department of Chemistry, Arizona State University, Tempe, AZ 85287 **[201]**

M. Ramsden, Department of Fermentation Development, Glaxochem Ltd., Ulverston, Cumbria, England **[137]**

James G. Rheinwald, Division of Cell Growth and Regulation, Dana-Farber Cancer Institute and Department of Cellular and Molecular Physiology, Harvard Medical School, Boston, MA 02115 **[113]**

Dennis R. Roop, Laboratory of Cellular Carcinogenesis and Tumor Promotion, National Cancer Institute, Bethesda, MD 20892 **[127]**

Loretta D. Schuman, Molecular Mechanisms of Tumor Promotion Section, Laboratory of Cellular Carcinogenesis and Tumor Promotion, National Cancer Institute, Bethesda, MD 20892 **[201]**

Nancy A. Sharkey, Molecular Mechanisms of Tumor Promotion Section, Laboratory of Cellular Carcinogenesis and Tumor Promotion, National Cancer Institute, Bethesda, MD 20892 **[201]**

B.J. Simpson, Department of Toxicology, Shell Internationale Petroleum Maatchappij, The Hague, The Netherlands **[393]**

Thomas J. Slaga, Department of Carcinogenesis, Science Park, The University of Texas M.D. Anderson Cancer Center, Smithville, TX 78957 **[xv,xix]**

Hugh L. Spitzer, American Petroleum Institute, Washington, DC 20006 **[xv,xix]**

Donald E. Stevenson, Shell Oil Company, Houston, TX 77210 **[xv,xix]**

James E. Strickland, Laboratory of Cellular Carcinogenesis and Tumor Promotion, National Cancer Institute, Bethesda, MD 20892 **[127]**

Masami Suganuma, Cancer Prevention Division, National Cancer Center Research Institute, Tokyo 104, Japan **[281]**

Takashi Sugimura, National Cancer Center, Tokyo 104, Japan **[281]**

Hiroko Suguri, Cancer Prevention Division, National Cancer Center Research Institute, Tokyo 104, Japan **[281]**

Arpad Szallasi, Molecular Mechanisms of Tumor Promotion Sections, Laboratory of Cellular Carcinogenesis and Tumor Promotion, National Cancer Institute, Bethesda, MD 20892 **[201]**

Bonita G. Taffe, Department of Environmental Health Sciences, Division of Toxicological Sciences, Johns Hopkins School of Hygiene and Public Health, Baltimore, MD 21205 and Laboratory of Human Carcinogenesis, National Cancer Institute, Bethesda, MD 20892 **[233]**

Kanji Takagi, Cancer Prevention Division, National Cancer Center Research Institute, Tokyo 104, Japan **[281]**

F.B. Thomas, Department of Toxicology, Shell Oil Company, Houston, TX 77002 **[393]**

Michael A. Trush, Department of Environmental Health Sciences, The Johns Hopkins School of Hygiene and Public Health, Baltimore, MD 21205 **[233]**

Robert Tucker, Department of Cell Physiology, Johns Hopkins Oncology Center, Baltimore, MD 21205 [127]

Barbour S. Warren, Molecular Mechanisms of Tumor Promotion Section, Laboratory of Cellular Carcinogenesis and Tumor Promotion, National Cancer Institute, Bethesda, MD 20892 [201]

William P. Watson, Environmental and Biochemical Toxicology Division, Shell Research Ltd., Sittingbourne Research Centre, Sittingbourne, Kent, England ME9 8AG [313]

Alan S. Wright, Environmental and Biochemical Toxicology Division, Shell Research Ltd., Sittingbourne Research Centre, Sittingbourne, Kent, England ME9 8AG [313]

Hiroshi Yamasaki, Program of Multistage Carcinogenesis, International Agency for Research on Cancer, 69372 Lyon Cedex 08, France [265]

Shigeru Yoshizawa, Cancer Prevention Division, National Cancer Center Research Institute, Tokyo 104, Japan [281]

Stuart H. Yuspa, Laboratory of Cellular Carcinogenesis and Tumor Promotion, National Cancer Institute, Bethesda, MD 20892 [127]

Preface

It has long been acknowledged that valuable scientific information concerning the etiology, the mechanisms of action, and the ultimate prevention of human cutaneous cancer can be obtained from both clinical and laboratory studies; therefore, a presentation of these studies by the world's leading scientists is especially relevant. This book, *Skin Carcinogenesis: Mechanisms and Human Relevance*, represents the most up-to-date knowledge of skin cancer and related scientific investigations. The skin is a major route of exposure to many environmental and industrial chemicals, as well as to radiation, and the effects of many potentially harmful agents on the skin of a variety of animal models have therefore been investigated. These studies not only provide knowledge pertaining directly to human skin cancer but provide insight into carcinogenesis in the general population.

This volume is a compilation of the proceedings of the conference "Dermal Carcinogenesis: Research Directions for Human Relevance" held in Austin, Texas Dec. 1–4, 1987. Included are chapters that discuss and evaluate mechanisms of carcinogenesis and the human relevance of animal studies in terms of risk assessment and future research needs. The skin as a target organ is discussed and the role of papillomaviruses is thoroughly analyzed, as are the metabolism of carcinogens and promoters in mouse skin and the importance and uniqueness of various model systems. The book also includes a comparative morphological evaluation of the effects of carcinogens and promoters. Tumor initiation and the consequences of exposure to initiating levels of carcinogens are examined, as well as cellular and biological aspects of promotion and progression. The biochemical and molecular aspects of promotion and progression are reviewed, including the roles of receptors and free radicals and the critical involvement of the arachidonic acid cascade in the process of tumor promotion. Finally, this volume addresses important considerations in using the skin model as an assay system. This assay system has become a valuable tool to both industry and governmental regulatory agencies. The data presented and the thorough examination of the most recent developments in dermal carcinogenesis further enhance man's understanding of the overall state of cancer research.

It is the general aim of this volume to carefully examine the important scientific role of dermal carcinogenesis and its significant influence on the entire field of carcinogenesis and cancer research. By compiling these findings, a valuable and in-depth resource is provided for the scientific investigator.

This volume will be of interest to cancer research scientists, dermatologists, toxicologists, pharmacologists, and biochemists, as well as radiation biologists and cellular and molecular biologists. Those in governmental administrative and regulatory agencies dealing with environmental health hazards will also find this volume helpful.

Thomas J. Slaga
Andre J.P. Klein-Szanto
R.K. Boutwell
Donald E. Stevenson
Hugh L. Spitzer
Bob D'Motto

Acknowledgments

The conference "Dermal Carcinogenesis: Research Directions for Human Relevance," on which this volume is based, was made possible by generous contributions from both academia and private industry. The conference organizers wish to sincerely thank Shell Oil Company, the R.J. Reynolds Tobacco Company, Harlan Sprague Dawley, Inc., Mobil Oil, Procter and Gamble, Rohm and Haas, and Allied Signal for their generous support. Also, contributions made by the American Industrial Health Council, the American Petroleum Institute, the Chemical Institute of Industrial Technology, EPA-ILSI Risk Science Institute–Cooperative Agreement, and The University of Texas M. D. Anderson Cancer Center Department of Carcinogenesis–Science Park are sincerely appreciated. Special thanks are extended to the Conference Organizing Committee: Thomas J. Slaga, Roswell K. Boutwell, Donald Stevenson, Byron Butterworth, Andre Klein-Szanto, John DiGiovanni, Bob D'Motto, and Jerry Smith. The details of conference organization were expertly directed by Karen Engel and her staff, Christie Hoy and LeNel Rice. For help in the preparation of this volume, I would especially like to thank Walter Pagel, director, and staff members Mary Markell and Edith K. Wilson of the Department of Scientific Publications at the University of Texas M. D. Anderson Cancer Center. Also, special thanks to Mary Slaga, a volunteer at Science Park, for assistance in final manuscript preparation.

Thomas J. Slaga

Introduction

In December 1987, the University of Texas M. D. Anderson Cancer Center in Science Park, Smithville, hosted the first conference on Research Directions for Human Relevance in Carcinogenesis. The first meeting of this series was entirely devoted to topics of cutaneous carcinogenesis. The program included invited lectures by leading scientists and physicians from the United States, Europe, and Japan.

This book represents the proceedings of that conference, including the discussions that followed each lecture. The major objective of this meeting was to bring together people from academia, regulatory agencies, industry, and public interest groups to discuss and evaluate the state-of-the-art knowledge on the skin as a target organ. Emphasis was placed on mechanisms, human relevance in terms of risk assessment, and future research needs.

Although a large part of the conference was devoted to describing and analyzing the latest developments in diverse but interrelated areas of basic science and clinical investigation, all authors made efforts to emphasize the human relevance of each experimental system.

The first part of this book includes overviews on chemical and viral carcinogenesis, genetic susceptibility, cutaneous bioassays, and the pathobiology of skin cancer. The use of the skin as an experimental model to study mechanisms of carcinogenesis is described in several chapters that contain the most recent advances in the cellular, biochemical, and molecular aspects of skin carcinogenesis. The final section includes a series of chapters devoted to the use of the skin as a bioassay for putative carcinogens, cocarcinogens, and promoters such as petroleum derivatives, tobacco products, and other environmentally relevant compounds.

Thomas J. Slaga
Andre J.P. Klein-Szanto
R.K. Boutwell
Donald E. Stevenson
Hugh L. Spitzer
Bob D'Motto

OVERVIEW

Skin Carcinogenesis: Mechanisms and Human Relevance, pages 3–15

Model Systems for Defining Initiation, Promotion, and Progression of Skin Neoplasms

R. K. Boutwell

McArdle Laboratory for Cancer Research, University of Wisconsin, Madison, Wisconsin 53706

Knowledge of the initiation and promotion components of carcinogenesis is very important in ascertaining carcinogenic hazards using animal assays that have a high degree of human relevance. There are a number of substances that at low levels of exposure do not elicit neoplasms of the skin of experimental animals. However, combinations of specific substances, if one is an initiator and it is followed by a promoter of cancer, cause many benign and malignant neoplasms. This observation, together with knowledge of the biology of this remarkable carcinogenic synergism, provides the basis for the design of tests for initiation and promotion.

In general, exposure of humans to carcinogens is at a level so low that the exposure is insufficient to cause cancer. However, humans are exposed to many different agents. The question that needs to be addressed is whether, among these combinations of different agents, there is synergism analogous to the initiation-promotion phenomenon in laboratory model systems.

The animal models can be easily adapted to assay for chemical, physical, or biological agents that may have human relevance. As shown by the data presented by Eastin in another chapter of this publication, the mouse model for initiation and promotion of skin neoplasms is readily and predictably standardizable for routine testing purposes. Initiation-promotion assays could be more informative of human risk than conventional tests in which maximally tolerated levels (plus perhaps two lower levels) of a substance are applied to the skin of mice for their entire life span.

To test for initiation, a single maximally tolerated level of test substance plus perhaps two lower levels need be applied only once to mouse skin. To reveal initiating potency of the test substance, an optimal-level dose of the very efficient promoting agent 12-O-tetradecanoylphorbol-13-acetate (hereafter referred to as TPA) is applied twice a week; if neoplasms do not appear after 1 year, it is likely that the test agent does not have initiating activity. Control mice treated with the potent initiator 7,12-dimethylbenz[a]anthracene (hereafter referred to as DMBA) followed by TPA will begin to show benign neoplasms within 6 weeks and malignant neoplasms within 20 weeks.

To test a substance for promoting activity, an amount of DMBA that is optimal for initiation is applied to the skin of the test animal. This is followed by twice-weekly (or more frequent) applications of several levels of the test substance.

In this chapter, several laboratory models for defining initiation, promotion, and progression of skin neoplasms are described. These models use both chemical and physical agents, and suitable species and strains are defined.

The chapter begins with a definition of terms that are used in describing aspects of skin carcinogenesis. This is followed by a discussion of the biology of multistage skin carcinogenesis. An understanding of the biology of the initiation and promotion procedure provides the background for the description of several models that may be appropriate to evaluate potential hazards for human skin.

DEFINITIONS

Cancer is a general term, commonly used, and is considered to be synonymous with malignant neoplasm. Cancer may develop in any tissue or organ.

A benign neoplasm is a heritably altered, relatively autonomous new growth of tissue that serves no physiological function.

A malignant neoplasm is a heritably altered, apparently autonomous new growth of tissue that differs from normal and benign growths in several ways. The primary distinguishing characteristics of malignant neoplasms are, first, the ability of the neoplasm to invade the surrounding normal tissue, and second, the ability of the malignant cells to migrate (metastasize) from the original site to distant sites where metastatic cancer may become established.

The word tumor is a general term, commonly used, and is considered to be synonymous with neoplasm. It is often preceded by the words benign or malignant. The word tumor is less precise than neoplasm, and the word tumor is used infrequently in this chapter.

A papilloma is a benign neoplasm of the skin. Papillomas originate in epidermal stem cells, especially those of the hair follicles, and are characterized by excessive production of keratin and a resemblance to human warts.

A carcinoma is a malignant neoplasm that originates in epidermal stem cells and may evolve from a papilloma or arise directly.

A carcinogen is an agent that causes a neoplasm by a two-step process involving initiation and promotion.

Initiation is accomplished in one or a few cells of a tissue that have been exposed to a carcinogen at a level that is insufficient to cause a neoplasm. A number of characteristics define the initiated cell, and these are described; included is the permanent nature of the change, which is attributable to specific changes in DNA that are caused by the initiating event.

Promotion involves a number of changes in an initiated cell, causing the initiated cell to grow faster than the surrounding normal cells and to develop into a visible neoplasm. As is true for agents that accomplish initiation, promoting agents alone do not or only rarely cause neoplasms to appear. However, following initiation, treatment with a promoting agent elicits both benign and malignant neoplasms.

Progression is a term that is applied to those changes in a benign neoplasm that result in malignancy and then in increased degrees of malignancy. The underlying changes, which occur at the molecular and genetic levels, are characterized by increased growth rate, increased independence from host support, invasive ability, and the potential for metastasis.

THE BIOLOGY OF INITIATION AND PROMOTION

A characteristic of experimental carcinogenesis of all organs, typified by skin, is the length of time that elapses from the first exposure to a carcinogen, be it chemical, physical, or viral, until a neoplasm appears. The induction time is dependent on a number of factors. Some carcinogens are potent, others vanishingly weak. The species and the strain within the species vary greatly, some being almost completely resistant to a given carcinogen while other species or strains develop neoplasms quickly. Age also determines susceptibility to carcinogenesis; the fetus at certain stages of development is sensitive, as are the newborn and the very young. The latter fact is proved in humans by the data on cancer mortality and age at the time of bombing in Hiroshima and Nagasaki. A major factor determining induction time is the dosage to which the animal is exposed. In all cases, increasing the level of exposure to either an initiator or a promoter both shortens the induction time and increases the incidence of neoplasms (1,2).

In some animal studies, the goal is to elicit neoplasms in the shortest possible time in order to ascertain the possible carcinogenicity of an agent. Hence, the maximally tolerated level of exposure is often employed. Irritation commonly accompanies these large doses of carcinogens. An inflammatory reaction is elicited in the skin, and the potent carcinogens are cytotoxic, i.e., they kill cells and cause skin wounds. These observations on cytotoxicity led to the investigation of the role of irritation in carcinogenesis. In this way, the first animal model that defined a role for wounding in the causation of skin cancer was reported in 1924 by Deelman (3). However, progress was slow, and it was another 20 years before the regimen now employed for initiation and promotion of skin tumors was established by Mottram (4). Specifically, Mottram applied a single application of benzo[a]pyrene to the skin of mice at a dose that did not elicit neoplasms. Multiple applications of croton oil, a very potent irritant, to the same site on the skin elicited many neoplasms, whereas the same regimen of croton oil to untreated skin elicited none.

It is interesting that for many years clinicians had associated irritation with the appearance of neoplasms in humans, and the word irritant was used synonymously with carcinogen. The tendency is retained by some clinicians, largely because a prominent pathologist, Cohnheim, asserted in 1880 that cancer arose by irritation of cells arrested at an embryonic stage. Hill, in 1761, used these words in attempting to explain the role of snuff in causing nasal cancer: "...whether the principles of the disorder were there before and the snuff only irritated the parts..." (5).

With a process as complex as carcinogenesis, it is advantageous to simplify investigations into the mechanism of the process by dividing it into components. However, in spite of the background information just presented, the model system devised by Mottram was not fully utilized for a number of years. Mottram and others chose croton oil for use in model systems because it is extremely irritating to skin. The active chemical component of croton oil, a phorbol ester called TPA, is now available. Only very small quantities of TPA, as small as 1 or 2 nmol, are required to promote skin tumors in some mice; these quantities cause minimal irritation.

By 1964 (2) the following facts had distinguished initiation and promotion as qualitatively different steps in skin carcinogenesis. For all carcinogens there is a dose sufficiently small that no skin tumors develop as a result of that dose, at least for practical purposes (Fig. 1, line 1). Some agents cause no cytotoxic or pleiotropic manifestations at initiating doses (6); examples include 7,12-dimethylbenz[a]anthracene (the most commonly used initiator), benzo[a]pyrene, and urethan. At initiating doses, the only defined consequence that is detectable (other than promotability) is the reaction of the initiator with nucleophilic sites; reaction with DNA resulting in permanent damage is probably the essential component of initiation (7). Current evidence indicates that initiation need only accomplish a heritable but unexpressed change in the DNA of a cell; no detectable change in the rate of DNA synthesis or cell division nor any change in enzyme activity is required. (The DNA of cells is monitored continually by enzymes that repair damage.) The initiated cell is not a dormant tumor cell. In the absence of a promoting stimulus, no tumors need result.

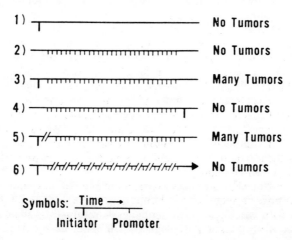

Figure 1. Schematic summary of the criteria that define initiation and promotion.

There also exist various agents known as promoters. These generally are not carcinogenic (Fig. 1, line 2), but when they are applied to initiated mouse skin repetitively over a period of weeks or months, many benign and some malignant tumors appear (Fig. 1, line 3), a remarkable synergistic action (2,8). However, if the treatment order is reversed, no tumors result (Fig. 1, line 4) (9). Clearly, a change is introduced into a cell by the initiator that is made manifest by treatment with the promoter.

In contradistinction to initiators, promoters cause a pleiotropic response; in other words, many changes in enzyme activity occur that are attributable to altered gene expression, and the tissues or cells exposed to the very potent promoters take on many of the morphologic characteristics of transformed tissues or cells (7).

There is another qualitative difference that distinguishes the action of an initiator from that of a promoter. An interval representing the greater part of a mouse's life may elapse after initiation and before promotion is begun, and yet tumors develop within 5 to 6 weeks after the beginning of promotion with TPA (Fig. 1, line 5) (10). In contrast, if intervals of 4 weeks elapse between applications of the promoter, promotion efficacy is lost (Fig. 1, line 6) (2). This phenomenon is one aspect of the reversibility of promotion.

The processes of initiation, promotion, and progression are diagrammed schematically in Figure 2. Normal cells are represented by the nine cells at the lower left; following exposure to a low, initiating dose of a carcinogen, one of them is shown with a dark nucleus that has sustained a permanent but unexpressed

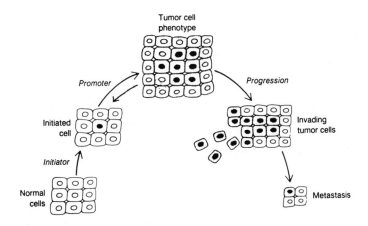

Figure 2. A simplified conception of the changes in cells produced by initiation (an unexpressed nuclear change), promotion (expression of the neoplastic phenotype), and progression (additional mutational changes leading to expression of the malignant phenotype).

change in its DNA. Exposure to a promoting agent causes changes in gene expression, resulting in many changes in the cytoplasm of the cells, including those responsible for an increased rate of cell division. Therefore, the number of all cells increases because of exposure to a promoting stimulus (see the uppermost drawing). After a sufficient exposure to a promoting agent, the changes in the initiated cells become irreversible, attributable to the defective DNA that was caused by the initiator. The irreversibly altered cells may progress to the malignant state (right, Fig. 2), and in the absence of continued exposure to the promoter, the uninitiated cells return to their original number.

PRELIMINARY TESTS FOR DOSE AND ACTIVITY

Rapid tests are advisable to evaluate the material in question.

Ames Test

It is reasonably certain that all initiators are mutagens or convert to mutagens. Many short-term tests exist to identify initiators/mutagens, one of which is the Ames test. The Ames test was designed to identify mutagens, and therefore potential initiators, with few false-negatives or false-positives (11). The relationship of short-term bioassay data on chemicals to their carcinogenic hazard to humans was reviewed by Pitot (12).

Inflammation

Some carcinogens/initiators and, in general, skin promoters cause an inflammatory reaction in the skin. A simple and useful assay for promoting activity was devised years ago. It was adopted by Hecker as a short-term assay for isolating TPA from croton oil. To do the assay, dissolve the test material in acetone (solvents will be discussed later) and apply a drop to a mouse ear. Only 2 or 3 mice are required plus untreated controls. The ears are observed for inflammation after about 12 h and again after 1 and 2 days. The response may range from a faint pink to a black, necrotic ear. A dose that results in an inflamed, red ear is near the maximum dose level that is suitable for long-term testing of a promoter by repeated application to the skin.

Hyperplasia

Without exception, promoting agents cause epidermal hyperplasia; 0.1 ml of a solution of the test agent should be applied to the shaved skin of the back of perhaps 2 to 6 mice. After 48 h, skin taken from the treated area is fixed, stained with hemotoxylin and eosin, and inspected for hyperplasia. If, compared with 2 or 3 cell layers from a control mouse, the epidermis shows increased numbers of cell layers, a dose level of a potential promoting agent has been found.

Miscellaneous Tests

There are a number of changes in mouse skin that have been associated with tumor promotion, including increases in the following responses: mitotic frequency, numbers of dark cells, ornithine decarboxylase activity, arachidonic acid cascade, oxygen-free radicals, and elimination of intercellular communication. Only rarely would the effort to establish one or more of the above assays be justified.

Intact Animal Toxicity

A preliminary test of perhaps 4 weeks during which the test substance is applied to the skin is essential to determine the maximally tolerable dose and frequency of application. The solvent to be used for the test substance should be applied to control animals, and an untreated group must be included in the preliminary test. Body weight must be checked because underweight animals tend to be resistant to carcinogenesis. Mild skin wounding is indicative of a near-maximum dose and frequency of application, and test dose levels should range downward. Systemic toxicity should be avoided because it may invalidate results.

Solvent

As a part of the preliminary animal testing, the choice of solvent, its volume, and the frequency of application must be established. A volatile solvent, low in toxicity, is preferable. Acetone is recommended because it evaporates rapidly, thereby diminishing toxic effects on the skin cells and leaving the test material in intimate contact with the skin. However, not all test substances are soluble in acetone in concentrations that may be required as determined by the preliminary tests for the appropriate dose level. A minimal quantity of a more polar solvent, such as alcohol, or of water may allow a mixture with acetone such that sufficient material is deposited on the skin. If nonvolatile solvents are used, the majority of the test substance is held away from the skin, becomes smeared over the animals and the cage, and frequently is cleaned from the skin by grooming and ends in the animal's stomach as it licks its paws (13). This is particularly true of solvents such as mineral oil. Although dimethyl sulfoxide is an excellent solvent for many materials, it should be used as a last resort and in minimal amounts, preferably mixed with acetone. Dimethyl sulfoxide affects cells and may complicate interpretation of the assay. Although its boiling point is higher, toluene is preferable to benzene if an aromatic hydrocarbon solvent must be used.

In some cases, the material must be tested without dilution or in water. In these cases, the material should be painted onto the shaved back with an artist's brush so that the material is in contact with the skin but only in a thin layer.

Guidelines for frequency of application are lacking. Generally, two to three times each week is appropriate. However, some 30 years ago I found that undiluted Tween 60 was an effective promoter when applied 12 times a week, at about 8 a.m. and 4 p.m., 6 days a week. At a rate of 5 times a week, it did not promote tumors. In industrial situations, substances may be in contact with human skin for more than 8 h a day, and therefore twice-weekly applications to mouse skin may not be an adequate test regimen.

The volume of solvent should be determined by the amount required to wet as much of the shaved back as possible without collecting near the bottom of the side of the animal. In the case of mice, 0.1 ml is usually the lowest volume and 0.2 ml is the maximum practical volume of volatile solvents such as acetone. It is most efficient to use as much of the back as possible, thereby putting the most possible cells at risk. If the material is not volatile, it should be painted onto the skin, and measuring the volume is then impractical and meaningless.

Species and Strain of Test Animal

In general, mice that have been bred for susceptibility to the initiation-promotion protocol are the test animals of choice. The subject has been reviewed by Slaga (14), who makes it clear that, although the SENCAR mouse model provides a good dose-response relationship for many initiators and promoters, other strains of mice may respond well to other promoters, for example benzoyl peroxide. One cannot generalize about the response of various strains to different initiators. Recently, Slaga has developed inbred strains of mice that are unusually susceptible to the initiation-promotion procedure, and these strains should be used.

EXAMPLES OF MODEL SYSTEMS

Initiation and Promotion by Chemicals

The standard mouse model for initiation and promotion is discussed by Eastin in another chapter of this book. Species other than the mouse are

Table 1. Promotion by Benzoyl Peroxide of Melanoma in Syrian Golden Hamsters

Treatment (20 hamsters/group)	Melanoma incidence (no./hamster, 16 mo.)
Control (1 ml acetone, 3 x/wk)	0
DMBA (i.p.,* 10 mg/kg, once)	0.6
Benzoyl peroxide (160 mg, 3 x/wk)	0
DMBA-benzoyl peroxide (80 mg, 3 x/wk)	2.2
DMBA-benzoyl peroxide (160 mg, 3 x/wk)	2.9

* i.p., intraperitoneally.

generally more resistant to the induction of papillomas and carcinomas by initiators and promoters. However, melanomas are induced in hamsters given initiation treatments of DMBA and promotion treatments of TPA (15,16) or benzoyl peroxide (17). Data from the latter experiment using benzoyl peroxide are shown in Table 1.

The melanomas in the experiment summarized in Table 1 were initiated by intragastrically administered DMBA. However, skin application of 2.5 mg of DMBA in 1.0 ml of acetone initiated European hamster skin so that melanomas, papillomas, and carcinomas of the skin were promoted by 40 nmol TPA in 0.5 ml acetone applied twice weekly for 25 weeks (16). There is a suggestion that promoting factors may be risk factors for human melanoma (18).

Recent reports show that human melanoma is occurring at an increasing frequency. Therefore, it is essential to improve the models for evaluating hazards that may act either by initiation or promotion together with sun exposure to increase the risk of human melanoma.

Initiation by Ultraviolet Light

In an excellent overview of ultraviolet radiation carcinogenesis, Fry (19) has reviewed the literature on initiation by ultraviolet light. He showed that carcinomas are promoted in mice by TPA following prior exposure to ultraviolet light. In one experiment, Fry found that exposure of hairless mice to a sunlamp three times a week for 12 weeks caused about a 2% incidence of carcinoma. In contrast, treating mice with 5 μg TPA three times a week for 52 weeks after an identical 12-week exposure to ultraviolet light caused about a 48% incidence of carcinoma (19). Fry also showed that combining the initiating properties of 8-methoxypsoralen and of ultraviolet light can increase the degree of initiation; TPA elicited more carcinomas in mice that had previously received initiation treatments with the combination. This is an important point that must be considered in estimating human hazard. A combination of chemicals may act together with sunlight to enhance the risk of human skin cancer at either the initiation or promotion phase of carcinogenesis and therefore is a matter of concern.

Initiation by Ionizing Radiation

There is only one substantial report in the literature in which ionizing radiation was found to initiate skin carcinomas in animals that were subsequently promoted with TPA. Jaffe and Bowden (20) exposed SENCAR mice to a single dose of 11.25 Gy of x-radiation followed by 8 nmol TPA for 60 weeks. A 6% incidence of carcinoma resulted in these mice, whereas none appeared in the control mice exposed to either x-radiation alone or TPA alone.

Proliferative State of Skin and Initiation

There are several studies in animals that show enhancement of skin tumor yield if the proliferative rate of the skin cells is elevated at the time of exposure to an initiator. It is conceivable that the human risk attendant to exposure to a low level of a potential carcinogenic/initiating hazard might be greater if the skin cells are multiplying faster than normal at the time of exposure.

In animals, the initiating potency of urethan, DMBA, and N-methyl-N'-nitro-N-nitrosoguanidine is enhanced by a single treatment of the skin with TPA or acetic acid within 24 h of initiation (21-23). Promotion was accomplished by multiple applications of TPA. The same phenomenon is true for tumors initiated with ionizing radiation (20).

Not only in animal assays must one control for the rate of cell proliferation at the time of initiation, there also may be increased risk for skin carcinogenesis in humans whose skin cells are proliferating at increased rates. Therefore, noncarcinogenic irritants, wound healing, and even warts caused by a papovavirus may result in increased sensitivity of human skin to initiating and promoting substances.

The Cocarcinogenesis Model

Thus far, we have discussed the model in which initiation followed by promotion yields tumors. However, initiating and promoting agents applied to mouse skin concurrently elicit many tumors (24). In fact, the initiation-promotion model was developed for research purposes and does not duplicate the usual real-life situations in which one is exposed concurrently to many agents that may initiate or promote cancer. Hence, consideration should be given to a test in which the skin of an appropriate species or strain of mice, e.g., SENCAR, is treated concurrently with a mixture of all the potential hazards that are of concern in a specific situation, according to the following format.

Appropriate levels of the mixture to be tested should be applied perhaps twice weekly to a control plus two test groups. The first test group is given DMBA once weekly at low initiating doses concurrently with the test material. The second test group is given TPA twice weekly at low promoting levels. In this assay, it is essential that the quantity of DMBA or TPA is sufficient to cause only a minimal initiating or promoting response, so that any augmenting effect of the test mixture can be seen. The DMBA and TPA should be administered on days that the test material is not administered. Of course, controls for DMBA, TPA, and solvent must be included. Although not yet validated, preliminary data indicate that this test may be the most rapid, sensitive, and therefore economical test for the detection of the possible initiating or promoting potential of a test substance.

SUMMARY

A number of items that must be considered in designing and choosing a suitable model for initiation and promotion testing have been described. Although these items may seem complex, tests for initiation and promotion are, in reality, quite simple and provide a rational approach to carcinogen testing.

Several tests have been described here and Eastin, elsewhere in this book, describes the validation of a simple and highly recommended test.

The processes involved in initiation and promotion are qualitatively different. The criteria for concern about possible human hazards as well as for regulation of initiators and promoters should be based on these qualitative differences. Realistic appraisal of the risk must be based on the level and nature of the potential hazard. In particular, it must be recognized that promoting action is reversible, that a threshold exists, and that promotion is readily inhibited. Therefore, animal tests that differentiate between potential initiators and promoters are essential to enable a logical assessment of human risk and the implementation of appropriate protective measures based on scientific facts.

OPEN FORUM

Question: Does turpentine act as a second-stage promoter?

Dr. R. K. Boutwell: Yes. Turpentine was used as a second-stage promoter in the first experiments that revealed that promotion consists of two stages. In addition, endogenously produced growth hormones are important. However, all living tissue is constantly exposed to mutagens that may facilitate progression to malignancy. Examples include background ionizing radiation, endogenously formed nitrosamines and natural mutagens/carcinogens in edible plants. In addition, TPA may cause mutational events via oxygen-free radicals.

Dr. S. C. Lewis: I would like to make a point of clarification about the influence of solvents. In our studies at Exxon and studies at the Kettering Institute, we got very mixed results concerning the impact of solvents. We have a theory about this that underscores the importance of careful selection of solvents. The carcinogenicity of benzo[a]pyrene was profoundly affected, depending on whether it was dissolved in toluene or mineral oil. However, there was no effect on either the tumor yield or latency of a refinery process product—heavy catalytic cycle oil—when dissolved in toluene or mineral oil. It may be mineral oil does not make a good solvent for pure benzo[a]pyrene because of the mineral oil's highly paraffinic nature but that the PAHs in heavy catalytic cycle oil (mostly aromatic) enjoyed a cosolvent benefit when dissolved in mineral oil. With that clarification, the choice of solvent is critical and probably should be influenced by the solute carcinogen to be studied.

Conventional bioassayists would prefer to not use any solvent at all. The lubricant oils can be used without a solvent because they are not irritating. However, we would occasionally like to be able to bioassay some materials that are fairly irritating. We have three options. We can dilute the material out in a solvent, introducing a new confounding variable; we can reduce the absolute dose, which probably has a cosmetic benefit (it reduces the treatment area so we do not see as much irritation over as broad an area, but significant irritation is probably still there); or we can reduce the frequency of treatment. Based on the data we saw, this latter option appears to be the most promising for relatively weakly active carcinogens. Many of these irritating materials turn out to be only weakly carcinogenic, with long latencies and comparably low tumor yields. Can you offer any comment on which of these or other options are appropriate?

Dr. Boutwell: Dilution with a volatile solvent to achieve a tolerable level of irritation is preferable. Our goal is to expose as many cells as possible to the test substance. One must experiment with the problem of frequency of application. Some promoting agents are effective only if applied to the skin twice daily (e.g., certain surface active agents). Others are more effective promoters when applied only once a week (e.g., chrysarobin).

REFERENCES

1. Verma AK, Boutwell RK. Effects of dose and duration of treatment with the tumor promoting agent TPA on mouse skin carcinogenesis. Carcinogenesis 1:271-276, 1980.
2. Boutwell RK. Some biological aspects of skin carcinogenesis. Prog Exp Tumor Res 4:207-250, 1964.
3. Deelman HT. The part played by injury and repair in the development of cancer. Zeitschrift für Krebsforschung 21:220-226, 1924.
4. Mottram JC. A developing factor in experimental blastogenesis. J Pathol Bacteriol 56:181-187, 1944.
5. Redmond DE. Tobacco and cancer: the first clinical report, 1761. N Engl J Med 282:18-23, 1970.
6. Slaga TJ, Bowden GT, Shapas BG, Boutwell RK. Macromolecular synthesis following a single application of polycyclic hydrocarbons used as initiators of mouse skin tumorigenesis. Cancer Res 34:771-777, 1974.
7. Miller EC, Miller JA. Searches for ultimate chemical carcinogens and their reactions with cellular macromolecules. Cancer 47:2327-2345, 1981.
8. Boutwell RK. The function and mechanism of promoters of carcinogenesis. CRC Crit Rev Toxicol 2:419-443, 1974.
9. Roe FJC. The effect of applying croton oil before a single application of 9,10-dimethyl-1,2-benzanthracene (DMBA). Br J Cancer 13:87-91, 1959.
10. Van Duuren BL, Sivak A, Katz C, Seidman I, Melchionne S. The effect of aging and the interval between primary and secondary treatment in two-stage carcinogenesis in mouse skin. Cancer Res 35:502-505, 1975.
11. McCann J, Ames BN. Detection of carcinogens and mutagens in the *Salmonella/* microsome test: Assay of 300 chemicals. Proc Natl Acad Sci USA 73:940-954, 1976.
12. Pitot HC. Relationship of bioassay data to their toxic and carcinogenic risk for humans. J Environ Pathol Toxicol 3:431-450, 1980.
13. Booth BA, Boutwell RK. Licking as a factor affecting dosage in skin carcinogenesis. Cancer Res 19:79-83, 1959.
14. Slaga TJ. Sencar mouse skin tumorigenesis model versus other strains and stocks of mice. Environ Health Perspect 68:27-32, 1986.
15. Goerttler K, Loehrke H, Schweizer J, Hesse B. Two-stage tumorigenesis of dermal melanocytes in the back skin of the Syrian golden hamster using systemic initiation with 7,12-dimethylbenz[a]anthracene and topical promotion with 12-O-tetradecanoylphorbol-13-acetate. Cancer Res 40:155-161, 1980.

16. Goerttler K, Loehrke H, Hesse B, Schweizer J. Skin tumor formation in the European hamster after topical initiation with DMBA and promotion with TPA. Carcinogenesis 5:521-524, 1984.
17. Schweizer J, Loehrke H, Lutz E, Goerttler K. Benzoyl peroxide promotes the formation of melanotic tumors in the skin of 7,12-dimethylbenz[a]anthracene-initiated Syrian golden hamster. Carcinogenesis 8:479-482, 1987.
18. Magnus K. Habits of sun exposure and risk of malignant melanoma. Cancer 48:2329-2335, 1981.
19. Fry RJM. Ultraviolet radiation carcinogenesis. In Slaga TJ (ed): Mechanisms of Tumor Promotion. Boca Raton, FL: CRC Press, 1984, pp 73-96.
20. Jaffe DR, Bowden GT. Ionizing radiation as an initiator in the mouse skin two-stage model of skin tumor formation. Radiat Res 106:156-165, 1986.
21. Hennings H, Bowden GT, Boutwell RK. The effect of croton oil pretreatment on skin tumor initiation in mice. Cancer Res 29:1773-1780, 1969.
22. Hennings H, Michael D, Patterson E. Enhancement of skin tumorigenesis by a single application of croton oil before or soon after initiation by urethan. Cancer Res 33:3130-3134, 1973.
23. Bowden GT, Boutwell RK. Studies on the role of stimulated epidermal DNA synthesis in the initiation of skin tumors in mice by methylnitronitrosoguanidine. Cancer Res 34:1552-1563, 1974.
24. Boutwell RK. Overview of tumor promotion. In Prostaglandins and Cancer: First International Conference. New York: Alan R. Liss, 1982, pp 183-188.

Skin Carcinogenesis: Mechanisms and Human Relevance, pages 17–24
© 1989 Alan R. Liss, Inc.

Relevance for Man of Skin Carcinogenicity in Experimental Animals

Paul Grasso

University of Surrey, Guildford, Surrey, England CR24AV

Skin cancer is but one type of neoplasia that afflicts humans and animals, and an assessment of the dermal carcinogenic potential of a chemical is one part of the current efforts to identify carcinogens, whether they act topically or systemically.

The use of laboratory animals, particularly rodents, for assessing the carcinogenic activity of chemicals is currently taken so much for granted that the objective for doing these tests tends to get blurred, if not lost sight of entirely. Indeed, many witty jokes have been directed at this seeming loss of objective, based on the theme that our work is more suitable to make this world a safer place for rats and mice than for man. To my mind, this is reflected in the recent tendency to warn the public that substance X is carcinogenic to animals, seemingly omitting any relevance for man. When I pointed out such a warning to a member of the public, the reaction was "I do not care what it does to your rats and mice. What does it do to me?" I am sure that I am not alone in this experience.

In fact, the whole object of carrying out animal tests is to discover whether chemicals carry a carcinogenic hazard for man. The suitability of animal models for this purpose rests principally on an empirical basis, but they are nonetheless valuable for it. In fact, dermal carcinogenesis gave the first indication that a human carcinogen, namely coal tar, was also carcinogenic to mice. This first experience was repeated with several other compounds (1), so that over the years, it has become accepted practice to assume that all substances that are carcinogenic in animals present a serious carcinogenic hazard to man.

On the face of it, there appears to be no strong argument against this assumption. But over the years, experience has shown that a number of confounding factors may make the interpretation of results difficult. These confounding factors can be grouped as dietary, hormonal, persistent injury, genetic (high background incidence of tumors, genetic drift) (see refs. 2-5 for reviews).

Of all these factors, the most controversial one is the question of persistent injury and development of neoplasia. The phenomenon of cancer production by repeated trauma is perhaps best illustrated by two examples—one concerning the production of sarcoma in the subcutaneous tissue of rodents and the other concerning the production of carcinoma in the urothelium in the same species.

The role of the tissue reaction to injury in the subcutaneous tissue was not appreciated until it was shown that the chemical used to induce trauma had little or no part in the production of tumors. Even biologically inert substances, such as metallic gold and silver, have been shown to produce tumors.

Then came the demonstration that it is the size of the material implanted rather than its chemical nature that is the critical factor in the production of these tumors. This situation was well defined by experiments carried out by Oppenheimer et al. (6) and Alexander and Horning (7), in which they showed that large pieces of cellophane implanted subcutaneously in rats induce a high incidence of tumors, smaller pieces induce fewer tumors, and the same amount of material in the shredded form produces no tumors at all.

The third, and to my mind, the most crucial point was the discovery that the large pieces induced a marked granulomatous reaction, whereas the smaller pieces induced much less of a reaction. Additional evidence of the importance of tissue reaction in the production of tumors came from the demonstration that removal of the plastic film after 5 months did not result in a regression of the thick granulomatous reaction. Instead, this persisted and led to the development of sarcoma (for reviews, see refs. 8,9). This was a watershed in experimental induction of tumors because it was clearly demonstrated that the reactive lesion induced by the implant was the determining factor in the production of these tumors.

Experience with other tissues led to the same conclusion. Thus Ball (10) showed that foreign bodies implanted in the bladder lead to the formation of carcinomata, and Flaks et al. (11) demonstrated conclusively that stone formation was the cause of the tumors found in animals treated with 4-ethylsulfonyl-naphthalene-1-sulfonamide, as acidification of the urine abolished stone formation and tumor development.

There are, of course, other organs that respond by producing tumors if subjected to frequent episodes of hyperplasia. The best example in this group is the thyroid gland, but other hormonally dependent organs are also affected (5).

I think this thumbnail sketch of cancer production in the rodent by agents that induce prolonged tissue hyperplasia establishes an important principle in the field of chemical carcinogenicity, namely that pathological changes induced by a chemical may produce cancer, with the chemical itself acting in a secondary role. This principle is beginning to be acknowledged in the field of toxicology and has led to the distinction between chemicals that are nongenotoxic but that, nevertheless, induce cancer through sustained tissue injury and those that are genotoxic. With the latter group of compounds, severe and sustained tissue damage is not necessary for the production of tumors.

The importance of this classification in toxicology cannot be overstressed, as it is a first step toward a distinction between cancer development from a chemical interaction with the genome as a primary event and cancer development as a result of a recognizable pathological mechanism. This distinction has implications in assessing hazard for man because for the latter group of chemicals, some form of a safety factor can be arrived at, which would give considerable reassurance that little or no hazard to man exists.

I must stress the safety factor in this assessment because in man cancer may be produced by pathological processes in much the same way as in animals. Examples in the literature that are well known but worth repeating include the hepatocellular tumors that develop in the cirrhotic liver (12), and squamous cell carcinoma that develops in chronic skin ulcers, whether they are produced as a result of defective circulation (the so-called varicose ulcers) or of tuberculous infection (lupus vulgaris) (13).

Thus in making this distinction the objective is not to dismiss some carcinogenic results as artifacts and deem others real. The tumors induced in animals are real enough, but the mode of their induction may be questionable if one takes into account not only the tumor data but also the experimental design and its execution in relation to human exposure to carcinogens.

What type of results would help us assess human risk? It is essential, first of all, to establish a causal link between the tumors induced experimentally and the test chemical. The best available evidence for this is a dose-response relationship coupled with a shortening of the latency period (14). This relationship has been demonstrated both by skin carcinogens and by systemic carcinogens (15,16).

Of course, a clear dose-response relationship involving several dose levels leaves no doubt whether the chemical concerned possesses a clear carcinogenic potential, but such ideal situations are unlikely to be reproduced in a common test protocol for a compound of unknown activity. This ideal situation is even more unlikely to be realized when the substance to be tested is a complex mixture such as a mineral oil. In such situations, it is not easy and may not be feasible to carry out classic dose-response studies. One has to look for other criteria to establish confidence in the results when one comes to assess human hazard.

Taking a lesson from protocols for systemic-acting carcinogens, one should, first of all, look into the structure-activity relationships. This can be done for a single chemical, and, from current evidence (17), one could get a good clue as to the potential of a chemical to act as a direct alkylating agent or to be metabolized by the skin (18,19). In the case of complex mixtures, a search should be made for expected carcinogens. I cannot overemphasize the importance of a chemical analysis in these instances. So much data has been collected in this field that a chemical profile can provide a good clue, but no more than that, to the likely hazard for man.

However, experience has also shown that the chemical analysis is by no means infallible, as it may miss some carcinogens or, on the other hand, may detect carcinogens that for some reason are not biologically available. This means that biological tests are essential. Here again, we can profit from the experience gained in other areas of chemical carcinogenicity. It is now customary to carry out comprehensive tests for genotoxicity on pharmaceuticals, agrochemicals, and food additives. There is, I think, a lot of merit in doing so. These tests provide us with a clue as to whether the genome is likely to be affected adversely. Aside from the problem of cutaneous cancer, a direct attack on the genetic material of the cell may have other equally undesirable consequences—mutagenic potential or a distortion of the immune response, for example. The problem that faces the toxicologist is what type of short-term test to employ in determining the genotoxic potential of the chemical or the complex mixture in question.

I think that the standard mutagenicity test battery is, with some reservations, adequate for single chemicals, but the same cannot be said at the moment for mineral oils and other complex mixtures. Some advances along this line have been made by Mobil Laboratories (20), but these procedures have not been around long enough for a proper appraisal of their potential. In any case, one needs a viable in vivo test to supplement the in vitro ones in order to confirm that the in vitro results are meaningful in terms of human risk, particularly if they are equivocal or borderline.

A number of short-term in vivo tests have been proposed for estimating the carcinogenic potential of a chemical applied topically. Two of these, Iversen's tetrazolium test (21) and the sebaceous gland suppression test, have been widely used. The former is now defunct to some extent, although it may well be worth a revival and reappraisal. The sebaceous gland suppression test (22) was a favorite at one time and is still in use in at least one large laboratory. These two tests have one important drawback—virtually nothing is known about how they work in relation to carcinogenesis.

There are other approaches: one measures unscheduled DNA synthesis (UDS), whereas the other measures polyploidy/aneuploidy in epidermal cells. The UDS test gives a measure of the DNA repair following the application of a test substance. In my view, this test has a lot to offer because it not only can be used in mice, but if ethical considerations could be satisfied, it might also be applied to man. This approach needs to be studied further, but I have no doubt that it will prove to be invaluable in the search for biological tools to assess human risk (23).

Another in vivo test that has been successfully employed in the British Petroleum laboratory at Surrey is the nuclear enlargement test. This change is consistently mentioned as prominent among early changes produced by a variety of carcinogens in target tissues. In fact, nuclear enlargement was first described by Page (24) in mouse skin treated with carcinogenic polycyclic aromatic hydrocarbons (PAHs). The significance of this phenomenon as an early indicator of carcinogenicity was systematically studied using an image-analyzing computer (Quantimet), and it was found that the application of benzo[a]pyrene induced nuclear enlargement in mouse skin to a much greater extent than that induced by hyperplastic agents, exemplified by croton oil (25). We also found that when a mixture of a hyperplastic agent and a carcinogen were painted on mouse skin, nuclear enlargement over and above that produced by croton oil was detected at a much lower concentration of the carcinogen than when the carcinogen was applied on its own (25).

Further investigation revealed that the type of nuclear enlargement produced by carcinogens was dose related (26) and produced by all the topical carcinogens we tried (27). These results gave us an empirical basis for attempting to investigate this approach on mineral oils. Results showed a good correlation between nuclear enlargement and the carcinogenic activity of mineral oils (Table 1).

Table 1. Nuclear Enlargement and Carcinogenic Activity of Mineral Oils

Oil code	Skin tumors	Mice	Nuclear area (mean, μm^2)	%Nuclei (>99 percentile)
N11	0	75	35.7	1.0
N1*	19	127	59.6†	29.0
N2*	4	127	52.0*	19.3
N3*	2	127	42.4	1.6
N4	1	100	40.7	3.3
N6	0	100	36.3	0.8
N8	0	100	41.8	0.4
N10	0	127	39.2	0.2
N12	1	127	43.1	2.2
N18	0	100	37.5	1.3

*Carcinogenic
†Significantly different from N11
From Ingram AJ, Grasso P, J Appl Toxicol 7:289-295, 1987. Copyright 1987, Journal of Applied Toxicology. Reprinted by permission of John Wiley & Sons, Ltd.

The crux of these investigations is that there seems to be a limit to the nuclear size attained when nongenotoxic agents that produce hyperplasia are applied to mouse skin, but this is exceeded when genotoxic carcinogens are applied.

This phenomenon was studied in some detail by Banerjee (28) in rat liver and by Ingram and Grasso (25) in skin. Both noted that the increase in size is due to DNA synthesis and is accompanied by a decrease in mitotic activity. This is thought to be indicative of a G2-block. Some work being carried out in the Robens Institute of Industrial and Environmental Health and Safety at the University of Surrey suggests that the nuclear enlargement by genotoxic agents is accompanied by aneuploidy.

A positive in vivo genotoxicity test of the type I have outlined will provide some basis for concern, and if results are strongly positive a standard carcinogenicity test may not be necessary. The short-term tests themselves may be sufficient to identify risk for man. Of course, if results of a carcinogenicity study are available, the tumor data will acquire much more relevance if supported by genotoxicity tests. I think that initiation and promotion tests should be considered to demonstrate genotoxicity.

I do not mean to diminish the value of a carcinogenicity study, but unless well conducted, it can create a greater confusion than would have prevailed if it had not been carried out at all. The criteria for a well-conducted test are not universally agreed on. In my view, they should be set after an irritancy test in the mouse strain that is intended to be used in the carcinogenicity study; the chemical concentration applied should be one that produces a minimum of hyperplasia; and careful note should be taken of any ulceration that develops after several months of treatment.

Cancers produced in mouse skin by test chemicals or mixtures of chemicals that are not genotoxic but that damage the epidermis should be considered to present a different kind of risk from agents or mixtures that are demonstrably genotoxic. With the latter, we have to acknowledge that, at present, we cannot give a reliable safe level of human exposure, and great caution needs to be exercised in arriving at an acceptable measure of human exposure. In the former, the tumor incidence cannot be dismissed as irrelevant. One can state, however, that if in man the exposure level is well below the level of exposure in the animal experiment, then the risk for man is negligible. It must not be forgotten, however, that persistent trauma in man may lead to cancer without the intervention of any chemical carcinogen in the agent causing the trauma. It must also be remembered that a large number of sources in our environment produce good initiating agents, so that tissue trauma may promote transformation after exposure to such agents.

OPEN FORUM

Dr. A.S. Wright: Dr. Grasso, I would like to reinforce your last point regarding the tumorigenic actions of croton oil and membrane implantation, i.e., chemical and physical agents that are not regarded as genotoxic. I do not think that your positive results with these agents are in conflict with the initiation-promotion model. Thus, the discovery of significant amounts of protein and DNA adducts in the tissues of unexposed human populations and laboratory animals suggests that some initiation may already have occurred. Second, I believe that cell transformation assays are undervalued both as procedures to discriminate between initiators and promoters and as systems to study carcinogenic mechanisms. We have worked with the C3H/10T1/2 system for 7 years. In our hands, this is the only in vitro assay that gives the anticipated results when tested with whole oils. However, the assay must be applied in the protracted exposure mode.

Dr. Kenneth Kraemer: Dr. Grasso, you mentioned using UDS and showed some results from humans. You mentioned you could also use it in rodents. Coming from a background of DNA repair work, I know that UDS primarily reflects excision repair, which is virtually nonexistent in rodents. I wonder how one would interpret your results. More recent studies, for instance, with ultraviolet (UV) radiation, show that UDS in rodents is about the level of xeroderma pigmentosum patients after UV, whereas the cell survival of rodent cells is normal. So there is a very poor correlation between the ability of these cells to show response to UV damage, for instance, and their excision repair, compared with normal cells.

Dr. Byron Butterworth: John DiGiovanni showed the results from the mouse studies in which we showed clear, strong chemical induction of UDS in mouse skin cells.

Dr. Kraemer: The primary method of dealing with UV photoproducts is not to remove them; that is, excision repair.

Dr. Butterworth: I think that the results that Dr. DiGiovanni presented indicates that UDS may be a very good indicator of chemical exposure.

Dr. Kraemer: Recent studies with UV from Bohr and Hanawalt have shown that different genes are repaired at different rates in rodent cells and in human cells. They interpret their data to say that essential genes, like dihydrofolate reductase genes in rodent cells, are repaired at a much higher rate than are nonessential genes. That may explain why the small level of excision repair is functioning. But it is clearly a different situation in rodent cells than in human cells.

Dr. Paul Grasso: If I am presented with a result that other experts say reflects DNA damage and repair, then as a pathologist I have to take notice of that, whatever the mechanism. This is what most toxicologists do.

REFERENCES

1. International Agency for Research on Cancer. Monographs on the Evaluation of the Carcinogenic Risk of Chemicals to Humans, Suppl. 1. Lyon, France: IARC, 1979.
2. Grasso P. Genetic, hormonal and dietary factors in determining the incidence of hepatic neoplasia in the mouse. In Popp JA (ed): Mouse Liver Neoplasia: Current Perspectives. Chemical Industry Institute of Toxicology Series. Washington, DC: Hemisphere Publishing Corp., 1984, pp 47-60.
3. Grasso P. Persistent organ damage and cancer production in rats and mice: Mechanisms and models in toxicology. Arch Toxicol [Suppl] 11:75-83, 1987.
4. Roe FJC. Food and cancer. Journal of Human Nutrition 33:405-415, 1979.
5. Lupulescu RA. Hormones and Carcinogenesis. New York: Praeger, 1983.
6. Oppenheimer BS, Oppenheimer ET, Stout AP. Carcinogenic effect of imbedding various plastic films in rats and mice. Surg Forum 4:672-678, 1953.
7. Alexander P, Horning E. Observations on the Oppenheimer method of inducing tumours by subcutaneous implantation of plastic films. In Wolstenholme GEW, O'Connor M (eds): Ciba Foundation Symposium on Carcinogenesis: Mechanisms of Action. London: Churchill, 1954, p 12.
8. Bischoff F, Bryson G. Carcinogenesis through solid state surfaces. In Homburger F, Karger S (eds): Progress in Experimental Tumour Research, Vol 5. New York: Basle, 1964, p 85.
9. Brand KG, Buoen LC, Johnson KH, Brand I. Etiological factors, stages, and the role of the foreign body in foreign body tumorigenesis: A review. Cancer Res 351:279-286, 1975.
10. Ball JK. The carcinogenic and co-carcinogenic effects of paraffin wax pellets and glass beads in the mouse bladder. Br J Urol 36:238-242, 1964.
11. Flaks A, Hamilton JM, Clayson DB. Effects of ammonium chloride on the incidence of bladder tumours induced by 4-ethylsulfonylnaphthalene-1-sulfonamide. JNCI 51:2007-2008, 1973.
12. Bassendine MF. Aetiological factors in hepatocellular carcinoma. In Williams R, Johnson P (eds): Clinical Gastroenterology: Liver Tumours. London: Balliere Tindall, 1987, pp 1-16.
13. Willis RA. Pathology of Tumours, 4th ed. Woburn, MA: Butterworth, 1967, p 259.

14. Druckrey H. Pharmacological approach to carcinogenesis. In Wolstenholme GEW, O'Connor M (eds): Ciba Foundation Symposium on Carcinogenesis: Mechanisms of Action. Boston: Little, Brown, 1959, pp 10-125.

15. Nesnow S, Triplett LL, Slaga TJ. Mouse skin tumour initiation-promotion and complete carcinogenesis bioassays: Mechanisms and biological activities of emission samples. Environ Health Perspect 47:255-268, 1983.

16. Peto R, Gray R, Brantom P, Grasso P. Nitrosamine carcinogenesis in 5120 rodents. In O'Neill IK, von Borstal RC, Miller CT, Long J, Bartsch H (eds): N-Nitroso Compounds. Lyon, France: International Agency for Research on Cancer, 1984. IARC Scientific Publication 57.

17. Golberg L (ed): Structure Activity Correlation as a Predictive Tool in Toxicology. Chemical Industry Institute of Toxicology series, Washington, DC: Hemisphere Publishing Corp., 1983.

18. Dipple A, Moschel RC, Bigger CAH. Polynuclear aromatic carcinogens. In Charles E. Searle (ed): Chemical Carcinogens, 2nd ed. Washington, DC: American Chemical Society, 1984, pp 41-129.

19. Lawley PD. Carcinogenesis by alkylating agents. In Charles E. Searle (ed): Chemical Carcinogens, 2nd ed. Washington, DC: American Chemical Society, 1984, pp 325-465.

20. Blackburn GR, Deitch RA, Schreiner CA, Mackerer CR. Predicting carcinogenicity of petroleum distillation fractions using a modified Salmonella mutagenicity assay. Cell Biology and Toxicology 2:63-84, 1986.

21. Iversen U, Iversen OH. The sensitivity of the skin of the hairless mouse to the tumourigenic action of coal tar in relation to the tetrazolium test. Acta Pathol Microbiol Scand [A] 80:612-614, 1972.

22. Bock FG, Mund R. A survey of compounds for activity in the suppression of mouse sebaceous glands. Cancer Res 18:887-892, 1958.

23. Honigsmann H, Brenner W, Tanew A, Ortel B. UV-induced unscheduled DNA synthesis in human skin: Dose response correlation with erythema time course and split dose exposure in vivo. Journal of Photochemistry and Photobiology [B] Biology 1:33-43, 1987.

24. Page RC. Cytologic changes in skin during the application of carcinogenic agents. Arch Pathol 26:800-813, 1938.

25. Ingram AJ, Grasso P. Nuclear enlargement and DNA synthesis in mouse skin treated with carcinogen and promoter. Exp Pathol 14:233-242, 1977.

26. Ingram AJ. Interaction of benzo[a]pyrene and a hyperplastic agent in epidermal nuclear enlargement in the mouse: A dose-response study. Chem Biol Interact 26:103-113, 1979.

27. Ingram AJ, Grasso P. Nuclear enlargement: An early change produced in mouse epidermis by carcinogenic chemicals applied topically in the presence of a promoter. J Appl Toxicol 5:53-60, 1985.

28. Banerjee MR. Mitotic blockage at G2 after partial hepatectomy during 4-dimethylaminoazobenzene hepatocarcinogenesis. JNCI 35:585-588, 1965.

Skin Carcinogenesis: Mechanisms and Human Relevance, pages 25–33

Human Model Systems
for Studies of Skin Cancer

Kenneth H. Kraemer

*Laboratory of Molecular Carcinogenesis, National Cancer Institute,
Bethesda, Maryland 20892*

Valuable information concerning the etiology, mechanism, and prevention of human cutaneous cancer may be obtained from clinical and laboratory studies of humans with genetic diseases that predispose them to skin cancer. Such studies provide knowledge pertaining directly to humans with these disorders and supply insights into carcinogenesis in the general population. These disorders thus may serve as model systems for cutaneous carcinogenesis. Three such disorders (1) will be discussed: the dysplastic nevus syndrome of familial cutaneous melanoma (DNS), basal cell nevus syndrome (BCNS), and xeroderma pigmentosum (XP).

REVIEW OF THE LITERATURE

Dysplastic Nevus Syndrome

Familial DNS is an autosomal dominant disorder in which affected individuals have a several-hundred-fold increased risk of developing malignant melanoma (2-4). Family members have clinically and histologically distinct pigmented lesions, or dysplastic nevi, which are markers of increased melanoma risk.

In familial DNS, individuals with dysplastic nevi have approximately a 150-fold increased melanoma risk. Family members who have had one cutaneous melanoma have about a 500-fold increased risk of developing another primary melanoma. In contrast, family members who are free of dysplastic nevi have nearly normal melanoma risk (3). Rarely, dysplastic nevi are precursors of melanoma. About 30,000 people in the United States have familial DNS (2,4). Close clinical follow-up and early removal of suspicious lesions appear to be beneficial in reducing melanoma mortality (3).

The nevi may be variegated tan, brown, and pink and often have areas of depigmentation. Coloration varies from lesion to lesion. Focal black areas suggest malignant melanoma. The lesions have an irregular shape and are frequently angulated. They are largely macular (flat) and may have a central papule. The border may fade into the surrounding skin. Nevi are frequently 5 to 10 mm in diameter or even larger. The number each patient has ranges from a few to more than 100, and they are mostly on the back and trunk, although they may appear on the scalp, breast, and buttocks. Nevi usually appear in childhood or adolescence, although new lesions may appear throughout adulthood.

Similar lesions are present in about 7% of the adult general population (5). A classification system has been proposed of putative melanoma risk categories in DNS (2-6) (Fig. 1). Under this system, sporadic DN without melanoma is type A. Familial DN without melanoma is type B. Type C is sporadic melanoma with DN and no family history of DN or melanoma. Approximately 50% of the newly diagnosed melanoma patients each year in the United States have DN. Type C thus may comprise approximately 10,000 patients per year (5). Their risk of subsequent melanoma is about 130-fold increased. Type D is familial DN with melanoma. This is subdivided into type D-1, which includes those with one family member with melanoma, and type D-2, those with more than one blood relative with melanoma. DNS type D-2 patients have the high melanoma risk cited above. Types A, B, and D-1 combined include about 12 million adults in the United States (5). Their melanoma risk is estimated as sevenfold increased. This is on the order of the increase in the number of people in the general population who sunburn easily and tan poorly (5).

Clinical and laboratory abnormalities found in familial DNS include a high frequency of cutaneous malignant melanoma. Linkage studies indicate a gene for DNS is on the short arm of chromosome 1 near the Rh locus (7). Laboratory

DYSPLASTIC NEVUS SYNDROME		MELANOMA IN KINDRED?	DYSPLASTIC NEVI IN TWO OR MORE BLOOD RELATIVES?	MELANOMA RISK	NUMBER OF PEOPLE AFFECTED
TYPE	DESCRIPTION				
A	Sporadic Dysplastic Nevi	−	−	LOW	MANY
B	Familial Dysplastic Nevi	−	+		
C	Sporadic Dysplastic Nevi with Melanoma	+	−		
D-1	Familial Dysplastic Nevi with Melanoma	+	+		
D-2		+ + *	+	HIGH	FEW

*AT LEAST TWO BLOOD RELATIVES WITH CUTANEOUS MELANOMA

Figure 1. Classification of kindreds with dysplastic nevus syndrome.

studies of skin fibroblasts and lymphoid cells reveal increased cell killing when exposed to UV light or nitroquinoline oxide (NQO) and hypermutability responses to UV (8,9) and to NQO (9). Chromosomal hypersensitivity to breakage by x-radiation in the G2 phase of the cell cycle was reported for cultured dermal fibroblasts and lymphocytes (10). These studies indicate that there is an abnormality in several cell types of familial DNS.

Basal Cell Nevus Syndrome

BCNS is an autosomal dominant disorder with a virtually 100% lifetime risk of multiple basal cell carcinomas. Multiple organ systems are involved (1). Affected patients also may have jaw cysts, pitting of the palms, and calcification of the falx in the brain. Several types of internal neoplasms have been found, including medulloblastoma (brain), ameloblastoma (bone), and ovarian fibromas. They also may have benign milia, lipomas, and fibromas; rib defects; brachymetacarpalism; ocular abnormalities; congenital hydrocephalus; mental retardation; or hypogonadism.

Sun exposure is important in development of the skin cancers. BCNS patients have a predisposition to develop only one type of skin cancer, basal cell carcinoma. BCNS patients have been found to be hypersensitive to development of cancers in skin regions receiving x-ray therapy. Several patients receiving therapeutic x-rays for medulloblastoma or for skin cancer have subsequently developed myriads of basal cell carcinomas in the fields of treatment.

Results of laboratory studies of cultured dermal fibroblasts show lifespan extension after transfection with pro-1 or v-myc genes (11). This suggests that the fundamental defect involves alteration of a gene involved in immortalization of cells, as normal cells transfected with these same genes do not undergo lifespan extension.

Cultured fibroblasts have normal survival following treatment with x-radiation. In view of the abnormal clinical radiosensitivity of their skin, BCNS patients may have an abnormal radiosensitivity limited to the epidermal cells. Recent advances in epidermal cell culture may make this hypothesis experimentally testable.

Xeroderma Pigmentosum

XP is an autosomal recessive disorder characterized by marked sun sensitivity, 1,000-fold increased risk of skin cancer (basal cell and squamous cell carcinoma and malignant melanoma), and defective DNA repair (1,12-15). Clinical symptoms are found in sun-exposed tissue (skin and anterior eye) and consist of freckling, atrophy, and premalignant (papular lesions, actinic keratoses, and keratoacanthomas) and malignant lesions. A minority of the patients also have progressive neurological abnormalities (15), such as mental deterioration and sensorineural deafness. Other neurologic symptoms include microcephaly, spasticity, ataxia, loss of neurons in the cerebral cortex, and demyelination of the dorsal columns. Conjunctivitis, acute blepharitis, exposure keratitis, corneal opacification, and benign lesions such as lip papillomas and symblepharon also may occur.

Symptoms often develop in early childhood, consisting of acute sunburn on minimal sun exposure. Interestingly, many patients progress to the stage of excessive freckling without having increased sensitivity to developing sunburns. Patients show signs of radiation damage (increased pigment alternating with decreased pigment, atrophy, and telangiectasia). At an early age, their skin has the appearance of that of a farmer or sailor with many years of sun exposure. Premalignant actinic keratoses develop on sun-exposed surfaces. There is a high incidence of skin cancers among these patients. In a recent large review, the median age at onset of skin cancers for XP patients was 8 years (15), a 50-year reduction in comparison with the general population.

We recently found that an oral retinoid, 13-*cis*-retinoic acid, is effective in preventing new malignant skin tumor formation in XP patients (16). The action of the retinoid was relatively rapid, with a reduction in tumor frequency within a few months. Similarly, tumor appearance resumed within a few months of stopping the medicine. Thus, in these patients the rapid effects suggest that the retinoid acted at a stage of tumor formation other than the first (initiation) step.

Laboratory studies have shown XP cells to be hypersensitive to UV, certain chemical carcinogens such as NQO and benzo[a]pyrene, and dietary tryptophan pyrolysis products (12,13,17,18). XP cells thus might be useful as human tester strains, analogous to bacterial tester strains.

Recent studies with plasmid vectors have yielded new insights into the DNA repair defect in XP (19-27). The plasmid vectors are used in a "host cell reactivation" assay. The plasmid is damaged in vitro with UV radiation or another DNA-damaging agent and then introduced into human cells. The cellular machinery acts upon the damaged DNA, performing repair, replication, or mutation. After 2 days of transient expression, the plasmid is harvested, and the alteration assayed. For DNA repair studies, a plasmid containing a bacterial gene, such as chloramphenicol acetyltransferase (*cat*), is utilized. The damaged plasmid is transfected into the cells, and subsequently *cat* activity is assayed (20-22). This type of experiment revealed that one photoproduct is sufficient to inhibit expression in the XP cells (20). Other experiments with a replicating shuttle vector plasmid, pZ189, indicated that that there is an abnormal UV mutagenic spectrum induced with XP cells and that dimer and nondimer photoproducts are mutagenic (23-27).

DISCUSSION

These diseases illustrate the usefulness of human cancer-prone genetic diseases as models for studies of skin cancer. Researchers could study patients with these diseases in order to explore cancer etiology and prevention and could obtain tissue and cell samples from them for investigations into mechanisms of carcinogenesis, mutagenesis, and survival. Risk assessors also might use information from these patients to determine threshold doses of environmental carcinogens and obtain cells that could be used as tester strains. Patients with genetic diseases predisposing them to cancer form a high-risk group in studies of agents that may cause cancer. Epidemiological studies have shown the more than 1,000-fold increased skin cancer risk in XP patients is due to UV exposure (14). Retrospective UV exposure studies in XP patients thus might afford a means of establishing a UV dose-response curve. Sun exposure and other environmental agents and drugs such as hormones or immunosuppressive agents appear to play a role in melanoma development in patients with DNS. Determination of exposure levels in DNS patients might provide indications of threshold levels in humans. XP patients have about a 20-fold increased frequency of brain tumors, but the carcinogenic mechanism involved has not yet been explained (14,15). Patients with BCNS have an increased susceptibility to x-radiation-induced skin cancer. Information about their x-ray exposure might be used to determine whether a threshold dose exists for x-radiation-induced skin cancer in humans.

Patients at high risk of development of certain forms of cancer provide models for studies of cancer prevention. Protection of XP patients from sun exposure early in life has prevented the formation of skin cancers and other cutaneous changes in a few patients (12,13). Demonstration of the chemopreventive effect of oral retinoids on development of new skin cancers has been achieved in a relatively short time by using a few XP patients with an extremely high frequency of skin cancer formation (16).

Although XP is a rare disorder (only a few hundred cases in the United States) (15), it has been estimated that more than 10 million people in the United States have dysplastic nevi (5). These individuals may be at increased cancer risk on exposure to certain environmental agents. Identifying the individuals at risk (in addition to pinpointing the agents of risk) may be necessary for adequate protection of the general population.

Cells from individuals with cancer-prone genetic diseases often have defects in important pathways involved in cancer prevention in normal individuals. Determination of the precise nature of the defects may give insights into carcinogenesis in the general population. XP cells have defective DNA repair. Damaged plasmids propagated in XP cells generate an abnormal mutagenic spectrum that is a subset of the normal spectrum (24,27). This subset may be particularly important in the development of skin cancers. Cells from patients with BCNS appear to have a partial defect in genes controlling cell lifespan (11). Cells from patients with DNS have an abnormal frequency of chromosome breakage after x-irradiation (10).

By virtue of these defects, such cultured human cells might be useful as tester strains for environmental carcinogens. For example, XP cells have been shown to be hypersensitive to cytotoxic effects of many environmental carcinogens, including those found in the diet (18). Plasmid vectors, with in vitro damage followed by transfection into appropriate human cells, might be usable for assessment of the effects of DNA-damaging agents.

OPEN FORUM

Dr. F. F. Becker: What type of UV radiation did you use in the results that gave the rather surprising transitions?

Dr. Kenneth Kraemer: The studies I showed were all done with germicidal radiation—254 nm. We are planning to do studies at longer wavelengths, such as those in natural sunlight.

Dr. Becker: So the various photoproducts that Haseltine and others have identified as mutational and lethal, but that are not necessarily found after solar radiation, might change those results?

Dr. Kraemer: We have done a series of experiments to see which of these lesions are mutagenic in this assay system. In addition to the studies I showed, we did a similar study, irradiating first and then treating with a photoreactivating enzyme that specifically removes the cyclobutane dimers but leaves the other photoproducts intact. In that study we found the mutation frequency declined and survival increased. That told us that the cyclobutane dimers were important for survival and also as a cause of mutations; however, there were still some mutations. When we examined the mutation sites, the same hot spots that we found initially were still present. The dinucleotides at all these mutational hot spots involved either 5'-TC or CC sequences. These sequences are the very ones that can form both the dimers and the 6,4-lesions. We collaborated with Dr. Doug Brash who measured the frequencies of the 6,4-photoproducts and the dimers at those sites. We found we could efficiently remove the cyclobutane dimers by photoreactivation. After removal, the hot spots were still preserved as hot spots. The interpretation is that, whatever the lesion, both the dimer and the 6,4 lesions were mutagenic at the same dinucleotides in the sequence. Except for the TT dimer (the major photoproduct), which is weakly mutagenic, we think the others are all mutagenic. We have not done these studies at longer UV wavelengths yet.

Dr. Michael Fry: A characteristic change when cells in culture are transformed from a cell strain to a cell line is from a diploid state to aneuploidy. In the case of basal cell nevus syndrome cells, when you transfected cells with an oncogene, were there chromosome changes?

Dr. Kraemer: That's not my data—it is Dr. Nancy Colburn's—so I cannot answer that.

Question: Does sunscreen provide protection against xeroderma?

Dr. Kraemer: The xeroderma patients that we selected for our clinical study had already developed large numbers of tumors. We have been following other xeroderma patients who were diagnosed very early in life, before severe progression. For this relatively small number of patients, a program of protection from sunlight exposure has been instituted, using chemical sunscreens and clothing that covers or shades the body, including the eyes. One patient has lived in Fort Lauderdale, Florida all her life. She is now 15 years old and has just a small amount of freckling, with no evidence of any other sun damage and no cancers. So a complete regimen of sun protection can be effective. On the other hand, the patients I described in the retinoid study were protected from sun exposure once the diagnosis was made, but they continue to develop tumors. From a mechanistic standpoint, many of their cells have presumably undergone initiation. It is the tumor progression that we have halted by the retinoid treatment. The sunscreens do not seem to be able to stop progression by themselves.

Question: Do you have any idea what proportion of non-induced skin cancer is due to the inherited distribution of melanocytes, namely, in persons of Celtic background.

Dr. Kraemer: The other point is that, of the so-called sporadic melanomas, about half those individuals have dysplastic nevi. That is an area of active research right now.

Dr. Fry: Although UV is not accepted as the etiological factor for melanoma, the figure that Dr. Kraemer gave for incidence was about 12 per 100,000, whereas in Texas or Arizona, it is more like 27 or 30 per 100,000. Thus, both geographical and genetic factors are important.

Dr. Jerry Smith: Has any clinical hypersensitivity been demonstrated to environmental xenobiotics other than radiation? If so, what are they? Has any resistance been seen?

Dr. Kraemer: The xeroderma pigmentosum cells are hypersensitive to many of the xenobiotics, including the benzpyrene derivatives and the diol epoxides, which have been studied extensively. Some clinical evidence was provided by one of our patients who smoked for half his lifetime, and died in his early thirties with lung cancer.

Dr. Terrence J. Monks: Dr. Kraemer, one or two of the patients you were treating with retinoic acid seemed to be nonresponsive. Is that a general phenomenon? Is there perhaps a polymorphism in response?

Dr. Kraemer: Of the five patients we showed, one was an apparent nonresponder. However, when we stopped the retinoids, the rate of tumors increased above the rate during treatment. Interestingly, he had the fewest number of tumors to begin with. We have two additional patients that we attempted to begin the same protocol with, but they were unable to tolerate the high dose that we were using because of elevated liver function test and triglycerides. Now we are using a lower dose regimen. They are still under observation.

Dr. R. K. Boutwell: We have used many promotion inhibitors—retinoids, protease inhibitors, non-steroidal anti-inflammatory agents, steroidal anti-inflammatory agents, cyclooxygenase inhibitors, and difluoromethyl ornithine. We determine dose-response levels for inhibition of these agents in our system. We then apply them at levels that are not maximal for inhibition of promotion. When we test combinations at these levels, we observe synergistic inhibition of promotion. Combining several inhibitors at levels at which no toxicity is seen for each alone may be one way to overcome toxicity in xeroderma pigmentosum patients.

REFERENCES

1. Kraemer KH. Heritable diseases with increased sensitivity to cellular injury. In Fitzpatrick TB, Eisen AZ, Wolff K, Freedberg IM, Austen KF (eds): Dermatology in General Medicine. New York: McGraw Hill, 1987, pp 1791-1811.
2. Greene MH, Clark WH Jr, Tucker MA, Elder DE, Kraemer KH, Guerry D IV, Witmer WK, Thompson J, Matozzo I, Fraser MC. Acquired precursors of cutaneous malignant melanoma: The familial dysplastic nevus syndrome. N Engl J Med 312:91-97, 1985.
3. Greene MH, Clark WH Jr, Tucker MA, Kraemer KH, Elder DE, Fraser MC. The prospective diagnosis of malignant melanoma in a population at high risk: Hereditary melanoma and the dysplastic nevus syndrome. Ann Intern Med 102:458-465, 1985.
4. Kraemer KH, Greene MH, Tarone RE, Elder DE, Clark WH Jr, Guerry D IV. Dysplastic naevi and cutaneous melanoma risk. Lancet 2:1076-1077, 1983.
5. Kraemer KH, Tucker MA, Tarone RE, Clark WA, Elder DE. Cutaneous melanoma risk in dysplastic nevus syndrome types A and B. N Engl J Med 315:1615-1616, 1986.
6. Kraemer KH, Greene MH. Dysplastic nevus syndrome: Familial and sporadic precursors of cutaneous melanoma. Dermatologic Clinics 3:225-237, 1985.
7. Greene MH, Goldin LR, Clark WH Jr, Lovrien E, Kraemer KH, Tucker MA, Elder DE, Fraser MC, Rowe S. Familial malignant melanoma: An autosomal dominant trait possibly linked to the Rh locus. Proc Natl Acad Sci USA 80:6071-6075, 1983.
8. Perera M, Um KI, Greene MH, Waters HL, Bredberg A, Kraemer KH. Hereditary dysplastic nevus syndrome: Lymphoid cell hypermutability in association with increased melanoma susceptibility. Cancer Res 46:1005-1009, 1986.
9. Howell JN, Greene MH, Corner RC, Maher VM, McCormick JJ. Fibroblasts from patients with hereditary cutaneous malignant melanoma are abnormally sensitive to the mutagenic effect of simulated sunlight and 4-nitroquinoline 1-oxide. Proc Natl Acad Sci USA 81:1179-1183, 1984.
10. Sanford KK, Tarone RE, Parshad R, Tucker MA, Greene MH, Jones GM. Hypersensitivity to G2 chromatid radiation damage in familial dysplastic nevus syndrome. Lancet 2:1111-1115, 1987.
11. Shimada T, Dowjat WK, Gindhart TD, Lerman MI, Colburn NH. Lifespan extension of basal cell nevus syndrome fibroblasts by transfection with mouse pro or v-myc genes. Int J Cancer 39:649-655, 1987.
12. Kraemer KH, Slor H. Xeroderma pigmentosum. Clin Dermatol 3:33-69, 1985.
13. Cleaver J, Kraemer KH. Xeroderma pigmentosum. In Scriver CR, Beaudet AL, Sly WS, Valle D (eds): The Metabolic Basis of Inherited Disease. Sixth Edition. New York: McGraw Hill (in press).
14. Kraemer KH, Lee MM, Scotto J. DNA repair protects against cutaneous and internal neoplasia: Evidence from xeroderma pigmentosum. Carcinogenesis 5:511-514, 1984.
15. Kraemer KH, Lee MM, Scotto J. Xeroderma pigmentosum: Cutaneous, ocular and neurologic abnormalities in 830 published cases. Arch Dermatol 123:241-250, 1987.
16. Kraemer KH, DiGiovanni JJ, Moshell AN, Tarone RE, Peck GL. Prevention of skin cancer in xeroderma pigmentosum with the use of oral isotretinoin. N Engl J Med 318:1633-1637, 1988.

17. Kraemer KH. Cellular hypersensitivity and DNA repair. In Fitzpatrick TB, Eisen AZ, Wolff K, Freedberg IM, Austen KF (eds): Dermatology in General Medicine. New York: McGraw Hill, 1987, pp 165-173.
18. Protic-Sabljic M, Whyte DB, Kraemer KH. Hypersensitivity of xeroderma pigmentosum cells to dietary carcinogens. Mutat Res 145:89-94, 1985.
19. Kraemer KH, Protic-Sabljic M, Bredberg A, Seidman MM. Plasmid vectors for study of DNA repair and mutagenesis. Curr Probl Dermatol 17:166-181, 1987.
20. Protic-Sabljic M, Kraemer KH. One pyrimidine dimer inactivates expression of a transfected gene in xeroderma pigmentosum cells. Proc Natl Acad Sci USA 82:6622-6626, 1985.
21. Protic-Sabljic M, Kraemer KH. Reduced repair of non-dimer photoproducts in a gene transfected into xeroderma pigmentosum cells. Photochem Photobiol 43:509-513, 1986.
22. Protic-Sabljic M, Kraemer KH. Host cell reactivation by human cells of DNA expression vectors damaged by ultraviolet radiation or by acid-heat damage. Carcinogenesis 10:1765-1770, 1986.
23. Protic-Sabljic M, Tuteja N, Munsen P, Hauser J, Kraemer KH, Dixon K. UV-induced cyclobutane pyrimidine dimers are mutagenic in mammalian cells. Mol Cell Biol 6:3349-3356, 1986.
24. Bredberg A, Kraemer KH, Seidman MM. Restricted mutational spectrum in an UV-treated shuttle vector propagated in xeroderma pigmentosum cells. Proc Natl Acad Sci USA 83:8273-8277, 1986.
25. Brash DE, Seetharam S, Kraemer KH, Seidman MM, Bredberg A. Photoproduct frequency is not the major determinant of ultraviolet mutation hotspots or coldspots in human cells. Proc Natl Acad Sci USA 84:3782-3786, 1987.
26. Seidman MM, Bredberg A, Seetharam S, Kraemer KH. Multiple point mutations in a shuttle vector propagated in human cells: Evidence for an error-prone polymerase activity. Proc Natl Acad Sci USA 84:4944-4948, 1987.
27. Seetharam S, Protic-Sabljic M, Seidman MM, Kraemer KH. Abnormal ultraviolet mutagenic spectrum in DNA replicated in cultured fibroblasts from a patient with the skin cancer-prone disease, xeroderma pigmentosum. J Clin Invest 80:1613-1617, 1987.

Skin Carcinogenesis: Mechanisms and Human Relevance, pages 35–42
© 1989 Alan R. Liss, Inc.

The Role of Papillomaviruses in Human and Animal Epithelial Neoplasia

Ronald S. Ostrow and Anthony J. Faras

Institute of Human Genetics and Department of Microbiology, University of Minnesota Medical School, Minneapolis, Minnesota 55455

This chapter presents a brief overview of some of the recent and ongoing work in this laboratory on the role that papillomaviruses (PV) play in the development of benign epithelial tumors and their progression to malignancy in both humans and animals. For a more detailed history of studies that have been done to date, the reader is referred to several excellent recent reviews (1-3). Papillomaviruses are the only known viruses that can produce epithelial tumors with a malignant potential. The types of benign tumors that the general population is most familiar with are the common hand wart and the plantar wart of the feet. These lesions may be unsightly or annoying, but the associated human papillomaviruses (HPVs), HPV 1, HPV 2, and HPV 4, present little significant danger to the patient. However, there are approximately 51 known HPV genotypes, which appear to form defined groups with different biological activities. Some types are found basically in the oral or genital mucosa, some are cutaneous in nature, some are relatively benign, and some are closely associated with malignancies in each of these target regions.

An etiological role for papillomaviruses in primary and metastatic carcinomas is most clearly evidenced in the rare skin disease called epidermodysplasia verruciformis (EV). These patients develop disseminated, flat wart-like lesions—usually associated with HPV 5—and have a one in three chance of developing carcinomas on sun-exposed areas of the skin. The next most convincing evidence for the role of HPV in advanced neoplasia concerns the association of several types of HPV DNA with the entire continuum of benign to premalignant to malignant neoplasia of the genital tract. About 80% of primary and metastatic lesions of the genital tract are associated with HPVs 16, 18, 31, 33, or 35—and occasionally with the relatively benign HPV types 6 and 11. Some of these HPV types are also associated with the entire range of oral neoplasia as well as with some cutaneous carcinomas in situ. Advancements in the field of molecular biology have permitted the sensitive detection of the nucleic acid footprint of these viruses and furthered understanding of some of their biological properties, even in the absence of an in vitro culture system for growing these viruses. In addition, the use of animal model systems—such as rabbit and bovine models, and, recently in our laboratory, nonhuman primates who have naturally occurring or experimentally induced benign or malignant lesions—has served to enhance our understanding of some of the mechanisms involved in the development of malignancies.

METHODS

For filter hybridization, total cellular DNA was extracted from the tissues and processed as described previously (4-6). Briefly, minced tissue was digested with sodium dodecyl sulfate (SDS) and protease. Then salt precipitation of the cellular proteins and a series of phenol and chloroform extractions were performed. Cellular RNA was removed with RNase A, extracted with protease and phenol, and concentrated with ethanol. Total cellular DNA, either native or cleaved with appropriate restriction endonucleases, was electrophoresed in an agarose gel and transferred to nitrocellulose filters. Nick-translated ^{32}P-labeled HPV DNA probes were then hybridized under conditions of high stringency (1 M NaCl, 50% formamide, 10% dextran sulfate) or low stringency (1 M NaCl, 30% formamide, 10% dextran sulfate) at 37°C and washed at appropriate salt and temperature conditions. Autoradiography was performed with the aid of an intensifying screen.

For discrimination between viral circular and linear episomal DNA, or integrated viral DNA, two-dimensional gel electrophoresis was employed (7). Essentially, total cellular DNA was electrophoresed for 11 h at 4°C and 50 V in the first dimension in a submarine gel apparatus containing 0.4% agarose gel in TBE buffer (0.09 M Tris-HCl, 0.09 M boric acid, 0.003 M EDTA) containing 0.5 μg/ml of ethidium bromide. The lane containing the sample DNA was removed, turned 90°, and laid at the top of a new gel bed. A parallel lane was exposed to ultraviolet light and photographed. Fresh 1.2% agarose was then poured over the bed and allowed to solidify. The DNA was electrophoresed in this second dimension for 18 h at 24°C and 55 V. A measured grid on a clear plastic film was then placed on the gel, and the stained DNA was photographed. The gels were denatured in alkali, and the DNA was transferred to nitrocellulose for hybridization as described above.

Tissues fixed in formalin and embedded in paraffin as routinely performed for histological examination were used for in situ hybridization as described elsewhere in more detail (8-10). Briefly, 5-μm sections were made from paraffin blocks, deparaffinized, and treated consecutively with solutions of HCl, triethanolamine, salt, digitonin, protease, ribonuclease, paraformaldehyde, and graded ethanols. HPV DNA that had been radiolabeled using tritiated deoxynucleotide triphosphate precursors in a nick-translation reaction was added to the tissue in hybridization solution (0.6 M NaCl, 50% formamide, 10% dextran sulfate) and heat denatured at 80°C. After being incubated at room temperature, the slides were washed and dipped in Kodak nuclear track emulsion and allowed to expose for approximately 30 days. The slides were then developed, counterstained with hematoxylin, and examined for the presence of silver grains over nuclei by light microscopy.

RESULTS

Our laboratory had determined not only that HPV 5 DNA was associated with primary carcinomas of patients with EV but also that the viral DNA was associated with rare metastatic tumors in these patients, indicating close linkage between the malignant state and the presence of HPV 5 DNA. During these early studies, it was determined by agarose gel electrophoresis and filter hybridization that the viral DNA was largely episomal in nature. Recent studies employing genital tumors and cell lines derived from genital tumors have shown that interruption of specific HPV genes either by integration or by genetic mutation and deletion was usually associated with the malignant state. Our laboratory has used the technique of two-dimensional gel electrophoresis to better separate large amounts of episomal viral DNA from smaller amounts of viral DNA that has become integrated into the host chromosomal sequences. Such analyses have found a portion of HPV 5 DNA apparently integrated, as indicated by the comigration of viral and cellular nucleic acid sequences (Fig. 1). The molecular cloning and characterization of the HPV-cellular DNA junction sequences is in progress.

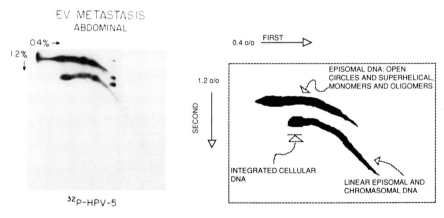

Figure 1. Two-dimensional gel electrophoresis of a cellular DNA extract from a metastatic tumor of an EV patient. (A) Cellular DNA was electrophoresed first in 0.4% agarose and then at right angles in 1.2% agarose, transferred to nitrocellulose, and hybridized to labeled HPV 5 DNA. This method separates circular and superhelical extrachromasomal viral DNA from linear and integrated viral DNA as indicated in (B). Abbreviations: EV, epidermodysplasia verruciformis; RhPV, rhesus monkey papillomavirus; HPV, human papillomavirus. (Reprinted with permission of Virology, from Kloster et al. Virology 166:30-40, 1988.)

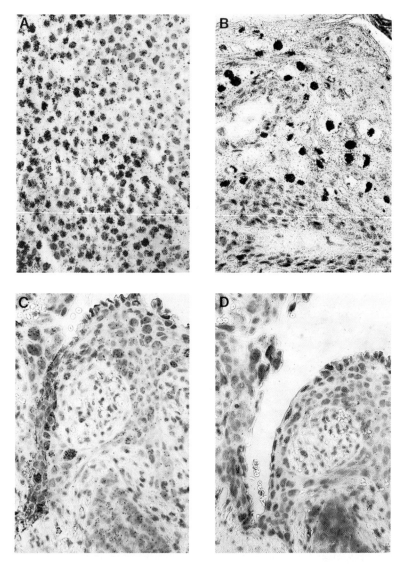

Figure 2. In situ hybridization using nonhuman primate papillomavirus DNA probes. Tissues were exposed for 21 days after hybridization under stringent conditions with either RhPV 1 (A,C) or PV from a colobus monkey, CgPV 2 (B,D). Samples shown are (A) a lymph node metastasis from which the RhPV 1 DNA was isolated, (B) the benign wart from which the CgPV 2 DNA was isolated, (C,D) a laryngeal carcinoma of a colobus monkey. Abbreviations: RhPV, rhesus monkey papillomavirus; CgPV, colobus monkey papillomavirus. (Reprinted with permission of Virology, from Kloster et al. Virology 166:30-40, 1988.)

RHESUS
LYMPH NODE METASTASIS

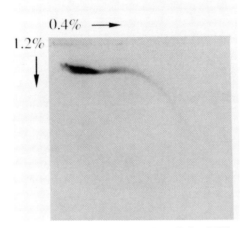

Figure 3. Two-dimensional gel electrophoresis of a cellular DNA extract from a rhesus monkey's lymph node metastasis. Cellular DNA was electrophoresed first in 0.4% agarose and then at right angles in 1.2% agarose, transferred to nitrocellulose, and hybridized to a labeled rhesus papillomavirus type 1 (RhPV 1) DNA. (Reprinted with permission of Virology, from Kloster et al. Virology 166:30-40, 1988.)

Integrated DNA from HPV 11, normally considered to be a more benign HPV of the oral-genital mucosa, has also been detected in a primary anal carcinoma and metastatic tumors of an immunosuppressed renal transplant patient by this laboratory. We and others have shown a very close correlation between the presence of various HPVs, but particularly HPV 16 and 18, in mucosal oral and genital high-grade neoplasias. Our finding of HPV 11 in malignant tumors may indicate that even HPVs with low-to-moderate oncogenic potential can contribute to the malignant phenotype, given the appropriate environment, which may include immunosuppression or other cofactors.

These kinds of findings are paralleled in several animal model systems. Our laboratory and others have shown that cottontail rabbit papillomavirus (CRPV) is capable not only of inducing benign warts in rabbits but also of producing malignant tumors in up to 25% of wild rabbits and up to 70% of domestic rabbits. Our recent studies of primary and metastatic tumors of these animals indicate that, unlike benign tumors, these malignant tumors contain integrated CRPV DNA, as determined by two-dimensional gel electrophoresis (data not shown). Similarly, using both filter and in situ hybridization techniques, we have detected novel PV DNAs in lesions of nonhuman primates, including warts and a laryngeal carcinoma of a colobus monkey and a lymph node metastasis from a primary penile carcinoma of a rhesus monkey (Figs. 2 and 3) (11). In the metastatic lesion integrated viral PV DNA also was detected.

DISCUSSION

Clearly, papillomavirus infection is associated with similar benign, pre-malignant, and malignant tumors in several species of animals and in humans. This has been shown both by experimentally induced lesions in animal model systems and by epidemiological studies. Although the possibility exists that in some human diseases, papillomaviruses may simply be a passenger in a cell that already has a malignant predisposition, the strong epidemiological correlations with specific types of HPV and the physical state of the HPV DNA have diminished this possibility. Continuing studies of malignant progression are in progress.

Published reports also have shown that a vaccine against a biosyntheti-cally derived bovine papillomavirus structural protein has been efficacious in preventing tumors in viral challenge studies (12,13). It is hoped that elucidation of the biological properties of these viruses will be useful in the treatment, cure, and prevention of HPV-induced neoplasia and that this information will be applicable to malignancies with different etiologies.

ACKNOWLEDGMENT

The work from our laboratory was supported by grants from the National Institutes of Health (CA25462) and the Minnesota Leukemia Research Fund.

OPEN FORUM

Question: Most of the viral DNA seems to be in one differential cell. Is that a trend?

Dr. Ronald Ostrow: Generally there seems to be a higher copy number of the virus in the more differentiated cells. However, decreased levels of viral DNA can be found right down to the basal cells. It has always been assumed that the basal cells may in fact be the target of the viral infection. In some of the more malignant conditions, the amount of virus present may be only one to five copies per cell, rather than the hundreds of copies that I showed here. In situ techniques show only a very few grains over some cell nuclei.

Question: Have you looked at leukoplakias that occur after tobacco use?

Dr. Ostrow: Not specifically. People have looked at leukoplakias and oral whitenings and have found papillomavirus DNA, at least in some cases. Cofactors are very important. In the case of EV, sunlight or ultraviolet light may be important cofactors. With domestic rabbits, painting warts with methylcholan-threne increases the cancer rate from 25% to 75%. Smoking is somewhat linked to increased genital cancer, but it is not known whether that reflects a life-style or whether it has a direct role.

Dr. Kenneth Kraemer: What is the role of interferon in therapy?

Dr. Ostrow: Interferon has had mixed results in therapy. In earlier studies, systemic or intralesional injections of interferon had remarkable results, particularly in patients severely afflicted with laryngeal papillomatosis. The lesions would regress. The person could breathe and would not need laser surgery as frequently. However, as soon as the treatment stopped, the lesions recurred. Last year at the annual papillomavirus meeting, Burroughs Wellcome indicated some of their most recent studies showed more long-lasting effects from interferon. So there is some hope that interferon can be used more efficaciously.

Question: What is known about the integration site?

Dr. Ostrow: The integration sites are very interesting. In the chromosome itself papillomaviruses appear to integrate relatively randomly, although there have been some associations with fragile sites within chromosomes noted. In one case, a papillomavirus (HPV 18) was found in one of its five integration sites in HeLa cells to be within 50 kb of the c-*myc* gene. However, this did not seem to significantly affect the rate of expression of the c-*myc* gene. We believe the integration, which involves the disruption of the viral genome, may be the important factor. The different integrations occur within a general region, but never at one particular site. Usually the genome opens some place within the E1 or E2 open-reading frames, which are important for integration and also for the positive and negative control functions of the virus itself. The autoregulation of the virus may be destroyed during this relatively rare integration event, resulting in a sudden loss of control of the replicative and tumorigenic properties of the virus.

Dr. Terrence J. Monks: Dr. Ostrow, do you know the nature of the mutagen you mentioned in the brachen fern. And regarding the species selectivity of the papillomavirus, I noticed the animal models that you showed (the rabbit, the monkeys, and the cattle) all seemed highly pigmented.

Dr. Ostrow: I do not know specifically what the brachen fern mutagen is. Concerning your second question, generally, we are talking about abnormal squamous cells, although recently adenosquamous tissue and adenocarcinomas have also been shown to be associated with papillomaviruses. I do not know that the pigmentation has that much to do with it.

REFERENCES

1. Ostrow R, Faras A. The molecular biology of human papilloma viruses and the pathogenesis of genital papillomaviruses and neoplasias. Cancer Metastasis Rev 6:383-395, 1987.
2. Pfister H. Biology and biochemistry of papillomaviruses. Rev Physiol Biochem Pharmacol 99:112-181, 1984.
3. Broker T, Botchan M. Papillomaviruses: Retrospectives and prospectives. Cancer Cells 4:17-36, 1986.

4. Okagaki T, Twiggs L, Zachow K, et al. Identification of human papillomavirus DNA in cervical and vaginal intraepithelial neoplasia with molecularly cloned virus-specific DNA probes. Int J Gynecol Pathol 2:153-159, 1983.

5   Southern E. Detection of specific sequences among DNA fragments separated by gel electrophoresis. J Mol Biol 98:503-517, 1975.

6. Ostrow R, Bender M, Seki T, et al. Human papillomavirus DNA in cutaneous primary and metastasized squamous cell carcinomas from patients with epidermodysplasia verruciformis. Proc Natl Acad Sci USA 79:1634-1638, 1982.

7. Wettstein F, Stevens J. Variable-sized free episomes of Shope papilloma virus DNA are present in all non-virus-producing neoplasms and integrated episomes are detected in some. Proc Natl Acad Sci USA 79:790-794, 1982.

8. Ostrow R, Manias D, Clark B, et al. Detection of human papillomavirus DNA in invasive carcinomas of the cervix by in situ hybridization. Cancer Res 47:649-653, 1987.

9. Blum H, Haase A, Vyas G. Molecular pathogenesis of hepatitis B virus infection: Simultaneous detection of viral DNA and antigens in paraffin-embedded liver sections. Lancet 2:771-775, 1984.

10. Haase A, Brahic M, Stowring L, Blum H. Detection of viral nucleic acids by in situ hybridization. In Maramorsch K, Koprowski H (eds): Methods in Virology, Vol. 7. New York: Academic Press, 1984, pp 189-226.

11. Kloster B, Manias D, Ostrow R, Shaver M, McPherson S, Rangen S, Faras A. Molecular cloning and characterization of the DNA of two papillomaviruses from monkeys. Virology 166:30-40, 1988.

12. Pilacinski W, Glassman D, Krzyzek R, Sadowski P, Robbins A. Cloning and expression in Escherichia coli of the bovine papillomavirus L1 and L2 open reading frames. Biotechnology 2:356-360, 1984.

13. Pilacinski W, Glassman D, Glassman K, et al. Development of a recombinant DNA vaccine against bovine papillomavirus infection in cattle. In Howley P, Broker T (eds): Papillomaviruses: Molecular and Clinical Aspects. New York: Alan R. Liss, 1985, pp 257-271.

BIOLOGICAL ASPECTS

Skin Carcinogenesis: Mechanisms and Human Relevance, pages 45–62

Morphological Evaluation of the Effects of Carcinogens and Promoters

A. J. P. Klein-Szanto

Department of Pathology, Fox Chase Cancer Center, Philadelphia, Pennsylvania 19111

The skin has played a crucial role in the development of new basic ideas about carcinogenicity of chemicals, structure-activity relationships, multistage carcinogenesis, and tumor progression. It has also been the organ of choice for the assessment of toxicity and carcinogenicity of numerous environmentally relevant compounds.

The acute and chronic effects of toxicants, carcinogens, and promoters on the different components of the skin are the subject of this review. To understand the morphological changes that take place in the skin after chemical exposure and during the development of different types of skin tumors, one must understand the normal morphology and differentiation patterns of skin components.

NORMAL SKIN STRUCTURE

The skin has three main components: the epidermis, a superficial lining of epithelial cells covering the body surface; the dermis, a richly vascularized connective tissue underneath the epidermis; and the cutaneous adnexa or appendages, a series of epithelial structures in the dermis that are connected to the epidermal surface (Fig. 1).

The number, composition, and thickness of these three components are extremely variable, and it is impossible to describe a single, normal cutaneous structural pattern. Not only does the skin differ from species to species but within each species numerous variations are determined by different topographical and physiological requirements as well. Additional variations can be caused by age, sex, hormonal status, and genetic constitution.

The epidermis is a stratified epithelium characterized by continuous replacement of the most superficial elements through proliferation and upward migration of the deeper layers. This is accomplished by cell division of the basal cells, cuboid or columnar cells that are separated from the dermis by a thin layer of proteinaceous material called basal lamina, and their subsequent migration and differentiation onto a layer of suprabasal cells that constitute the spinous layer. These cells are large and polyhedral with numerous intercellular junc-

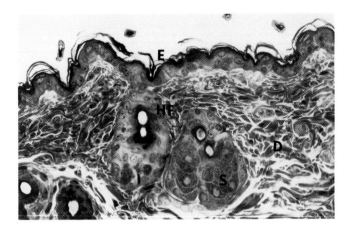

Figure 1. Normal murine skin showing hair follicle (HF) connected to the epidermis (E). Sebaceous gland (S) and dermis (D). Epon section, toluidine blue stain.

tions known as desmosomes and a large number of keratin bundles or tonofilaments. As these cells migrate closer to the surface they become flatter and lose many of their cytoplasmic organelles, the nuclei become smaller and condensed, and several irregular, electron-dense granules (keratohyalin granules) appear in the cytoplasm. These granules, now known to contain a histidine-rich protein called filaggrin, have an important role in aggregating and homogenizing keratin filaments, characteristics that begin to appear in this granular layer and are clearly seen in the most superficial layer, or horny layer. The latter is formed by extremely flat cells without nuclei but with a very homogeneous cytoplasm. This is the end stage of this migration and differentiation process. In addition to epithelial cells or keratinocytes, the epidermis contains several nonkeratinocytes or dendritic cells, i.e., Langerhans cells (bone-marrow derived cells that act as antigen-presenting cells), Merkel's cells (probably of neuroectodermal origin with neuroendocrine functions), and melanocytes (melanin-synthesizing cells of neural crest origin).

The dermis is a loose connective tissue compartment found between the epidermis and the subcutaneous adipose tissue. It contains the cutaneous adnexa and numerous nerves, as well as blood and lymphatic vessels.

The cutaneous adnexa are the hair follicles and the sweat and sebaceous glands. The hair follicles are an apparent downgrowth of the epidermis in which an ordered array of keratinized cells are gradually pushed upward in the form of hair shafts. The hair-producing cells are stratified into a large number of layers, finally giving rise to hair by a process of terminal differentiation analogous to but more complicated than the one described for the epidermis.

Two types of sweat glands have been described in mammals. Eccrine glands aid in thermoregulation by secreting water and salts. They are composed of a long, coiled secretory tubule and a connecting long excretory duct that ends in the epidermis. The apocrine glands secrete a proteinaceous material that originates from the loss of cytoplasm pieces from the glandular cells. Their function is not clear, but they are related to several accessory scent glands that produce attractant odors during the mating season in some species. The mammary glands are also modified apocrine glands. Sebaceous glands develop from the neck or infundibulum of hair follicles just as apocrine sweat glands do. They are composed of lipid-laden cells that completely disintegrate to form the sebaceous secretion or sebum. Sebum is discharged into the infundibulum of the hair follicles and spreads to the epidermal surface, where it helps in moisture retention of the epidermal horny layer.

EARLY MORPHOLOGICAL CHANGES INDUCED BY CARCINOGENS AND PROMOTERS

Carcinogens and promoters may produce immediate or acute effects, which are usually nonspecific, i.e., many physical or chemical agents without any carcinogenic or promoting abilities will produce similar alterations. Nevertheless, there are a few telltale signs that have been described as putative specific effects of promoters; these will be highlighted in this section.

The effects of early chemical changes induced in the skin can be divided into two categories: immediate, usually involutional, changes characterized by cutaneous damage and reactive changes that take place somewhat later as a response of the cutaneous components to the previous damage. Injury to the

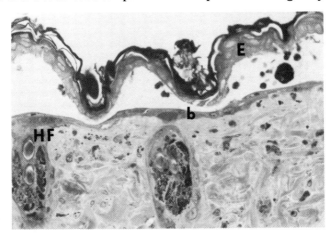

Figure 2. The necrotic epidermis (E) is being sloughed, and a few flattened basal cells (b) are starting the regenerative process. Regeneration is often accomplished by cells migrating from the hair follicles (HF). The skin was treated with 15% H_2O_2 48 h before biopsy. Epon section, toluidine blue stain.

epidermal cells can be seen as massive necrosis with erosion and ulcerations. This type of hyperacute involutional change is seen when very high doses of chemicals, including promoters, are used (Fig. 2). Moderate epidermal damage involving a smaller population of epidermal keratinocytes is seen with the usual doses of promoters or a single complete carcinogenic dose of chemicals such as polycyclic hydrocarbons (1,2). In these cases, areas of microerosion and necrosis of individual basal keratinocytes or groups of keratinocytes can be seen (Fig. 3C).

With usual promoting doses of phorbol esters, very few cells manifest morphological changes indicative of sublethal or lethal damage (cytoplasmic and nuclear vacuolization, pyknotic nuclei) (Fig. 3E) (3). The number of damaged cells can be investigated by isolating basal cell keratinocytes and enumerating the number of cells stained with trypan blue. Using this technique 10%-30% of

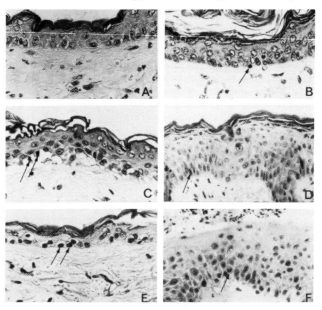

Figure 3. (A) Epidermal change 12 h after 2 µg TPA treatment. The epidermis shows a slight increase in thickness and cell size. (B) Ninety-six hours after 2 µg TPA treatment. The increase in thickness is still associated with hyperkeratosis. A few nonepithelial cells are seen in or near the basal layer (arrow). (C) Twelve hours after 20 µg TPA treatment. The epidermis shows marked intracellular edema and pyknotic nuclei (arrows) in the basal layer. An increase in thickness is also seen. (D) Ninety-six hours after 20 µg TPA treatment. The epidermis shows marked hyperplasia and some hyperbasophilic cells (arrow). (E) Twelve hours after 200 µg TPA treatment. Cytoplasmic vacuolization and pyknosis is prominent in the basal layer (arrows). An increase in thickness is not seen. (F) Ninety-six hours after 200 µg TPA treatment. The epidermis adjacent to an ulcerated area shows marked hyperplasia and mitosis (arrow). Intercellular edema is still seen in the basal layer. (A-F) Paraffin section, hematoxylin and eosin. (Reproduced from Klein-Szanto AJP et al. Carcinogenesis 5:1459-1465, 1984; used with permission.)

the cells exhibited trypan blue stain 12 to 48 h after single in vivo applications of the usual promoting doses of 12-O-tetradecanoylphorbol-13-acetate (TPA) (3). Most of the sublethally damaged cells initially react (in the first 12 h) with an increase in the cell volume due to aqueous inhibition of the cytoplasm and nucleus. Consequently, the whole epidermis increases in volume; this is detectable early as an increased epidermal thickness (Fig. 3A). Later, a regenerative burst adds to this increased thickness (Figs. 3A,D,F). This increase in the number of cells and cell layers, termed epidermal hyperplasia, can be differentiated from the earlier epidermal hypertrophy that is caused by an increase in the size but not in the number of keratinocytes. These changes can be evaluated by measurements of the epidermal thickness combined with measurements of the number of cell layers (2). An interesting parameter recently described as a good indicator of the carcinogenic effect of chemicals is the nuclear volume (see chapter in this volume by P. Grasso).

Most of these volumetric changes are nonspecific, and many noncarcinogenic and nonpromoting agents used in adequately high concentrations will produce sublethal or lethal damage and even reactive hyperplasia. Acetic acid, mezerein, cantharidin, and ethyl phenylpropiolate are examples of such agents. According to Argyris (4,5), the difference between these agents and efficient tumor promoters resides in the fact that the latter are able to maintain their hyperplasiogenic action after multiple topical applications (Figs. 4A and B and 5), whereas acetic acid and mezerein, for example, are unable to produce prolonged epidermal hyperplasia during protracted treatment. Closely related to and supporting this idea is the fact that TPA induces epidermal hyperplasia in hamsters after a single application but that this hyperplasia is not maintained after multiple treatments (6). In addition, TPA is not a tumor promoter in hamster skin (7). These findings seem to indicate that the capacity to sustain a chronic hyperplastic state is an important factor in tumor promotion and a good morphological indicator of promoter efficiency that could be used in eventual bioassays (8-10).

The induction of dark basal keratinocytes or dark cells (DC) (Fig. 6) is another good indicator of promoter efficiency. Although a certain level of DC induction is always associated with epidermal hyperplasia, only those agents that are effective promoters are able to induce a DC population of 10% or more in the basal layer. In addition to potent promoters, a group of compounds that are not complete promoters and thus seem to be an exception to the rule is able to induce a large percentage of DC. This group is composed of 3-O-methyl TPA and the calcium ionophore A23187, which are very effective if applied in stage I before mezerein (an incomplete promoter effective in stage II that does not induce high levels of DC) in a multistage promotion protocol (9).

In another study, it was shown that fluocinolone acetonide and tosyl phenylalanine chloromethyl ketone inhibit stage I promotion and inhibit the production of DC, which are normally induced in large quantities by the stage I promoter (11). Retinoic acid, on the other hand, does not inhibit tumorigenesis if applied during stage I and does not decrease the number of DC. When applied without TPA, retinoic acid is able to induce DC. This correlates with its weak first-stage

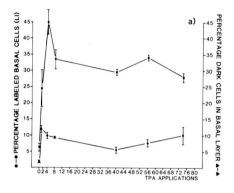

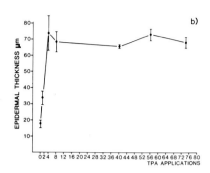

Figure 4. Evaluation of TPA-induced epidermal hyperplasia. (a) Percentage of labeled epidermal basal cells and dark cells in basal layer; (b) epidermal thickness (except horny layer); (c) number of hair follicles per length of epidermal surface. All points are significantly different from the respective values for acetone-treated epidermis (P<.05, Student's t-test). Points, means; bars, SE. (Reproduced from Aldaz CM et al. Cancer Res 45:2753-2758, 1985; used with permission.)

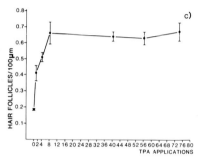

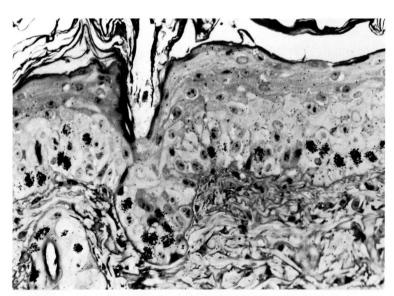

Figure 5. Sustained hyperplasia after TPA application. Note high labeling index after a single injection of tritiated thymidine 1 h before the mice were killed. Epon section, toluidine blue stain. Abbreviation: TPA, 12-O-tetradecanoylphorbol-13-acetate.

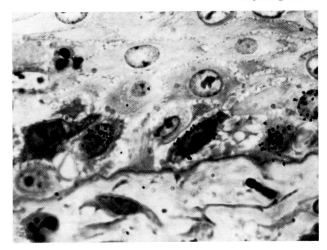

Figure 6. TPA-induced dark basal keratinocytes. Note numerous grains on these cells. Autoradiography after single-pulse tritiated thymidine injection. Epon section, toluidine blue stain. Abbreviation: TPA, 12-O-tetradecanoylphorbol-13-acetate.

and complete promoting capacities (12). These studies suggest that DC are important in stage I of promotion, and that production of DC could be an initial and crucial event in the series of phenomena leading to tumor promotion. In addition, other effective promoters such as benzoyl peroxide, lauroyl peroxide (1), and chrysarobin (Kruszewski F, DiGiovanni J, personal communication) are effective inducers of DC. Regenerative hyperplasia produced by skin abrasion is also a very good DC inducer in the epidermis. Argyris (13) has described abrasion as an effective, although not extremely potent, promoting stimulus.

In addition to the epidermis, other skin components also react when topically treated with chemical agents. Some carcinogens and promoters applied in sufficiently high concentrations are able to totally or partially destroy hair follicles, causing alopecia (14,15). This could be visualized as hypoplasia, atrophy, or even complete absence of these appendages. Sebaceous glands are similarly affected, especially by some carcinogenic chemicals (16,17).

An interesting phenomenon that seems to contradict the previously described effects is that TPA applied repetitively in the usual promoting doses will cause follicular neogenesis (18,19). It is important to note that these studies were carried out in the tail skin, a peculiar area of the integument, which offers a good model for the studies but at the same time is characterized by an unusual scale-interscale regimentation with particular features. In the dorsal skin, the presence of follicular neogenesis was not directly observed; in our studies, a tendency to atrophy and epidermoid metaplasia of the follicles was the rule. Nevertheless, when the follicles were counted in histological sections, there was an obvious increase with respect to those of the untreated controls (Fig. 4C) (20).

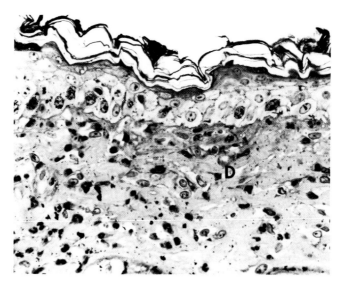

Figure 7. An increased number of inflammatory cells is seen in the papillary dermis (D) a few days after promoter application. Epon section, toluidine blue stain.

Taking into account that differences in strains, doses, and administration schedules can also contribute to this variation, we speculate that a double effect of TPA, which holds true for the epidermis as well—i.e., enhancement of differentiation (metaplasia and hyperorthokeratinization) and dedifferentiation (follicular neogenesis starting from the infundibular region)—constitutes the basis for promoter-induced alterations of epithelial skin components.

Inflammation of the dermis is a well-known effect of most promoters and some carcinogens and has been used by some investigators as an essential parameter (congestion) in biological assays to investigate the putative promoting potential of chemicals (21). The early dermal inflammatory reaction is mainly perivascular and perifollicular. Numerous polymorphonuclear leukocytes are seen distributed in diffuse fashion throughout the papillary dermis (Fig. 7). After repetitive applications, the infiltrates become predominantly lymphocytic and decrease in magnitude, further indications of tissue adaptation to toxic effects. Fibrosis and fibroblastic proliferation of the dermis are also noted during protracted promoter application, resulting in a thickened dermis and increased cellularity (Fig. 8B) (20). Using biochemical techniques, investigators have found increased synthesis and destruction of dermal collagen during this process (22,23).

An increased number of mast cells has also been noted both in promoter- (Fig. 8C) and carcinogen-treated skin (20-24). An interesting observation of Takigawa et al. (25) focused on the destruction of Langerhans cells after

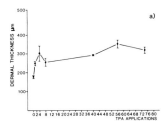

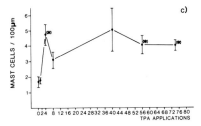

Figure 8. Evaluation of TPA-induced dermal changes after chronic TPA treatment, according to (a) dermal thickness from the basement membrane to the subcutaneous adipose tissue; (b) total dermal cellularity per microscopic field; and (c) number of mast cells per length of epidermal surface. All the data in (a) and (b) and asterisks in (c) represent statistically significant differences from the respective values in acetone-treated controls ($P<.05$ by Student's t-test). Points, means; bars, SE. (Reproduced from Aldaz CM et al. Cancer Res 45:2753-2758, 1985; used with permission.)

promoter application. As has been observed after psoralen-ultraviolet A treatments, it can be speculated that croton oil and TPA decrease the number and/or impair the immunodefensive functions of Langerhans cells, thus enhancing the possibilities for malignant expression.

LATE MORPHOLOGICAL CHANGES INDUCED BY CHEMICAL CARCINOGENESIS PROTOCOLS

The evaluation of the final deleterious effects of chemical carcinogenesis protocols is based on the number and type of cutaneous neoplasms produced. Interestingly, few preneoplastic lesions of the skin, which are common in humans (e.g., solar keratosis), have been described in laboratory animals. In rodents, a large number of papillomas and other benign tumors precede the appearance of cutaneous malignancies, especially when multistage protocols are used. This indicates that at least for these experimental approaches, papillomas should be considered premalignant lesions (26,27). Similar observations have been made with respect to keratoacanthomas. These tumors are clearly premalignant in rodents (28-30).

EXPERIMENTALLY INDUCED SKIN TUMORS

Since Yamagiwa and Ishikawa (31) produced the first chemically induced skin cancers in rabbits by protracted topical applications, a large number of investigators have induced skin tumors in mice, rats, hamsters, guinea pigs, and other animals. Although some tumor types are more frequent in certain strains or species, the general morphological characteristics of these tumors are similar in the different species, including man. In addition, some chemical carcinogens will preferentially induce specific tumor types, but as a general rule, tumor morphology is independent of the experimental protocol used to induce the tumors, and many different carcinogens will produce the same tumor types.

Papilloma

Papillomas are benign epithelial tumors seen frequently after chemical carcinogen exposure, especially in two-stage carcinogenesis protocols of mouse skin. They are probably the most common skin tumors seen by cancer researchers. Papillomas are cauliflower-like structures with either a narrow or a broad base consisting of a series of folds united by common stalks to the underlying skin (Fig. 9). Each of these folds consists of a central connective tissue core covered by an epidermis-like epithelium. The epithelium is usually thick and has numerous mitoses in the germinative layers; a high, although variable, labeling

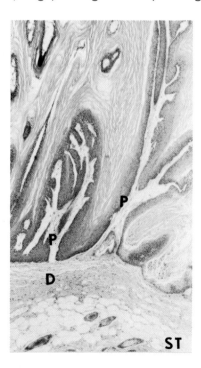

Figure 9. Papilloma of murine skin produced by two-stage carcinogenesis protocol. Abbreviations: ST, subcutaneous tissue; D, dermis; P, papillomatous components.

index; distinct spinous and granular layers; and a thick, usually orthokeratotic, horny layer. Areas of cellular atypia can be seen in many of these tumors.

Papillomas seem to arise from metaplastic or hyperplastic hair follicles, especially from the infundibular area. Papillomas may regress or continue their progression toward carcinomas. Papilloma regression has been well documented (32) in two-stage carcinogenesis, but the possibility that many of the regressions are due to accidents such as torsion of the pedicle, biting, and infection has not been excluded. Confluency into larger, usually malignant, tumors is also a distinct possibility. Most of the papillomas induced by two-stage carcinogenesis protocols have the potential to progress to carcinomas. Extensive chromosome analyses, as well as the frequent presence of atypical foci or clear-cut microcarcinomas in these lesions, support this possibility (26,27). Papillomas produced by complete carcinogenesis protocols do not regress and eventually give rise to carcinomas. However, it is generally accepted that most carcinomas produced with these protocols arise de novo from nonpapillomatous skin.

Keratoacanthoma

Keratoacanthomas (KA) are similar in all species, including man. They appear often after exposure to UV light or complete carcinogens. They are rarely seen in two-stage carcinogenesis experiments. As does its human counterpart, murine KA starts as an intradermal growth of epithelial prolongations originating in the hair follicles (33,34). It usually acquires a cup-shaped architecture with a central horny crater and a papillomatous exophytic component, as well as an endophytic component of deeply penetrating epithelial cords that usually does not invade the panniculus carnosus. Regression of murine KA does not seem to be common. Conversely, conversion to squamous cell carcinoma seems widely accepted by numerous authors (28-30).

Squamous Cell Carcinoma

Squamous cell carcinomas (SCC) have been induced in many different species using UV light, ionizing radiation, or chemical carcinogens. These tumors originate from preexisting lesions such as papillomas, KA, and preneoplastic lesions, or from apparently normal or hyperplastic epidermis. Histologically, they are usually well differentiated, with massive production of horny material (Fig. 10). Less-differentiated SCC variants, including spindle cell carcinoma (35), are less common. Metastasis to regional lymph nodes and distant sites, especially the lungs, is a late occurrence. Practically all SCC will metastasize after 1 year (Fig. 11) (36).

Other Tumors

Basal cell carcinomas (BCCs) are frequent in the rat. With protocols of complete and two-stage chemical carcinogenesis, the incidence of BCC is higher

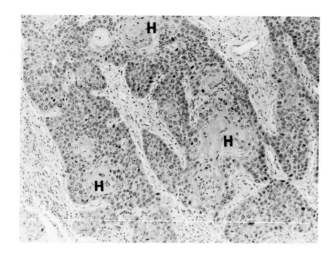

Figure 10. Squamous cell carcinoma of mouse skin produced by DMBA initiation and TPA promotion. Paraffin-embedded section with hematoxylin and eosin stain. Abbreviations: DMBA, dimethylbenz[a]anthracene; TPA, 12-O-tetradecanoylphorbol-13-acetate; H, horny pearls.

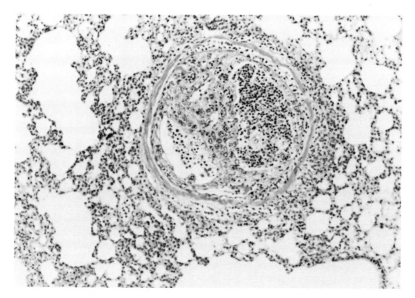

Figure 11. Metastatic embolus in the lung from a chemically induced squamous carcinoma. Paraffin-embedded section stained with hematoxylin and eosin.

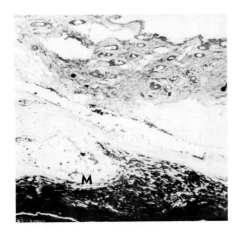

Figure 12. Murine subcutaneous melanoma (M) induced by complete carcinogenesis with DMBA. Paraffin-embedded section with hematoxylin and eosin stain. Abbreviation: DMBA, dimethylbenz[a]anthracene.

than that of SCC (37). Since rats are rarely used in experimental cutaneous oncology, the literature on rodent BCC is not abundant. BCC in rats is frequently of the nodular type, and the histological variants resemble those seen in man (38). BCC are occasionally seen in mice (39). Other adnexal tumors such as sebaceous ones, adenomas, and trichoepitheliomas have been described in rats, mice, and hamsters (38,40,41).

Melanotic tumors, a generic term that includes both benign and malignant tumors, have been produced by topical carcinogenic treatment of the skin in hamsters, guinea pigs, gerbils, and mice (42). Most chemically induced melanotic tumors are less aggressive than are human malignant melanomas.

Most lesions in hamsters and mice resemble dermal blue nevi or intradermal melanocytic tumors (Fig. 12) (43-45). Although there are reports of hamster melanotic tumors metastasizing spontaneously or after transplantation into syngeneic hosts (44-47), the progression to malignancy of most lesions is probably very slow, if it takes place at all. Similar conclusions can be reached about murine melanotic lesions. Nevertheless, in a recent report, Berkelhammer and Oxenhandler (48) reported the production of metastatic malignant melanomas in C57Bl/6 mice with dimethylbenz[a]anthracene (DMBA) and croton oil. Guinea pigs treated with DMBA develop melanomas of the nodular type, some of which eventuate in regional and distant metastases (49,50).

In summary, studies of the effects of carcinogens and tumor promoters on the skin have helped elucidate carcinogenesis mechanisms in the progression of benign lesions such as papillomas to melanomas and squamous cell carcinomas.

OPEN FORUM

Dr. S. C. Lewis: Is there any differential response of the rat to different classes of carcinogens? Specifically, does the rat respond with papillomas and carcinomas to polynuclear aromatic-type carcinogens as opposed to the more exotic organics?

Dr. A. J. P. Klein-Szanto: The experiments I have seen lately are complete carcinogenesis experiments with DMBA and methylcholanthrene, which have been the classic carcinogens producing basal cell carcinomas. There seems to be some kind of dose-related effect. Lower doses of DMBA result in basal cell carcinomas; higher doses result in squamous cell carcinomas without basal cell carcinomas, implying that the higher dose is toxic to the stem cells for the basal cell carcinomas.

Dr. Stuart Yuspa: You showed variable risk for progression, with different slopes for papillomas to carcinomas. Do you think this is predetermined at the initiation state or random? What determines that?

Dr. Klein-Szanto: We used continuous applications in our experiment. I suspect this has something to do with it. When TPA is not applied during 50 weeks, the results are different. Papillomas regress or the yield is lower; however, we have not studied the chromosomal changes in that type of protocol.

Dr. Yuspa: Have you increased the dose of initiator to see whether the slopes change?

Dr. Klein-Szanto: No.

Dr. A. Balmain: Dr. Klein-Szanto, you mentioned the different morphologies of the papillomas that you observed during initiation and promotion. Have you seen any consistent changes depending on the particular initiator used? In other words, do papillomas induced with N-methyl-N'-nitro-N-nitrosoguanidine (MNNG) look slightly different than those induced with DMBA? Molecular evidence indicates that these two substances may not have similar types of mutations in these tumors. Also, is there any difference in the frequency of progression depending on the initiating agent used?

Dr. Klein-Szanto: I do not know. We have not really looked at other initiators in detail. However, the type of protocol clearly influences the type of tumors induced by MNNG. The types of tumors resulting when MNNG, for example, is used as a complete carcinogen are remarkably different than those resulting from an initiation-promotion protocol.

Dr. John DiGiovanni: There are some data on the ratio of carcinomas to papillomas that arise under the influence of different skin tumor initiators. With MNNG, one often sees a higher ratio of carcinomas to papillomas. This is very reproducible. DMBA results in a tremendous number of papillomas; however, MNNG always results in a low number of papillomas, most of which become carcinomas.

Question: Are the absolute numbers about the same?

Dr. R. K. Boutwell: We have compared DMBA, benzo[a]pyrene, methylcholanthrene, and dibenzanthracene as complete carcinogens as well as initiators in the same experiment, and there is a remarkable difference in the ratio of papillomas to carcinomas, even among various hydrocarbons. With benzo[a]pyrene, you do not see many papillomas but you can certainly induce carcinomas. Certainly DMBA results in more absolute numbers of papillomas than all the other hydrocarbons.

Dr. P. H. Craig: How were the doses normalized? Were they normalized on a weight basis? Do you think there might also be a difference in the degree of metabolism or the degree of activation?

Dr. Boutwell: In that particular experiment, which was either complete carcinogenesis or initiation-promotion, 25, 10, and 1 µg were applied to the skin to determine a dose-response curve for DMBA. The other carcinogens were applied equimolar to the 25 µg levels of DMBA. DMBA was by far the most effective on a molar basis, particularly for papillomas. Originally, Berenblum used benzo[a]pyrene because that was the more readily available hydrocarbon.

REFERENCES

1. Klein-Szanto AJP, Slaga TJ. Effects of peroxides on rodent skin: Epidermal hyperplasia and tumor promotion. J Invest Dermatol 79:30-34, 1982.
2. Klein-Szanto AJP. Morphological evaluation of tumor promoter effects on mammalian skin. In Slaga TJ (ed): Mechanisms of Tumor Promotion, Vol. II. Boca Raton, FL: CRC Press, 1984, pp 41-72.
3. Klein-Szanto AJP, Chiba M, Lee SU, Conti CJ, Thetford D. Keratinocyte damage produced by 12-O-tetradecanoylphorbol-13-acetate in rodent epidermis. Carcinogenesis 5:1459-1465, 1984.
4. Argyris TS. Analysis of the epidermal hyperplasia produced by acetic acid, a poor promoter, in the skin of female mice initiated with DMBA. J Invest Dermatol 80:430-435, 1983.
5. Argyris TS. Nature of epidermal hyperplasia produced by mezerein, a weak tumor promoter, in initiated skin of mice. Cancer Res 43:1768-1773, 1983.
6. Sisskin EE, Barrett JC. Hyperplasia of Syrian hamster epidermis induced by single but not multiple treatments with 12-O-tetradecanoylphorbol-13-acetate. Cancer Res 41:346-350, 1981.
7. Hasper F, Miller G, Schweizer J. Histological, proliferative, and biochemical alterations in dorsal epidermis of the Syrian golden hamster induced by 12-O-tetradecanoylphorbol-13-acetate and the calcium ionophore A23187. Cancer Res 42:2034-2039, 1982.
8. Klein-Szanto AJP, Major SK, Slaga TJ. Induction of dark keratinocytes by 12-O-tetradecanoylphorbol-13-acetate and mezerein as an indicator of tumor-promoting efficiency. Carcinogenesis 1:399-406, 1980.
9. Klein-Szanto AJP, Slaga TJ. Numerical variation of dark cells in normal and chemically induced hyperplastic epidermis with age of animal and efficiency of tumor promoters. Cancer Res 41:4437-4440, 1981.
10. Slaga TJ, Klein-Szanto AJP, Triplett L, Yotti L, Trosko JE. Skin tumor promoting activity of benzoyl peroxide, a widely used free radical generating compound. Science 213:1023-1025, 1981.
11. Slaga TJ, Klein-Szanto AJP, Fischer SM, Weeks CE, Nelson K, Major S. Studies

on the mechanism of action of antitumor promoting agents: Their specificity in two-stage promotion. Proc Natl Acad Sci USA 77:2251-2254, 1980.

12. Fischer S, Klein-Szanto AJP, Adams LM, Slaga TJ. The first stage and complete promoting activity of retinoic acid but not the analog RO-10-9359. Carcinogenesis 6:575-578, 1985.

13. Argyris TS, Slaga TJ. Promotion of carcinomas by repeated abrasion in initiated skin of mice. Cancer Res 41:5193-5195, 1981.

14. Cramer W, Stowell RE. The early stages of carcinogenesis with 20-methylcholanthrene in the skin of the mouse. II. Microscopic tissue changes. JNCI 2:379-402, 1942.

15. Liang HM, Cowdry EV. Changes in hair follicles after a single painting of methylcholanthrene in ice. Cancer Res 14:340-345, 1954.

16. Bock FC, Mund R. Evaluation of substances causing loss of sebaceous glands from mouse skin. J Invest Dermatol 26:479-481, 1956.

17. Bock FC, Mund R. A survey of compounds for activity in the suppression of mouse sebaceous glands. Cancer Res 18:887-892, 1958.

18. Schweizer J. Neogenesis of functional hair follicles in adult mouse skin selectively induced by tumor-promoting phorbol esters. Experientia 35:1651-1653, 1979.

19. Schweizer J, Marks F. Induction of the formation of new hair follicles in mouse tail epidermis by the tumor promoter TPA. Cancer Res 37:4195-4201, 1977.

20. Aldaz CM, Conti CJ, Gimenez IB, Slaga TJ, Klein-Szanto AJP. Cutaneous changes during prolonged application of 12-O-tetradecanoylphorbol-13-acetate mouse skin and residual effects after cessation of treatment. Cancer Res 45:2753-2758, 1985.

21. Hecker E. Isolation and characterization of the cocarcinogenic principles from croton oil. Methods in Cancer Research 6:439-484, 1971.

22. Marian B. Enhancement of collagen-degrading enzymes in the dermis after one topical application of tumor-promoting phorbol esters. Carcinogenesis 7:723-726, 1986.

23. Marian B. Chronic 12-O-tetradecanoylphorbol-13-acetate treatment prevents restoration of collagen loss associated with its inflammatory effect on mouse skin. Cancer Lett 34:273-282, 1987.

24. Farnoush A, Mackenzie IC. Proliferation of mast cells in normal and DMBA-treated mouse skin. J Oral Pathol 13:359-365, 1984.

25. Takigawa M, Komura J, Ofriji S. Early fine structural changes in human epidermis following application of croton oil. Acta Derm Venereol (Stockh) 58:31-36, 1978.

26. Conti CJ, Aldaz CM, O'Connell JF, Klein-Szanto AJP, Slaga TJ. Aneuploidy, an early event in mouse skin tumor development. Carcinogenesis 7:1845-1848, 1986.

27. Aldaz CM, Conti CJ, Klein-Szanto AJP, Slaga TJ. Progressive dysplasia and aneuploidy are hallmarks of mouse skin papillomas: Relevance to malignancy. Proc Natl Acad Sci USA 84:2029-2032, 1987.

28. Canfield PJ, Greenoak GE, Reeve VE, Gallagher CH. Characterization of UV induced keratoacanthoma-like lesions in HRA/Skh-1 mice and their comparison with keratoacanthomas in man. Pathology 17:613-616, 1985.

29. Hannuksela M, Stenbäck F, Lahti A. The carcinogenic properties of topical PUVA: A lifelong study in mice. Arch Dermatol Res 278:347-351, 1986.

30. Holland JM, Fry RJM. Neoplasms of the mouse integument and arde. In Foster HL, Small JD, Fox JG (eds): Experimental Biology and Oncology. New York: Academic Press, 1982, pp 513-528.

31. Yamagiwa K, Tshikawa K. Uber die atypische Epithelwucherung. Verh Jpn Pathol Ges 4:136-148, 1914.

32. Burns FJ, Albert RE, Altshuler B. Cancer progression in mouse skin. In Slaga TJ (ed): Mechanisms of Tumor Promotion, Vol II. Boca Raton, FL: CRC Press, 1984, pp. 18-39.

33. Ghadially FN. Comparative morphological study of keratoacanthoma of man and similar experimentally produced lesions in rabbit. J Pathol Bacteriol 75:441-453, 1958.

34. Ghadially FN. The role of the hair follicle in the origin and evolution of some cutaneous neoplasms of man and experimental animals. Cancer 14:801-816, 1961.

35. Morison WL, Jerdan MS, Hoover TL, Farmer ER. UV radiation-induced tumors in haired mice: Identification as squamous cell carcinomas. JNCI 77:1155-1162, 1986.

36. Patskan GJ, Klein-Szanto AJP, Phillips JL, Slaga TJ. Metastasis from squamous cell carcinomas of sencar mouse skin produced by complete carcinogenesis. Cancer Lett 34:121-127, 1987.

37. Schweizer J, Loehrke H, Hesse B, Goerttler K. 7,12-Dimethylbenz[a]anthracene/12-O-tetradecanoyl-phorbol-13-acetate-mediated skin tumor initiation and promotion in male Sprague-Dawley rats. Carcinogenesis 3:785-789, 1982.

38. Zackheim HS. Experimental basal cell carcinoma in the rat. In Maibach L (ed): Models in Dermatology, Vol. I. Karger: Basle, 1985, pp 89-97.

39. Johnson WD, Robertson KA, Pounds JG, Allen JR. Dehydroretronecine-induced skin tumors in mice. JNCI 61:85-89, 1978.

40. Goerttler K, Loehrke H, Hesse B, Schweizer J. Skin tumor formation in the European hamster (Cricetus cricetus L.) after topical initiation with 7,12-dimethylbenz[a]anthracene (DMBA) and promotion with 12-O-tetradecanoylphorbol-13-acetate (TPA). Carcinogenesis 5:521-524, 1984.

41. Rice JM, Anderson LM. Sebaceous adenomas with associated epidermal hyperplasia and papilloma formation as a major type of tumor induced in mouse skin by high doses of carcinogens. Cancer Lett 33:295-306, 1986.

42. Pawlowski A, Lea PJ. Nevi and melanoma induced by chemical carcinogens in laboratory animals: Similarities and differences with human lesions. J Cutan Pathol 10:81-110, 1983.

43. Ghadially FN, Ghadially R, Lalonde J-M. A comparative ultrastructural study of cutaneous blue naevi of humans and hamsters. J Submicrosc Cytol 18:417-432, 1986.

44. Kanno J, Matsubara O, Kasuga T. Histogenesis of the intradermal melanocytic tumor in BDF1 mice induced by topical application of 9,10-dimethyl-1,2-benzanthracene (DMBA) and 12-O-tetradecanoylphorbol-13-acetate (TPA). Acta Pathol Jpn 36:1-14, 1986.

45. Rappaport H, Pietra G, Shubik P. The induction of melanotic tumors resembling cellular blue nevi in the Syrian white hamster by cutaneous application of 7,12-dimethylbenz[a]anthracene. Cancer Res 21:661-666, 1961.

46. Goerttler K, Loehrke H, Schweizer J, Hesse B. Two-stage tumorigenesis of dermal melanocytes in the back skin of the Syrian golden hamster using systemic initiation with 7,12-dimethylbenz[a]anthracene and topical promotion with 12-O-tetradecanoylphorbol-13-acetate. Cancer Res 40:155-161, 1980.

47. Vesselinovitch SD, Mihailovich N, Richter WR. The induction of malignant melanomas in Syrian white hamsters by neonatal exposure to urethane. Cancer Res 30:2543-2547, 1970.

48. Berkelhammer J, Oxenhandler RW. Evaluation of premalignant and malignant lesions during the induction of mouse melanomas. Cancer Res 47:1251-1254, 1987.

49. Pawlowski A, Haberman HF, Menon IA. Junctional and compound pigmented nevi induced by 9,10-dimethyl-1,2-benzanthracene in skin of albino guinea pigs. Cancer Res 36:2813-2821, 1976.
50. Pawlowski A, Haberman HF, Menon IA. Skin melanoma induced by 7,12-dimethylbenzanthracene in albino guinea pigs and its similarities to skin melanomas of humans. Cancer Res 40:3653-3660, 1980.

Skin Carcinogenesis: Mechanisms and Human Relevance, pages 63–80
© 1989 Alan R. Liss, Inc.

Epidermal Tumor Promotion by Damage in the Skin of Mice

*Thomas S. Argyris**

Department of Pathology, State University of New York, Health Sciences Center, Syracuse, New York 13210

Two-stage skin carcinogenesis involves initiation treatment of the epidermis with a subcarcinogenic dose of a carcinogen, usually dimethylbenz[a]anthracene (DMBA), followed by multiple applications of a tumor promoter, such as 12-O-tetradecanoylphorbol-13-acetate (TPA), usually twice weekly until tumors appear (1). The hallmark of tumor promotion is the appearance of an epidermal hyperplasia. This form of epidermal growth is characterized by epidermal thickening due to an increase in the number of cell layers. There is an increased amount of mitotic activity in the basal layer of the epidermis, and the suprabasal cells are greatly enlarged (2). Epidermal hyperplasia also characterizes the response of the epidermis to a wide variety of damaging stimuli, from mechanical to irradiation damage (3). Therefore, the role of damage in the production of epidermal tumors had been investigated long before the two-stage skin carcinogenesis regimen became popular (for review, see ref. 3). In general it was found that wounding did often enhance tumor production in the skin of mice.

EPIDERMAL TUMOR PROMOTION IN MICE BY DAMAGE IN SKIN GIVEN INITIATION TREATMENTS

Hennings and Boutwell (4), Clark-Lewis and Murray (5), and ourselves (6), using slightly different two-stage skin carcinogenesis protocols, demonstrated that full-thickness wounds in DMBA-treated mouse skin results in the appearance of tumors (Fig. 1), thus showing that full-thickness wounds are a sufficient condition for epidermal tumor promotion in mice. One cannot conclude, however, that the regenerative epidermal hyperplasia at the wound edge, where the tumors appear, is by itself a sufficient condition for the promotion of epidermal tumors. The reason is that, in addition to the regenerative epidermal hyperplasia, there is a massive connective tissue growth, the formation of the granulation

---

* Address for correspondence: 1525 Dolphin Drive, Aptos, CA 95003.

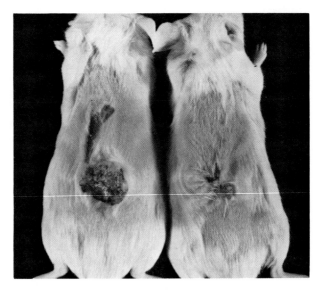

Figure 1. Papillomas on the back skin of CD-1 female mice given dimethylbenz-[a]anthracene as initiator and repeated full-thickness wounds as promoters.

tissue. The regenerating epidermal tissue sits on top of the granulation tissue. Therefore it may receive cues from the granulation tissue that enable epidermal tumor promotion. That connective tissue underlying the epidermis can influence it by a variety of cues is well known (7). To demonstrate that regenerative epidermal hyperplasia is sufficient for epidermal tumor promotion in initiation-treated mouse skin, one must demonstrate that the regenerating epidermis by itself, without any underlying regenerating connective tissue, can support tumor promotion. This requires that we produce a regenerative epidermal hyperplasia without the associated granulation tissue formation. This can be done by removing the epidermis by abrasion, which leads to its regeneration from the underlying hair follicles, without any massive connective tissue regeneration (8). The epidermis is hyperplastic for at least 10 days, and then gradually returns to its normal thickness by about 21 days after abrasion.

The skin of mice given DMBA was repeatedly abraded every 21 days, and after about six cycles of abrasion papillomas and carcinomas appeared in the abraded area (Figs. 2 and 3). Therefore, regenerative epidermal hyperplasia is sufficient for epidermal tumor promotion (6,9). Because the number of tumors that appear along the wound edge or in the abraded area is much less than that seen on the back of a mouse following the application of a chemical tumor promoter, it is often concluded that full-thickness wounds and abrasion are weak tumor promoters. This conclusion is incorrect because the abraded area is much

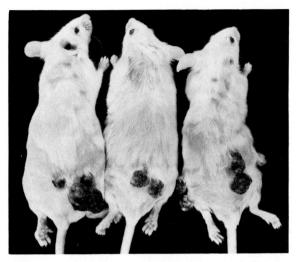

Figure 2. Papillomas on the back skin of SENCAR mice treated by dimethylbenz[a]anthracene as initiator and repeated abrasion as promoter. (Reprinted with permission from Argyris TS, CRC Crit Rev Toxicol 14:211-258, 1985. Copyright CRC Press, Inc., Boca Raton, FL.)

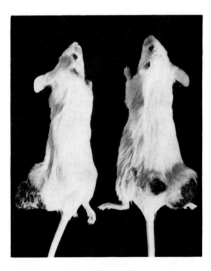

Figure 3. Carcinomas on the back skin of SENCAR mice treated by dimethylbenz[a]anthracene as initiator and repeated abrasion as promoter. (Reprinted with permission from Argyris TS, CRC Crit Rev Toxicol 14:211-258, 1985. Copyright CRC Press, Inc., Boca Raton, FL.)

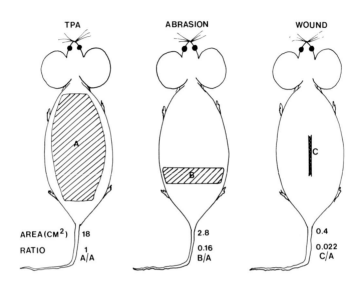

Figure 4. Diagrammatic sketch of the area of skin given promotion treatments of TPA, abrasion, or full-thickness wounds. (From Argyris TS, CRC Crit Rev Toxicol 14:211, 1985, with permission, copyright, CRC Press, Inc., Boca Raton, FL.)

smaller than that to which a chemical promoter is applied. Figure 4 shows that the area to which a chemical tumor promoter is applied is about 18 cm², that abraded is about 2.8 cm², and that wounded is 0.4 cm². Clearly, if we want to compare the efficiency of abrasion or wounding for promotion with that of a chemical promoter such as TPA, we must normalize the data we get after abrasion or wounding to an area equivalent to that treated by TPA. If we do this we find that both abrasion and wounding produce as many tumors as TPA. This is shown for wounding in Table 1. The actual number of papillomas per mouse are many fewer than that after treatment with TPA, but when normalized to the area treated by TPA, the number of tumors is equal. Table 1 also shows that delaying tumor promotion by wounding for up to a year following initiation does not affect the efficiency of tumor promotion. This is also true for chemical tumor promoters (1). Thus, promotion by damaging stimuli need not follow soon after initiation in order for tumor promotion to occur. Another important fact about promotion by damage is the demonstration by Hennings and Boutwell (4) that a single wound 4 cm in length made on the backs of tumor-susceptible mice 6 weeks after treatment with DMBA leads to the appearance of both papillomas and carcinomas. Thus under the proper circumstances a single wounding is a sufficient condition for the appearance of tumors. This, to the best of my

Table 1. The Effect of Varying the Time between Initiation of CD-1 Female Mouse Skin with 200 nmoles of Domethylbenzanthracene and Promotion by Repeated Wounding Every 14 Days

No. of mice	Age mice initiated	Time post-initiation mice wounded	No. of times skin cut	Mice with tumors	No. of tumors	Tumors/ mouse	Normalized tumors/ mouse
32	2 months	7 days	6*	8	11	0.34†	14.5‡
18	2 months	3 months	6	5	5	0.28	11.9
27	2 months	6 months	6	10	14	0.52	22.1
22	2 months	12 months	6	5	6	0.27	11.4

* Full-thickness skin wounds 2 cm long were made. Wounds were reopened every 14 days
† The area of skin promoted by wounding was 0.4 cm².
‡ The number of tumors if the area promoted by wounding was 17 cm² as it was after the application of chemical promoters such as TPA.

knowledge, has never been demonstrated for TPA. Thus, for those individuals who may have a genetic predisposition to carcinogenesis, a single traumatic event could be all that is necessary for tumor promotion to occur.

We can conclude that a regenerative epidermal hyperplasia is a sufficient condition for epidermal tumor promotion in the skin of mice. Does this mean that all regenerative epidermal hyperplasias are sufficient conditions for epidermal tumor promotion in the skin of mice? There is not sufficient evidence to answer this question, but current evidence suggests that some regenerative epidermal hyperplasias are not capable of supporting tumor promotion. Furstenberger et al. (10) claim that if one gently rubs the back of mice with fine cosmetic sandpaper one can produce a regenerative hyperplasia. If one periodically continues the rubbing of the skin with the cosmetic sandpaper, one can sustain the epidermal hyperplasia. This regimen applied to initiation-treated skin of mice does not result in epidermal tumor promotion. Similarly, plucking hair follicles in mouse skin in the resting phase initiates hair follicle growth. In addition, the epidermis undergoes a regenerative epidermal hyperplastic growth due to the damage to the surrounding epidermis caused by the hair plucking (11). The epidermal hyperplasia persists for at least 10 days, and then the epidermis slowly returns to its normal thickness by about 21 days after plucking. We have plucked DMBA-treated (200 nmol) CD-1 female mouse skin eight times, and no epidermal tumors have appeared (unpublished observations). Thus there may be some situations in which regenerative epidermal hyperplasias are not a sufficient condition for epidermal tumor promotion. Of course, we cannot rule out the possibility that if Furstenberger et al. (10) had extended their cosmetic paper abrasion for a longer period of time, or if we had continued our plucking for many more times, epidermal tumors would have appeared.

The question arises as to what are the characteristics of the epidermal regenerative hyperplasias that are successful in tumor promotion. To begin to answer this question, we have examined the growth characteristics of the regenerative epidermal hyperplasia produced by abrasion.

THE GROWTH KINETICS OF THE REGENERATIVE EPIDERMAL HYPER-PLASIA PRODUCED BY ABRASION

Normal mouse epidermis (Fig. 5) is approximately two cell layers in thickness, whereas the regenerative hyperplasia caused by abrasion has at least four cell layers, and the epidermal cells are much enlarged (Fig. 6). Thus this hyperplasia is characterized by a considerable increase in epidermal mass. How is this epidermal growth brought about? Within 3 days after abrasion, the epidermal mass, as measured by changes in epidermal wet weight and protein, exceeds that of the normal epidermis (Fig. 7). Epidermal growth continues and reaches its maximum, approximately six times that of normal, at about 5 days after abrasion. Gradually by 21 days after abrasion, epidermal wet weight and protein return toward normal levels. Figure 7 also shows that the increase in epidermal mass is due to an increase in the number of cells, as shown by the increase in total DNA, and to an increase in epidermal size, as indicated by the increases in epidermal wet weight and protein that are beyond the level of the increase in total DNA. These results are expected from Figure 6. There is no information on how the increase in epidermal cell size is brought about except that, associated with the increase in epidermal wet weight and protein, there is

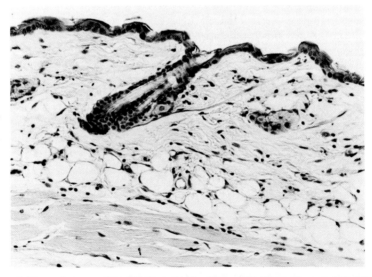

Figure 5. Normal mouse skin. H&E, magnification x 195. (From Argyris TS, CRC Crit Rev Toxicol 14:211, 1985, with permission, copyright CRC Press Inc., Boca Raton, FL.)

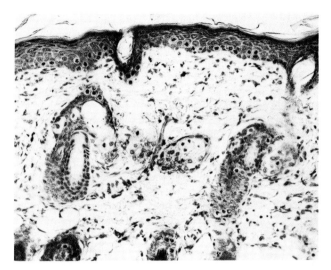

Figure 6. Regenerative epidermal hyperplasia 6 days following abrasion. H&E, magnification x 195. (From Argyris TS, CRC Crit Rev Toxicol 14:211, 1985, with permission, copyright, CRC Press, Inc., Boca Raton, FL.)

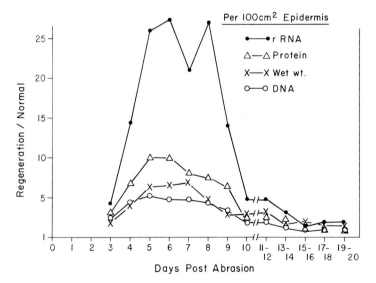

Figure 7. Epidermal wet weight, total protein, DNA, and ribosomal RNA in regenerating mouse epidermis following abrasion. (From Argyris TS, CRC Crit Rev Toxicol 9:151, 1981, with permission, copyright CRC Press, Inc., Boca Raton, FL.)

a massive increase in the number of ribosomes per cell (Fig. 7). Just what the relationship is between the massive accumulation of ribosomes and the increase in cell size deserves investigation because it may give us a clue as to the mechanism for increasing epidermal cell size during epidermal hyperplastic growth.

In contrast to our almost total ignorance of the mechanism by which cell enlargement is brought about during regenerative epidermal hyperplastic growth, we have some information as to how the increase in epidermal cell number is achieved. There is a large increase in epidermal mitotic activity seen by 3 days after abrasion. Mitotic activity remains high until about 10 days after abrasion and then begins, gradually, to return toward normal levels (12). But at the end of the regenerative cycle, at 21 days, it is still slightly above normal, even though epidermal thickness is normal. The increase in epidermal mitotic activity is not due to an increase in the number of epidermal cells entering the cell cycle because the growth fraction in normal epidermis is essentially 1, or 100% (13). That is, all the basal epidermal cells are cycling, although not all at the same rate (14). Therefore the increase in the epidermal basal cell proliferative activity must be due to a decrease in the cell cycle time of the basal cells. This is in fact what occurs. Morris has shown that most basal cells in normal mouse epidermis require about 121-175 h to go through the cell cycle (13). Three days after abrasion the basal epidermal cells traverse the cell cycle in just 11 h. During the next few days, when the epidermal hyperplastic growth is at its maximum, the cell cycle remains short. It begins to increase as the hyperplastic epidermis returns to its normal size. Morris has also shown that the drastic reduction in the length of the cell cycle during regenerative epidermal hyperplastic growth following abrasion is almost completely accounted for by the decrease in the length of the G1 phase of the cell cycle (13). This phase, which usually requires 120-150 h in normal mouse epidermis, is completed in just 2-4 h during the growth phase of the regenerative epidermal hyperplasia following abrasion. This means that the required replication of the cellular constituents necessary for the orderly progression of the epidermal cells through the cell cycle is accomplished in an astonishingly short period of time.

Another method that the epidermis might use to increase its mass during its regenerative growth following abrasion would be to decrease the rate of epidermal cell differentiation or keratinization. The rate of epidermal cell differentiation can be approximately determined by measuring the transit time of the epidermal cells; that is, the time required for the basal cells to reach the top layer of the epidermis. In normal epidermis it usually requires about 8 days for the basal cells to reach the top layer of the epidermis (13). Following abrasion the transit time is actually reduced to about 2 days. Therefore, the growth of the epidermis following abrasion occurs not only without the help of a decrease in the rate of epidermal cell differentiation, but actually in spite of an increase in that rate.

Epidermal regeneration following the removal of the epidermis by abrasion is quite different from the kind of regeneration that occurs in other types of organs, such as in the liver after partial hepatectomy or the kidney following unilateral nephrectomy. This difference is shown in a diagramatic fashion in Figure 8. In A, the growth kinetics are depicted for normal growth of cells in

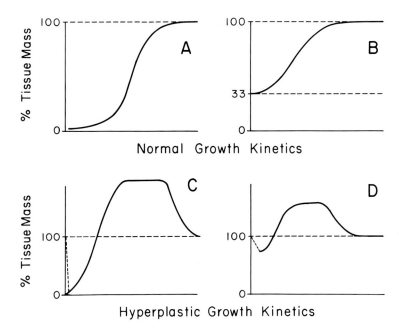

Figure 8. Idealized drawing to show normal and hyperplastic growth kinetics. (A) Normal growth kinetics, such as for cells in culture. (B) Normal regenerative growth kinetics such as for regenerating liver following partial hepatectomy. (C) Hyperplastic growth kinetics, following the removal of the entire epidermis by abrasion, with epidermal regeneration occurring from the underlying hair follicles. (D) Hyperplastic growth kinetics following treatment of the epidermis with a chemical that causes some epidermal destruction. (From Argyris TS, CRC Crit Rev Toxicol 9:151, 1981, with permission, copyright, CRC Press, Inc., Boca Raton, FL.)

culture or organs during embryonic development. In B, we see that similar kinetics occur, for example, after the removal of two-thirds of the liver following partial hepatectomy. The liver regenerates its mass, and once this is achieved growth ceases. Similar kinetics would be seen if one kidney were removed. The remaining kidney would grow to restore the lost mass and then stop growing. But, as we see in C, the regeneration of the epidermis following its removal by abrasion exhibits quite different growth kinetics. The epidermis regenerates quickly, but restoration of epidermal mass does not signal the end of the regenerative process. Epidermal growth continues, resulting in a massive overshoot followed by a gradual decrease in epidermal mass to its normal amount. If epidermal mass is only partly reduced, as happens after, for example, tape stripping, the kinetics of epidermal growth are similar to that following abrasion, except that the overshoot is less (D). Thus, compared to the regenerative growth of other organs, epidermal hyperplastic growth does not show "normal" growth kinetics. It is no wonder that early investigators of regenerative epidermal hyperplastic growth viewed it as a kind of preneoplastic growth.

Why does this massive overshoot in epidermal growth occur? We do not have an answer to this important question, but we do offer the following speculation. We have already pointed out that during regenerative epidermal hyperplastic growth there is a massive increase in ribosomes, usually 4-5 times that seen in normal epidermal cells. This massive accumulation of ribosomes is probably much more than is needed for cell replication in the basal layer and for epidermal cell keratinization or differentiation in the suprabasal layers (3). We speculate that this large increase in epidermal ribosomes results in unbalanced growth. This is supported by the fact that protein/cell is 2-3 times above normal, as we have indicated in Figure 7. In order for growth to be brought into proper balance, the epidermal cells will continue to proliferate until ribosome numbers are reduced. Thus we envision that the abnormal buildup of ribosomes acts as a driving force that keeps the epidermal cells proliferating (15). There are a number of lines of evidence to support this speculation. Fibroblasts grown in 10% serum-containing medium show optimal growth characteristics, accompanied by a synthesis of rRNA. If one removes the fibroblasts and places them in a 0.5% serum-containing medium, growth and the synthesis of rRNA cease (16). If one grows fibroblasts in a 10% serum-containing medium for a few hours and then transfers them to a 0.5 % medium, some of the fibroblasts continue to enter DNA synthesis and presumably divide. The longer one keeps the fibroblasts in 10% serum-containing medium before transferring them to a 0.5% serum medium, the greater the number of fibroblasts that continue to divide. The authors suggest that those cells that continue to divide are those that have accumulated a certain number of ribosomes. Thus the accumulation of ribosomes acts as an inertial force that permits the fibroblasts to divide in an environment that is normally not supportive of cell proliferation.

If Chinese hamster cells are placed in a medium that contains actinomycin D at a dosage that inhibits rRNA synthesis but not mRNA or tRNA synthesis, the cells will not divide. If, however, the cells are allowed to synthesize rRNA and thus accumulate ribosomes before they are exposed to actinomycin D, then a fair number of the cells will continue to divide, even though they are in an environment that is unsupportive of DNA synthesis and cell division (17).

Thus the evidence suggests that the accumulation of ribosomes, as well as the network of other linked metabolic changes, appears to keep cells dividing. Epidermal hyperplastic growth differs from normal growth in that the ribosome accumulation and the other linked metabolic changes persist, resulting in the maintenance of high epidermal proliferative activity. This in turn leads to epidermal overgrowth, that is, the formation of the epidermal hyperplasia. Eventually the numbers of ribosomes are reduced, and the epidermis returns to its normal thickness.

We may next ask what characteristics of the epidermal hyperplasias are not sufficient conditions for epidermal tumor promotion, but there is not enough information to answer this question. Detailed analysis of the growth kinetics of

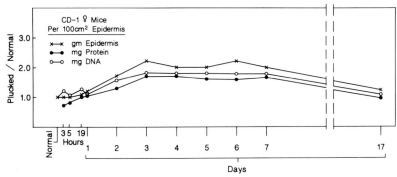

Figure 9. The changes in epidermal wet weight, total protein, and DNA following plucking of CD-1 mouse skin.

regenerative hyperplasias that do not support the evolution of tumors in initiation-treated skin of mice is badly needed. But we do offer the following suggestion. The kinetics of epidermal growth following plucking are shown in Figure 9. It can be seen that the increases in epidermal wet weight, protein, and DNA are much less than that seen after abrasion. Not shown is the fact that the amount of RNA per cell is also much less than after abrasion (unpublished observations). Perhaps epidermal hyperplasia following plucking is not a sufficient condition for epidermal tumor promotion because the amount of epidermal growth is not enough. A certain critical amount of epidermal hyperplastic growth must be achieved in order for it to be a sufficient condition for epidermal tumor promotion. If so, then we would expect that the amount of epidermal hyperplastic growth following the application of the tumor promoter TPA should be similar to that seen after abrasion. This has been shown to be the case (18). Moreover, we have shown that the accumulation of ribosomes and the changes in the cell cycle and transit times are similar to those that occur after abrasion (for review, see ref. 3).

IS THE EPIDERMAL HYPERPLASIA PRODUCED BY CHEMICAL TUMOR PROMOTERS A REGENERATIVE HYPERPLASIA?

We have shown that a single application of 17 nmol of TPA, a dosage that results in strong tumor promotion, will produce detectable histological evidence of epidermal damage within 18 h. The damage is characterized by the appearance of nuclear pyknosis, cytoplasmic vacuolization, and breakdown of nuclear components (18). This epidermal damage is not necessarily uniform over the entire back of the mouse. It persists for a few days and then is no longer evident at the light microscope level. Thus clearly the epidermal hyperplasia produced by 17 nmol of TPA is a regenerative epidermal hyperplasia. Do lower doses of

TPA, which result in less tumor promotion, also result in a regenerative epidermal hyperplasia? The answer to this question is not known. It is our impression from preliminary work that lower doses of TPA do result in damage, but less than that seen after 17 nmol of TPA. As we shall discuss below, acetic acid and mezerein also damage the epidermis. In addition, we have made preliminary observations of the effects of turpentine, ethyl phenylpropiolate, and cantharidin and have found that after one application of these substances at a dosage that has been reported in the literature as weakly tumor promoting, some damage appears in the epidermis. It is our working hypothesis that all chemicals that promote epidermal tumorigenesis produce a regenerative epidermal hyperplasia. But we keep an open mind.

We may now ask whether the epidermal damage seen after the first application of 17 nmol of TPA is also seen following each subsequent application of TPA. After a few applications of TPA evidence for epidermal damage is no longer evident at the light microscope level. This does not necessarily mean that damage is not being produced by TPA. It might be evident at the electron microscope or biochemical level. We have referred to the loss of evidence for epidermal damage at the histological level as evidence for an adaptive response of the epidermis to the toxic effects of TPA (18). Adaptation of the skin to toxic effects of chemicals extends beyond substances that are tumor promoters (3).

The adaptive response of skin to the toxic effects of TPA can be quite remarkable. If one applies 170 nmol of TPA, 10 times the optimal dose for tumor promotion, twice weekly on the skin of CD-1 female mice treated with DMBA, a marked skin ulceration occurs. Figure 10 shows a section of mouse skin treated with a few applications of 170 nmol of TPA. Massive leukocytic infiltration is obvious, as is the degeneration of the epidermis and hair follicles. The dermis is separating from the underlying fatty tissue and will be exfoliated. If one persists with the application of 170 nmol of TPA, a remarkable situation unfolds. Damage is reduced, and soon the entire back of the mouse is covered by a very thick regenerative epidermal hyperplasia (Fig. 11). Continued treatment with 170 nmol of TPA results in the appearance of many tumors (Fig. 12). Thus the adaptive response of the skin to the toxic effects of TPA can be quite impressive. It is also clear that the assumption that when a tumor promoter results in massive ulceration tumor promotion will not occur need not be correct.

We may next ask whether the epidermal hyperplasia produced by weak tumor promoters is a regenerative epidermal hyperplasia, and if so, why these tumor promoters promote weakly. We have shown that 1 day following the application of 667 μmol of acetic acid, a dosage that promotes optimally (19), the toxic effect of acetic acid on the epidermis is characterized by loss of staining, along with an inflammatory response. Within a day or two the epidermis again stains, and it is hyperplastic (20). However, this regenerative epidermal hyperplasia is unlike that produced by abrasion or TPA. First, the increase in epidermal mass is less. Second, although the number of cell layers actually approaches that seen after TPA application, the cells are not as hypertrophic, and the nuclei are not enlarged. They are thin, and nucleoli are not easily seen. Third, epidermal mitotic activity is less (20). Continued application of acetic acid

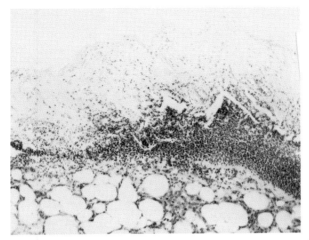

Figure 10. CD-1 female mouse skin after three applications of 170 nmol TPA. Note epidermal, hair follicle, and dermal degeneration. Also note massive leukocytic infiltration between dermis and fatty layer of the skin and separation of the dermis from the panniculus adiposus. Hematoxin and eosin x 195. (From Argyris TS, CRC Crit Rev Toxicol 14:211, 1985, with permission, copyright, CRC Press, Inc., Boca Raton, FL.)

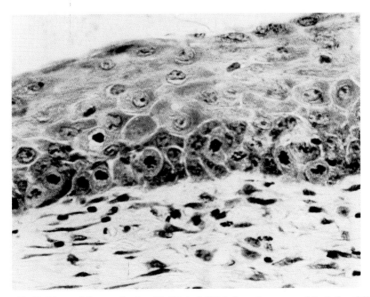

Figure 11. Epidermal hyperplasia of initiated CD-1 female mouse skin 1 day following the 10th application of 170 nmol TPA. Hematoxylin and eosin x 195.

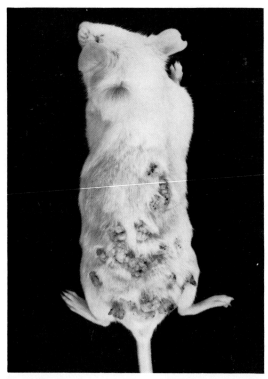

Figure 12. Epidermal tumors promoted by the repeated application of 170 nmol of TPA in CD-1 female mouse skin given initiation treatments of dimethylbenz[a]anthracene. (From Argyris TS, CRC Crit Rev Toxicol 14:211, 1985, with permission, copyright, CRC Press, Inc., Boca Raton, FL.)

does not result in an increase in the thickness of the epidermis. To the contrary, there is a decrease in epidermal thickness, to the point that in many areas the skin appears normal. Interestingly, as one continues the application of the acetic acid, the loss of epidermal stainability is always seen 1 day after its application. Thus, unlike the case following TPA applications, the skin does not show a decrease in the toxic effects of acetic acid with prolonged application. It would seem, then, that the reason acetic acid is not a strong promoter at this dosage is that it cannot produce and sustain a strong epidermal hyperplasia.

Mezerein is also considered to be a weak tumor promoter. The application of 17 nmol in mouse skin initiated with DMBA results in mild epidermal damage, characterized by nuclear pyknosis and cytoplasmic vacuolization. However, in contrast to acetic acid, it produces a strong hyperplasia. The amount of epidermal growth and the kinetics of its production are very similar to those produced by TPA (21). Continued treatment with mezerein, however, results in a decrease in the amount of epidermal hyperplasia. Again, mezerein is a weak promoter because it does not sustain the epidermal hyperplasia. In addition we learn another important lesson. One cannot be certain that if the first application of a substance produces a strong hyperplasia it will continue to do so upon repeated application (21). Conversely, one should not assume that if the first application of a substance produces little or no hyperplasia, continued application will not result in the appearance of an epidermal hyperplasia.

POSSIBLE IMPLICATIONS FOR CARCINOGENESIS IN MAN

Damage-induced epidermal hyperplasia may be a sufficient condition for epidermal tumorigenesis in man. The time between initiation and promotion can probably be varied without affecting tumor promotion. A single damaging stimulus may be a sufficient condition for epidermal tumor promotion in man, if the individual has a predisposition for epidermal tumors.

Chemical tumor promoters probably promote by producing a lasting regenerative epidermal hyperplasia. A weak chemical promoter can be as dangerous as a strong tumor promoter, since in man the promotion of a single neoplasm is unacceptable.

Probably a wide range of damaging stimuli that can induce a regenerative epidermal hyperplasia can promote tumorigenesis. It would not be surprising if epidermal tumor promotion could occur by a mixture of these damaging stimuli. The damaging stimuli may not have to be applied in an orderly schedule to be effective—for example, every 2-3 days, as is done in experimental situations. Just what interval of time can transpire before the next application of a promoting stimulus fails to sustain epidermal hyperplasia is unknown.

One cannot be certain that a chemical that, after one application, produces a strong hyperplasia will continue to do so upon repeated applications. Nor can one be certain that a substance that does not produce an epidermal hyperplasia after one application will not do so after many applications. It may also be possible that a substance that does not produce an epidermal hyperplasia will be able to sustain one produced by another substance. Clearly the ability to predict whether or not a substance will promote epidermal tumorigenesis with certainty is an extremely difficult goal to achieve.

ACKNOWLEDGMENTS

This research was supported by NIH grants AM 18219 and AG 01324.

OPEN FORUM

Dr. J. Michael Holland: Dr. Argyris, if, by removing epidermis, you are removing most of the cells that are potentially initiated, where do you think the papillomas originate? Could you speculate on the potential significance of that?

Dr. Thomas Argyris: Years ago, people used radiolabeled DMBA and methylcholanthrene, and this was found in the resting hair follicles themselves, especially in the mouths of the hair follicles. That is where I believe the regeneration occurs, and that is where many initiated cells are. That is not to say that there aren't any in the epidermis.

Dr. Holland: I have come to the same conclusion, as have many others (Glucksman A. Cancer Res 5:385, 1945). If that is true, then how do you explain your negative results with plucking?

Dr. Argyris: My bias is that the damage stimulus is not sufficient to produce a really good long-lasting hyperplasia, but this is pure speculation.

Dr. Norma Scribner: In the experiments where you studied the hyper-plastic response with TPA and acetic acid, I noticed that the initiating agent was DMBA. Did you do any experiments in which you did not apply an initiator, and, if so, did you see the same hyperplastic response?

Dr. Argyris: Your question is: Have I ever applied TPA or acetic acid onto skin not given an initiator and seen the growth parameters I have mentioned? The answer is yes. You see them in both cases in the same way.

Question: Do you think that the inflammatory process might explain the difference between promoting hyperplasia and nonpromoting hyperplasias? Nonpromoting hyperplasias are either very mild or very drastic, so maybe your wounding system elicits a strong inflammatory component and this is playing a role.

Dr. Argyris: This could very well be the case.

Dr. Thomas J. Slaga: Today you pointed out that when you compare the abrasion with TPA promotion by normalizing the area of the skin given a pro-moter, the results are equal or possibly even better. It may be even much better when you are considering the question that Mike Holland was talking about— that every time you abrade you are taking out that clone of cells that is already expanding, so the next abrasion wipes that out. So you are, in a way, starting over from the hair follicles. If there was some way to prevent that—and I know there isn't—this type of promotion would be much better than TPA.

Dr. Argyris: That is very possible. We tried to abrade the skin without getting below the basal layer. We were never successful, so I do not have any answer to your question.

Dr. Andrew T. Huang: When you abrade the mouse skin, you remove the epidermal cells. People who study carcinogen dose response to tumor initiation show the amount of carcinogen binding to epidermal DNA is proportional to the number of papillomas. When you remove the epidermal cells, you also remove initiated cells. How can you explain this?

Dr. Argyris: If I understood your question correctly, Dr. Huang, you are asking how can one have tumor promotion following abrasion if, in fact, we remove by abrasion the epidermis that contains the initiated cells.

When an initiator is applied to mouse skin, both the epidermal and the cells of the resting hair follicle, especially those at the mouths of the hair follicles, are initiated. When we abrade, the epidermis is removed, but the hair follicle remains. The regeneration of the epidermis occurs from these hair follicles. Many of the cells of the regenerating hair follicles were initiated. Therefore, the regenerated epidermis now has many initiated cells.

Question: It is possible to stimulate proliferation by just removing the horny layer. It used to be done years ago with Scotch tape stripping, but that does not seem to have a promoting effect. Can you explain this?

Dr. Argyris: There is not much evidence. If one were to measure the growth that occurs after the tape stripping, I think you would find that the hyperplasia produced is not as much as after abrasion or TPA. I think this is the reason tape stripping is not a successful tumor promoting method.

Dr. Allan Balmain: I was very interested in your results with mezerein, where you suggest that there is a quantitative difference in the degree of persistent hyperplasia that you see there as opposed to with TPA. Doesn't that go against the ideas that mezerein is a second-stage promoter and that persistent hyperplasia is supposed to be the most important thing? Second, do you believe in first- and second-stage promotion?

Dr. Argyris: I do not think there is enough evidence for me to take a stand one way or another.

Dr. Slaga: I can answer the first question. If you pretreat with one application of TPA and follow it with mezerein, you do get a persistent hyperplasia. If you just apply mezerein repetitively, the hyperplasia is reduced. But if you give TPA first, it somehow continues and you get a sustained hyperplasia. We have shown that in several publications.

Dr. Argyris: Under those operational conditions, I agree. But it is conceivable that if we knew enough about how to handle mezerein, we could administer it in such a way that it could eventually act as a first-stage promoter—if you knew what dose to put on every time you applied it. From the operational point of view, if you apply TPA and then mezerein, everything works well. That is important as far as "adaption" is concerned. I believe the epidermis treated by TPA has adapted in some way that allows mezerein to do whatever is necessary.

Dr. G. Tim Bowden: Do you see primitive dark cells when you use abrasion or Scotch tape?

Dr. Argyris: I have not looked with an electron microscope for dark cells. At the light microscope level, we see their equivalent—basophilic, small, dark, densely staining cells—with abrasion. I do not know whether you see these following Scotch tape stripping.

REFERENCES

1. Boutwell RK. The function and mechanism of promoters of carcinogenesis. CRC Crit Rev Toxicol 2:419-443, 1974.
2. Argyris TS. The regulation of epidermal hyperplastic growth. CRC Crit Rev Toxicol 9:151-200, 1981.

3. Argyris TS. Regeneration and the mechanism of epidermal tumor promotion. CRC Crit Rev Toxicol 14:211-258, 1985.
4. Hennings H, Boutwell RK. Studies on the mechanism of skin tumor promotion. Cancer Res 30:312-320, 1970.
5. Clark-Lewis I, Murray AW. Tumor promotion and the induction of epidermal ornithine decarboxylase activity in mechanically stimulated mouse skin. Cancer Res 38:494-497, 1978.
6. Argyris TS. Tumor promotion by abrasion induced epidermal hyperplasia in the skin of mice. J Invest Dermatol 75:360-362, 1980.
7. Wessells NK. Differentiation of epidermis and epidermal derivatives. N Engl J Med 277:21-33, 1967.
8. Argyris TS. Kinetics of epidermal production during epidermal regeneration following abrasion in mice. Am J Pathol 83:329-340, 1976.
9. Argyris TS, Slaga TJ. Promotion of carcinomas by repeated abrasion in initiated skin of mice. Cancer Res 41:5193-5195, 1981.
10. Furstenberger G, Marks F. Growth stimulation and tumor promotion in skin. J Invest Dermatol 81(Suppl):157-161, 1983.
11. Silver AF, Chase HB, Arsenault CT. Early anagen initiated by plucking compared with early spontaneous anagen. Advances in Biology of Skin 9:265-289, 1969.
12. Argyris TS. Kinetics of regression of epidermal hyperplasia in the skin of mice following abrasion. Am J Pathol 88:575-582, 1977.
13. Morris R, Argyris TS. Epidermal cell cycle and transit times during hyperplastic growth induced by abrasion or treatment with 12-O-tetradecanoylphorbol-13-acetate. Cancer Res 43:4935-4942, 1983.
14. Morris R, Fischer SM, Slaga TJ. Evidence that a slowly cycling subpopulation of adult murine epidermal cells retains carcinogen. Cancer Res 46:3061-3066, 1986.
15. Argyris TS. Ribosome accumulation and the regulation of epidermal hyperplastic growth. Life Sci 24:1137-1148, 1979.
16. Kazem-Mostafapour M, Green H. Effects of withdrawal of a serum stimulus on the protein synthesizing machinery of cultured fibroblasts. J Cell Physiol 86:313-320, 1975.
17. Epifanova OI, Aduladze MK, Zosimooskaya AI. Effects of low concentrations of actinomycin D on the initiation of DNA synthesis in rapidly proliferating and stimulated cell cultures. Exp Cell Res 92:23-30, 1975.
18. Argyris TS. The nature of epidermal growth produced by the first application of 12-O-tetradecanoylphorbol-13-acetate on the skin of mice initiated with dimethylbenzanthracene. J Invest Dermatol 77:230-234, 1981.
19 Slaga T, Bowden GT, Boutwell RK. Acetic acid: A potent stimulator of mouse epidermal macromolecular synthesis and hyperplasia but with weak promoting activity. JNCI 55:983-987, 1975.
20. Argyris TS. An analysis of the epidermal hyperplasia produced by acetic acid, a weak tumor promoter, in the skin of mice initiated with dimethylbenzanthracene. J Invest Dermatol 80:430-435, 1983.
21. Argyris TS. Nature of the epidermal hyperplasia produced by mezerein, a weak tumor promoter, in initiated skin of mice. Cancer Res 43:1768-1773, 1983.

Skin Carcinogenesis: Mechanisms and Human Relevance, pages 81–93

Mouse Skin Papillomas as a Stage in Cancer Progression

F. J. Burns

Institute of Environmental Medicine, New York University Medical Center, New York, New York 10016

Mouse skin has been used extensively as a model system for studying the progression of normal epidermal cells to squamous carcinoma. Evidence is accumulating that this progression occurs in discrete genetic steps, perhaps involving the activation of carcinogen-specific oncogenes (1,2). The mouse skin papilloma has been the key lesion in these studies because the papilloma is a benign clonal growth of cells that have experienced at least one of the genetic alterations necessary to produce a full-fledged cancer cell (3-8). Balmain and others have found that papillomas initiated with 7,12-dimethylbenz[a]anthracene (DMBA) and promoted with 12-O-tetradecanoylphorbol-13-acetate (TPA) have a specific mutation in the H-*ras* oncogene (9). Some papillomas are presumably subject to additional cancer-relevant alterations, because even without further treatments some papillomas progress to carcinomas (10-13).

Some papillomas are dependent on the continuation of promotion; these papillomas regress when the treatment is stopped. Still others may acquire autonomy and may persist without the need for further promotion (14-16). Presumably, a number of alterations are necessary to convert a papilloma cell to a cancer cell. These alterations may be produced by action of a carcinogen, or they may occur spontaneously (Fig. 1). It is a major task of carcinogenesis research to identify these changes and to determine when they occur in the progression of the disease.

In the multistage theory of carcinogenesis, each stage is the result of independent genetic alterations, and the probability of a cancer cell is the product of the probabilities of the individual alterations (17-19). These ideas can be formulated into a simple mathematical framework as follows. Assume that the transition to cancer requires n stages and that the transition probability per unit time for any given stage can be written as

$$K_i = a_i + b_i d, \qquad (1)$$

where a_i is the spontaneous transition rate, b_i is the dose coefficient of the ith transition, and d is the dose rate or concentration of the carcinogen. If a_i and b_i

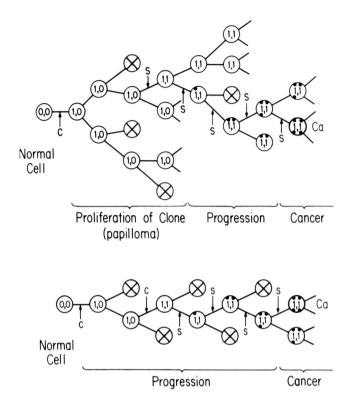

Figure 1. Diagram of the multistage hypothesis with proliferation. Progression to cancer requires the accumulation of multiple events, some being caused by action of the carcinogen (labeled C) and some occurring spontaneously (labeled S). Cells may multiply into clones (upper panel) probably in response to action of promoters, thereby increasing the number of cells at risk for the next step in the progression to cancer. Progression may occur without clonal expansion (lower panel), but this may require higher doses of a carcinogen.

are constants and the dose rate is constant, the cumulative probability of the ith transition is given by $K_i t$ where t is elapsed time. The cumulative probability per unit time of cancer occurrence can be written as the product of the probabilities of the individual transitions, i.e., the product of n expressions of the type shown in equation 1. The product can be simplified by assuming that, for m transitions, the spontaneous rate is negligible in comparison to the carcinogen-induced rate, i.e., $a_i << b_i d$. With this assumption, the cumulative probability simplifies to

$$H(t,d) = (\text{constant})d^m t^n, \tag{2}$$

where n is the total number of transitions and m is the number of carcinogen-dependent transitions.

The stages and transitions are speculative but certainly encompass the idea of carcinogenic progression as it is currently understood (20-22). If the exponent on the power function of time is really the number of stages in carcinogenesis, it should be constant and independent of carcinogen dose at least in a given organ system (23). The exponent sometimes varies, but this can usually be handled by invoking clonal expansion as a determinant of cancer onset. A normal cell may follow at least two different routes to cancer: it may undergo n alterations in sequence without clonal expansion of intermediate stages, or in any one or all of the intermediate stages, it may undergo clonal expansion by action of promoters or as a result of normal proliferative activities in the tissue. Some mouse skin papillomas may progress to carcinomas either spontaneously or as a result of the action of carcinogens (2).

In the experiments described here, mice were observed every other week, and the progress of individual tumors was charted (24). Regression of tumors and progression of benign lesions to malignancy were noted. Animals were killed when moribund or when tumors exceeded 1.0 cm³ in size. Representative papillomas and all carcinomas were confirmed histologically. For each observation interval, the number of new tumors was divided by the average number of mice alive to obtain the rate of tumor occurrence. These rates were added cumulatively to obtain the yield of tumors as a function of time.

Figure 2 shows the yield of papillomas and carcinomas in 63 mice receiving

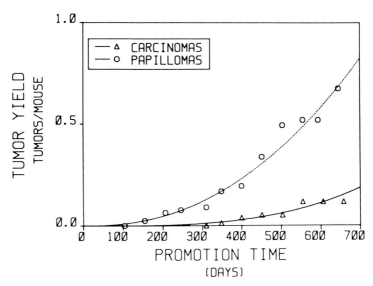

Figure 2. The yield of skin papillomas and carcinomas in 63 mice treated with 5 µg TPA in 0.2 ml acetone three times weekly. The data were fitted with a power function exponent of 2.8.

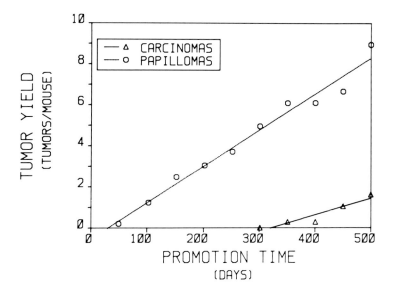

Figure 3. The yield of papillomas and carcinomas in mouse skin after a single topical treatment with 128 µg BaP at 56 days of age followed by 5.0 µg TPA three times a week. Linear curves were fitted to the data, indicating an average temporal displacement of about 340 days.

only 5.0 µg TPA three times weekly. Median survival was 550 days, and there were 7 mice alive at 650 days. Papilloma formation began at 150 days, and new papillomas were observed up to 650 days. All carcinomas arose from papillomas. The conversion of papillomas to carcinomas was initially evident at 350 days and seemed to maintain a reasonably constant ratio of about 7:1 thereafter. No tumors were observed in 40 acetone-treated mice during the same period of time.

Figure 3 shows the papilloma and carcinoma yield after a single tumor-initiating dose of 128 µg benzo[a]pyrene (BaP) followed by TPA three times a week. The temporal pattern is typical of that for other initiating doses of BaP. Papillomas were first observed at about 50 days, and new papillomas continued to appear at a fairly steady rate thereafter. The best-fitting power function exponent (n) for the papilloma data was about 1.5, which is low in comparison to the value of 5.5 for carcinoma yield in the same mice. The latter high exponent may be a result of the long lag period for papillomas to progress to cancer. The average time for this progression is about 450 days.

The dose-response relationship for papilloma induction at 200 days for BaP applied topically is shown in Figure 4. The regression line shown is consistent with the linear, no threshold action of BaP as an initiator. On the other hand, as a whole carcinogen the action of BaP is clearly nonlinear. These

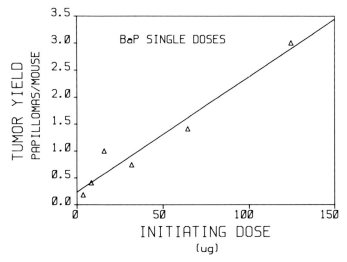

Figure 4. The yield of papillomas at 200 days of promotion as a function of the initiating dose of BaP followed by promotion with 5.0 µg TPA three times a week. A linear function is shown fitted to the data.

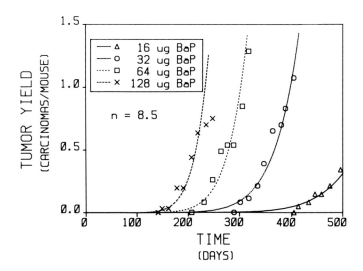

Figure 5. Carcinoma yield for different weekly doses of BaP as indicated. Topical BaP was started at 56 days of age. The average fitted power function exponent was 8.5.

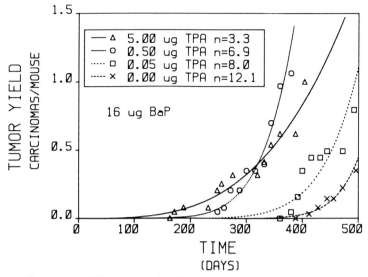

Figure 6. Carcinoma yield in mouse skin for topical treatments with TPA as indicated. BaP was applied weekly on Mondays and the indicated doses of TPA were given topically in 0.2 ml acetone on Wednesdays and Fridays.

data are shown in Figures 5 and 6. Mouse skin was exposed to weekly topical doses of BaP in 0.2 ml acetone. As the BaP dose was increased from 16 μg weekly to 128 μg weekly, the cancer yield curves were displaced progressively to earlier times without losing their power function shapes. The power function time exponent (n) shown fitted to the data was 8.5.

Adding twice weekly doses of a promoter, such as TPA, to the weekly doses of BaP had the effect of displacing the cancer yield to the left as if the dose of BaP were larger. At 5.0 μg TPA, the leftward displacement seemed to saturate and the exponent decreased, perhaps a result of TPA toxicity.

A dose-effect relationship for carcinoma induction by repeated weekly BaP exposure can be produced by considering the tumor yield at a specific point in time, e.g., 400 days. The functions in Figure 5 are so steep that substantial extrapolation of the fitted curves is necessary to obtain responses at a given time for all dose rates. The results are shown in Figure 7, in which the data have been fitted with a power function dose exponent (m) of 3.7. Based on these data, the cumulative probability of skin cancer can be written as

$$H(t,d) = C \; d^{3.7} t^{8.5}, \tag{3}$$

for regular weekly doses, d, of BaP in acetone.

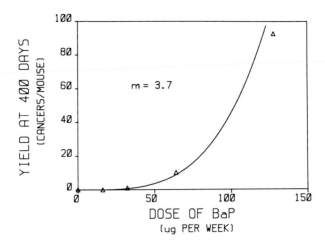

Figure 7. Cancer yield in mouse skin as a function of the weekly dose of BaP applied topically. These data are based on the fitted curves in Figure 5 extrapolated when necessary. The best-fitted power function dose exponent is $m = 3.7$.

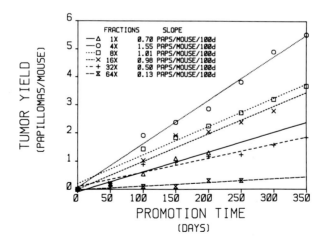

Figure 8. The yield of papillomas for an initiating dose of BaP given in various numbers of weekly fractions as indicated. In each group, tumor promotion with 5.0 μg TPA three times a week was started 1 week after the final BaP application. Time is measured from the beginning of tumor promotion. The slopes of the best-fitting straight lines are shown in the key. Abbreviation: PAPS, papillomas.

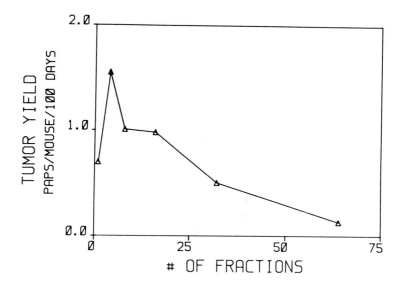

Figure 9. The papilloma yield as measured by the slopes in Figure 8 is shown as a function of the number of fractions. In each group, tumor promotion with 5.0 μg TPA three times a week was started 1 week after the final BaP application. Abbreviation: PAPS, papillomas.

Subdividing the initiating dose into various numbers of small fractions causes an increase in the initiating activity per unit dose at early times and a decrease at later times. Shown in Figure 8 are data on the number of papillomas for 64 μg BaP divided into various weekly fractions as indicated. A peak occurred at about four weekly fractions; for greater numbers of fractions the tumor yield decreased progressively. This trend is shown in Figure 9, where yield has been plotted against number of fractions (number of weeks). No ready explanation for these findings is available except that older mice tend to be more resistant to the action of carcinogens on skin than younger mice.

One of the most striking aspects of adding the action of a promoter to that of a carcinogen is the change in the shape of the dose-response curve. The promoter accelerates the occurrence of carcinomas in the sense that many more cancers are produced at the same point in time for combined exposure than for exposure only to the carcinogen. More important, the dose-response power function relationship becomes linear, which means that the promoter has a proportionately greater effect at lower doses. Cancer yield as a function of the amount of topically applied BaP with and without promotion with 5.0 μg TPA is shown in Figure 10. Similar data are shown in Figure 11 for topical application

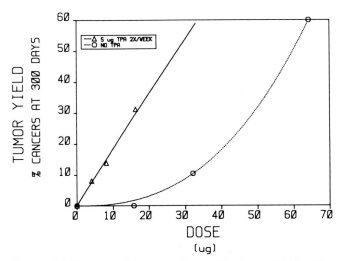

Figure 10. Tumor yield in mouse skin exposed to weekly doses of BaP on Monday with or without 5.0 µg TPA on Wednesdays and Fridays. The treatments were started at 56 days of age. The best-fitting power function dose exponents are $n = 0.97$ and 2.53 for the groups with and without TPA, respectively.

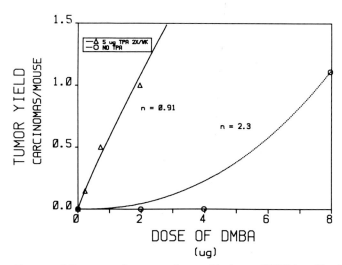

Figure 11. Tumor yield in mouse skin exposed to weekly doses of DMBA on Mondays with or without 5.0 µg TPA on Wednesdays and Fridays. The treatments were started at 56 days of age. The best-fitting power function dose exponents are $n = 0.91$ and 2.30 for the groups with and without TPA, respectively. All treatments were stopped at 170 days.

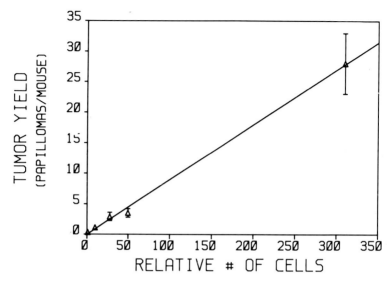

Figure 12. The yield of papillomas in adult mice treated with DMBA transplacentally. Tumor promotion with 5.0 µg TPA three times a week was begun at 56 days of age. The papilloma yield was determined after 13 weeks of promotion. The relative number of cells was estimated by counting cells per area on sections and comparing average sizes at the time of exposure. The best-fitting straight line is shown.

of DMBA for 170 days either with or without TPA as indicated. For DMBA alone the data are insufficient for estimating the value of the dose exponent. The exponent for BaP is shown. The leftward displacement is more pronounced for DMBA than for BaP when TPA is added as a cocarcinogenic promoter.

In experiments in which mice were exposed in utero to various doses of DMBA given intragastrically to the mothers, the yield of papillomas induced by TPA applications on the adult skin showed linearity with dose and with number of cells at risk in the skin at the time of exposure. Figure 12 shows how the yield of tumors in the adult offspring of DMBA-treated pregnant female mice varies with the number of skin cells in the test mice at the time of exposure. The data reflect exposures at 9, 12, and 15 days of embryonic growth and in the adult. The number of papillomas per mouse is essentially proportional to the number of cells at risk at the time of exposure. Absolute numbers were not determined, although the area of back skin treated in the adult was estimated on histological sections to contain about 8×10^6 cells. For each cell in the differentiating epidermal basal layer of the 9-day mouse fetus, there are about 10 cells in the 12-day fetus, 27 cells in the 15-day fetus, 63 cells in the 18-day fetus, and 428 cells in the adult epidermal basal layer. In arriving at these numbers, it was assumed that the relevant cells are contained in a monolayer covering the outer surface of the animal, that shape is not significantly changed by the growth, and that the number of cells is proportional to surface area.

A cell exposed to tumor-initiating agents can survive and be transmitted in its initiated state to progeny during the considerable amount of proliferation and growth occurring from a 9-day-old embryo to an adult (25,26). Linearity between number of cells and number of papillomas implies that the initiated cells did not expand into clones any larger than the clone size for developmental proliferation of normal epidermal cells. Apparently, having undergone initiation conferred no growth advantage until TPA was applied.

The ideas outlined here are an attempt to define more precisely the distinction between carcinogen-induced and spontaneous events and the role of clonal growth in carcinogenesis. The loss of the dose-squared dose-response relationship in the presence of tumor promotion needs to be explained. One possible explanation is that clonal growth of a cell exposed to a tumor-initiating agent amplifies the number of cells at risk for the next transition so greatly that additional carcinogen action is unnecessary. The cells progress to cancer under the influence of the spontaneous transition mechanism. Because of the greater number of such cells at risk, the dose-response relationship for initiating agents, which is linear, becomes limiting. The exponent on the time function (n) represents the total number of events in the cancer progression, unless significant clonal growth occurs. If clonal growth of an intermediate stage is involved in cancer progression, the time exponent represents an upper limit on the number of events. Clonal growth may affect the value of the time exponent in a way that relates to the growth rate of the clone. To the extent that clonal growth of initiated cells is stimulated by the action of promoters, these ideas emphasize the importance of promotion and promoters in determining the temporal functions of cancer incidence. Even more important for risk assessment, promoters have a profound effect on the dose-response relationship, even eliminating the need for multiple events. Linear cancer risk extrapolation in the presence of promoters may be realistic rather than conservative (27).

REFERENCES

1.   Harper JR, Roop DR, Yuspa SH. Transfection of the EJ rasHa gene into keratinocytes derived from carcinogen-induced mouse papillomas causes malignant progression. Mol Cell Biol 6:3144-3149, 1986.
2.   Hennings H, Shore R, Mitchell P, Spangler EF, Yuspa SH. Induction of papillomas with a high probability of conversion to malignancy. Carcinogenesis 6:1607-1610, 1985.
3.   Burns FJ, Vanderlaan M, Snyder E, Albert R. Induction and progression kinetics of mouse skin papillomas. In Slaga TJ, Boutwell RK, Sivak A (eds): Carcinogenesis: A Comprehensive Survey, Vol. 2. Mechanisms of Tumor Promotion and Cocarcinogenesis. New York: Raven Press, 1978, pp 91-96.

4. Slaga TJ, Bowden GT, Scribner JD, Boutwell RK. Dose-response studies on the ability of 7,12-dimethylbenz[a]anthracene and benz[a]anthracene to initiate skin tumors. JNCI 53:1337-1340, 1974.

5. Slaga TJ, Fischer SM, Nelson K, Gleason GL. Studies on the mechanism of skin tumor promotion: Evidence for several stages in promotion. Proc Natl Acad Sci USA 77:3659-3663, 1980.

6. Burns F, Vanderlaan M, Sivak A, Albert R. The regression kinetics of mouse skin papillomas. Cancer Res 36:1422-1427, 1976.

7. O'Connell JF, Klein-Szanto AJP, DiGiovanni DM, Fries JW, Slaga TJ. Enhanced malignant progression of mouse skin tumors by the free-radical generator benzoyl peroxide. Cancer Res 46:2863-2865, 1986.

8. Klein-Szanto AJP, Nelson KG, Shah Y, Slaga TJ. Simultaneous appearance of keratin modifications and gamma-glutamyltransferase activity as indicators of tumor progression in mouse skin papillomas. JNCI 70:161-168, 1983.

9. Balmain A, Ramsden M, Bowden GT, Smith J. Activation of the mouse cellular Harvey-ras gene in chemically induced benign skin papillomas. Nature 307:658-660, 1984.

10. Scribner JD, Scribner NK, McKnight B, Mottet NK. Evidence for a new model of tumor progression from carcinogenesis and tumor promotion studies with 7-bromomethylbenz[a]anthracene. Cancer Res 43:2034-2041, 1983.

11. Reddy AL, Caldwell M, Fialkow PJ. Studies of skin tumorigenesis in PGK mosaic mice: Many promoter-independent papillomas and carcinomas do not develop from pre-existing promoter-dependent papillomas. Int J Cancer 39:261-265, 1987.

12. Kruszewski FH, Conti CJ, DiGiovanni J. Characterization of skin tumor promotion and progression by chrysarobin in SENCAR mice. Cancer Res 47:3783-3790, 1987.

13. Aldaz CM, Conti CJ, Klein-Szanto AJP, Slaga TJ. Progressive dysplasia and aneuploidy are hallmarks of mouse skin papillomas: Relevance to malignancy. Proc Natl Acad Sci USA 84:2029-2032, 1987.

14. Jaffe DR, Williamson JF, Bowden GT. Ionizing radiation enhances malignant progression of mouse skin tumors. Carcinogenesis 8:1753-1756, 1987.

15. Roe FJC, Carter RL, Mitchley BCV, Peto R, Hecker E. On the persistence of tumour initiation and the acceleration of tumour progression in mouse skin tumorigenesis. Int J Cancer 9:264-273, 1972.

16. Peto R, Roe FJC, Lee PN, Levy L, Clack J. Cancer and aging in mice and men. Br J Cancer 32:411-426, 1975.

17. Armitage P, Doll R. The age distribution of cancer and a multistage theory of carcinogenesis. Br J Cancer 8:1-12, 1954.

18. Berenblum I. Frontiers of Biology, Vol. 34. Carcinogenesis as a Biological Problem. Amsterdam/Oxford: North Holland, 1974.

19. Whittemore A, Keller J. Quantitative theories of carcinogenesis. Society for Industrial and Applied Mathematics Review 20:1-30, 1978.

20. Iannaccone PM, Gardner RL, Harris H. The cellular origin of chemically induced tumors. J Cell Sci 29:249-269, 1978.

21. Andrews EJ. The morphological, biological, and antigenic characteristics of transplantable papillomas and keratinous cysts induced by methylcholanthrene. Cancer Res 34:2842-2851, 1974.

22. Herlyn D, Elder DE, Bondi E, Atkinson B, Guerry D IV, Koprowski H, Clark WH Jr. Human cutaneous nevi transplanted onto nude mice: A model for the study of the lesional steps in tumor progression. Cancer Res 46:1339-1343, 1986.

23. Druckrey H. Quantitative aspects of chemical carcinogenesis. In Truhart R (ed): Potential Carcinogenic Hazards from Drugs: Evaluation of Risks. UICC Monograph Series, Vol. 7. New York: Springer-Verlag, 1967, pp 60-78.

24. Burns FJ, Albert R, Altshuler B, Morris E. Approach to risk assessment for genotoxic carcinogens based on data from the mouse skin initiation-promotion model. Environ Health Perspect 50:309-320, 1983.

25. Vesselinovitch SD, Rao RVN, Mihailovich N. Neoplastic response of mouse tissues during perinatal age periods and its significance in chemical carcinogenesis. NCI Monograph No. 51, Bethesda, MD: National Cancer Institute, 1979, pp 239-250.

26. Napalkov V. Transplacental Chemical Carcinogenesis. Proceedings of the 11th International Cancer Congress, Florence, Italy, Vol. 3. New York: American-Elsevier, 1974, pp 300-306.

27. Crump IKS, Hoel DG, Langley CH, Peto R. Fundamental carcinogenic processes and their implications for low dose risk assessment. Cancer Res 36:2973-2979, 1976.

Skin Carcinogenesis: Mechanisms and Human Relevance, pages 95–100

Malignant Conversion: The First Stage in Progression from Benign to Malignant Tumors

Henry Hennings

Laboratory of Cellular Carcinogenesis and Tumor Promotion, National Cancer Institute, Bethesda, Maryland 20892

Multiple stages in the induction of benign and malignant tumors have been clearly defined experimentally in the mouse skin model (for reviews, see refs. 1 and 2). Although tumors can be induced by repeated topical applications of a carcinogen (3), initiation-promotion-conversion protocols have been most useful in delineating stages in tumor development (4-6). In a typical experiment, the first stage, initiation, is accomplished with a single exposure to a low, initiating dose of a carcinogen, such as 7,12-dimethylbenz[a]anthracene (DMBA). Initiation, which may represent a single mutational event (7), causes a heritable change in some epidermal cells.

Without subsequent treatment, these initiated cells do not develop into tumors. Subsequently, repeated topical treatment of initiated mice with a tumor promoter such as 12-O-tetradecanoylphorbol-13-acetate (TPA) induces the formation of benign squamous papillomas. This second stage, promotion, is effective even when the first promoter treatment is delayed for several months after initiation, indicating the permanence of the mutation produced by initiation. In contrast, the tumor-promoting effects of individual TPA applications are reversible, as papillomas do not develop after insufficient exposure of initiated skin to promoters or when the interval between the individual promoter applications is too long. Promotion is characterized by the selection for the clonal expansion of initiated cells; mutational changes do not appear to be involved.

Although large numbers of papillomas can be induced in sensitive mice by DMBA initiation and TPA promotion, few of these benign tumors progress to malignancy. In fact, continued treatment with TPA after most papillomas have appeared does not alter their rate of conversion to malignant squamous carcinomas (4). However, the rate of malignant conversion can be significantly increased by treating papilloma-bearing mice with genotoxic agents such as 4-nitroquinoline-N-oxide (4-NQO) or urethane. The agents active in the third stage of epidermal carcinogenesis are likely to act via a genetic mechanism. Further stages in progression, involving increased independence of tumor growth and metastasis, have also been demonstrated in the mouse skin model (6). This manuscript describes the experimental evidence supporting a malignant conversion stage, as well as the heterogeneity that exists among papillomas in their potential for conversion to malignancy.

MATERIALS AND METHODS

Chemicals were purchased from the following sources: DMBA from Eastman (Rochester, NY), TPA from LC Services (Woburn, MA), 4-NQO from Sigma (St. Louis, MO), and urethane from MCB (Cincinnati, OH). SENCAR female mice were obtained from the NCI-DCT Animal Program (Frederick, MD); CD-1 female mice were purchased from Charles River Laboratories (Kingston, NY). Mice were shipped at 4–5 weeks of age. Mice were treated with the initiating agent DMBA at 7–8 weeks of age, in the resting phase of the hair growth cycle. Once-weekly promotion with TPA was begun 1 week later. The duration of promotion protocols varied; weekly treatments with the converting agents 4-NQO or urethane were begun 1 week after the last TPA treatment. Papilloma and carcinoma counts were recorded every 2 weeks, and mice were weighed once a month. Noninvasive, raised lesions were classified as papillomas if their diameter exceeded 1 mm and they had been present for at least 2 weeks. Suspected carcinomas, as well as any unusual lesions, were verified by pathological evaluation of tumor histology. Carcinomas that result from initiation-promotion protocols generally progress from papillomas (5). The percentage of papillomas that converted to carcinomas was calculated with the following formula:

Percent conversion = (Total carcinomas/total papillomas) x 100.

RESULTS AND DISCUSSION

Papilloma Heterogeneity

At least two types of cells are thought to result from initiation (8), as indicated in Figure 1. The majority of papillomas (those benign lesions that develop from promotion of type A initiated cells) (Fig. 1) do not convert to malignant carcinomas and may not have the potential for conversion to either a persistent benign lesion or a malignant tumor. In CD-1 mice, these TPA-dependent papillomas regress when treatment with the promoter is stopped (5,6). In SENCAR mice, all of the papillomas that spontaneously convert to malignancy (those that develop from promotion of type B initiated cells in Figure 1) are promoted by the first five applications of the promoter TPA (5). The non-progressing papillomas appear later, after continued TPA promotion. These results are shown in Table 1. Promotion for 5 weeks resulted in only 25%–35% of the maximum number of papillomas inducible by promotion for 10–40 weeks, but the number of carcinomas was identical regardless of the duration of promotion. Further support for the existence of subclasses of papillomas comes from studies of weak promoters such as mezerein, which is much less effective

STAGES IN CARCINOGENESIS

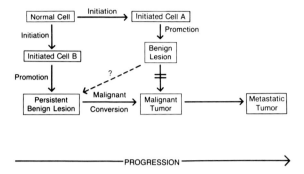

Figure 1. Stages in carcinogenesis.

Table 1. Papillomas with a High Frequency of Conversion to Carcinomas Are Induced by Short-Term Promotion with TPA*

Group	Weeks of promotion	Total papillomas	Total carcinomas	Percent conversion
1	5	189	25	13.2
2	10	582	24	4.1
3	20	748	24	3.2
4	40	734	20	2.7

* Groups of 30 SENCAR mice underwent tumor-initiating treatment with 20 µg DMBA and weekly promoting treatments with 2 µg TPA for 5, 10, 20, or 40 weeks. The experiment was terminated at week 52.
Abbreviations: TPA, 12-O-tetradecanoylphorbol-13-acetate; DMBA, 7,12-dimethylbenz[a]-anthracene.

than TPA as a promoter of papillomas but produces as many carcinomas as does TPA (5). Mezerein-promoted papillomas, as well as those promoted by short-term TPA treatment, do not regress when promoter treatments are stopped (data not shown). This persistence appears to characterize the subpopulation of papillomas with a high rate of spontaneous conversion to malignancy.

Induction of Malignant Conversion

The rate of spontaneous conversion of papillomas to carcinomas can be increased by treating papilloma-bearing mice with 4-NQO topically or with urethane intraperitoneally (4,6). After DMBA initiation and 10–12 weeks of TPA promotion, weekly exposure to the malignant converting agents for 10–30 weeks was necessary to accomplish an increase in the rate of conversion to malignancy. Although continued TPA treatment did not increase this first stage of progression, another promoter, benzoyl peroxide (9), was active as a converting agent. This result emphasizes the importance of comparing the mechanisms of action of these promoters, as well as chrysarobin (10), teleocidin (11), mezerein (5,12), and others, since the ratio of carcinomas to papillomas is much lower after TPA treatment than it is with the other promoters. A promoter that is especially effective in the production of carcinomas could act either by the selective induction of the subclass of papillomas that is likely to progress to carcinomas or by having additional activity in the malignant conversion stage.

When individual tumors were tracked from the development of papillomas until their conversion to carcinomas (5), all carcinomas appeared to arise in tumors with the gross appearance of papillomas. Foci of carcinoma in situ also have been seen frequently in initiation-promotion experiments (13,14). In a group of 40 CD-1 mice treated with acetone solvent instead of TPA after initiation, only three papillomas and no carcinomas developed in response to 40 weeks of urethane treatment (6). Thus, the papilloma stage appears to be necessary for carcinoma development with this treatment protocol. The clonal expansion of the population of initiated cells (with one critical mutation) to form a papilloma may be required to provide a large target population for a second genetic change induced by a converting agent.

To further establish that the properties of the malignant conversion stage differ from those of the promotion stage by TPA, we tested the effect of an established inhibitor of promotion, fluocinolone acetonide (FA), on malignant conversion (2). After initiation with DMBA and promotion with TPA, treatment

Table 2. Lack of Effect of Fluocinolone Acetonide on Malignant Conversion*

Stage of FA treatment	Total no. papillomas	Total no. carcinomas	Percent conversion
None	480	24	5.0
Promotion	64	4	6.3
Malignant conversion	392	23	5.9

* Groups of 40 Charles River CD-1 mice underwent tumor-initiating treatment with 50 µg DMBA and weekly promoting treatments with 10 µg TPA for 12 weeks. Malignant conversion of the resulting papillomas was accomplished with weekly intraperitoneal injections of 20 µg urethane from weeks 13 to 40. FA (1 µg/0.2 ml acetone) was applied topically 30 min before each weekly TPA treatment or 30 min before each urethane injection. The cumulative papilloma and carcinoma incidences at the time the experiment ended, at week 52, are shown.
Abbreviations: DMBA, dimethylbenz[a]anthracene; FA, fluocinolone acetonide; TPA, 12-O-tetradecanoylphorbol-13-acetate.

with 1 µg FA 30 min before each injection of urethane did not affect the number of carcinomas or the percent of conversion (Table 2). In contrast, FA given 30 min before each promoting treatment of TPA inhibited both papilloma and carcinoma formation by more than 80%. The rate of malignant conversion was unaffected by FA application during the promotion stage, indicating an equal inhibition of papillomas with a high or low risk of conversion to carcinomas.

As more agents are tested for activity in the malignant conversion stage of carcinogenesis, the mechanism of action of converting agents will be better understood. In addition to 4-NQO and urethane, hydrogen peroxide (15) and ionizing radiation (16) are active as converting agents. The chemical properties that are responsible for activity of converting agents are unclear because of the recent finding that some chemicals that are neither initiators nor promoters are active as converting agents (Slaga TJ, personal communication). Mechanistic studies will be simplified if conversion can be accomplished with fewer treatments. We have found that a single injection of the chemotherapeutic agent cisplatin, which initiates tumor development in mouse skin (17), increases the rate of malignant conversion by about twofold (Hennings H, Yuspa SH, unpublished results). In addition, work is under way on a cell culture model to study the possible cooperation between initiation by an activated Ha-*ras* oncogene and malignant conversion by chemical treatment (Yuspa SH, unpublished observations).

The results presented here summarize the evidence for heterogeneity of papillomas with regard to their potential for conversion to malignancy. The papilloma stage appears to be a prerequisite for carcinoma formation in initiation-promotion-conversion protocols. Malignant conversion is clearly distinct from TPA promotion, although other promoters may also be active as converting agents. A genetic mechanism for malignant conversion appears likely, since genotoxic agents are active as converting agents, but future studies will be required to determine the detailed mechanism.

ACKNOWLEDGMENTS

I thank Dr. Gary L. Knutsen of Pathology Associates, Inc., Ijamsville, MD, for histological evaluation of tumors and Roxana Rivas for assistance in typing the manuscript.

OPEN FORUM

Dr. Hiroshi Yamasaki: Your earlier results indicated there were at least two different kinds of initiated cells, but later you indicated that one single mutation may be enough. How do you reconcile this?

Dr. Henry Hennings: As a minimum, one mutation may be enough to give you papillomas. Perhaps the early papillomas resulting from a few TPA treatments already have two critical mutations.

REFERENCES

1. Slaga TJ. Mechanisms involved in two-stage carcinogenesis in mouse skin. In Slaga TJ (ed): Mechanisms of Tumor Promotion, Vol. II. Tumor Promotion and Skin Carcinogenesis. Boca Raton, FL: CRC Press, Inc., 1984, pp 1-16.
2. Hennings H. Tumor promotion and progression in mouse skin. In Barrett JC (ed): Mechanisms of Environmental Carcinogenesis, Vol. II. Multistep Models of Carcinogenesis. Boca Raton, FL: CRC Press, Inc., 1987, pp 59-71.
3. Shubik P. The growth potentialities of induced skin tumors in mice. The effects of different methods of chemical carcinogenesis. Cancer Res 10:713-717, 1950.
4. Hennings H, Shores R, Wenk ML, Spangler EF, Tarone R, Yuspa SH. Malignant conversion of mouse skin tumours is increased by tumour initiators and unaffected by tumour promoters. Nature 304:67-69, 1983.
5. Hennings H, Shores R, Mitchell P, Spangler EF, Yuspa SH. Induction of papillomas with a high probability of conversion to malignancy. Carcinogenesis 6:1607-1610, 1985.
6. Hennings H, Spangler EF, Shores R, Mitchell P, Devor D, Shamsuddin AKM, Elgjo KM, Yuspa SH. Malignant conversion and metastasis of mouse skin tumors: A comparison of SENCAR and CD-1 mice. Environ Health Perspect 68:69-74, 1986.
7. Quintanilla M, Brown K, Ramsden M, Balmain A. Carcinogen-specific mutation and amplification of Ha-*ras* during mouse skin carcinogenesis. Nature 322:78-80, 1986.
8. Scribner JD, Scribner NK, McKnight B, Mottet NK. Evidence for a new model of tumor progression from carcinogenesis and tumor promotion studies with 7-bromomethylbenz[a]anthracene. Cancer Res 43:2034-2041, 1983.
9. O'Connell JF, Klein-Szanto AJP, DiGiovanni DM, Fries JW, Slaga TJ. Enhanced malignant progression of mouse skin tumors by the free-radical generator benzoyl peroxide. Cancer Res 46:2863-2865, 1986.
10. Kruszewski FH, Conti CJ, DiGiovanni J. Characterization of skin tumor promotion and progression by chysarobin in SENCAR mice. Cancer Res 47:3783-3790, 1987.
11. Fujiki H, Suganuma M, Matsukura N, Sugimura T, Takayama S. Teleocidin from *Streptomyces* is a potent promoter of mouse skin carcinogenesis. Carcinogenesis 3:895-898, 1982.
12. Hennings H, Yuspa SH. Two-stage tumor promotion in mouse skin: An alternative explanation. JNCI 74:735-740, 1985.
13. Knutsen GL, Kovatch RM, Robinson M. Gross and microscopic lesions in the female SENCAR mouse skin and lung in tumor initiation and promotion studies. Environ Health Perspect 68:91-104, 1986.
14. Ward JM, Rehm S, Devor D, Hennings H, Wenk ML. Differential carcinogenic effects of intraperitoneal initiation with 7,12-dimethylbenz[a]anthracene or urethane and topical promotion with 12-O-tetradecanoylphorbol-13-acetate in skin and internal tissues of female SENCAR and BALB/c mice. Environ Health Perspect 68:61-68, 1986.
15. Rotstein J, O'Connell J, Slaga T. The enhanced progression of papillomas to carcinomas by peroxides in the 2-stage mouse skin model (abstract). Proceedings of the American Association for Cancer Research 27:143, 1986.
16. Jaffe DR, Williamson JF, Bowden GT. Ionizing radiation enhances malignant progression of mouse skin tumors. Carcinogenesis 8:1753-1755, 1987.
17. Barnhart KM, Bowden GT. Cisplatin as an initiating agent in two-stage mouse skin carcinogenesis. Cancer Lett 29:101-105, 1985.

CELLULAR AND MOLECULAR ASPECTS

Skin Carcinogenesis: Mechanisms and Human Relevance, pages 103–112
© 1989 Alan R. Liss, Inc.

Relevance of In Vitro Transformation Systems to Skin Carcinogenesis In Vivo

Ann R. Kennedy

*Department of Radiation Oncology, University of Pennsylvania
School of Medicine, Philadelphia, Pennsylvania 19104*

There are now many different systems for studying malignant transformation in vitro; the characteristics of these systems have been discussed in detail elsewhere (1). The process involved in the induction of transformation in vitro by radiation and chemical agents is highly subject to modification; in general, the agents that enhance or suppress skin carcinogenesis in animals also affect, in the same fashion, radiation- and chemical carcinogen-induced transformation in vitro (1-3). While the mechanisms involved in the multiple stages of carcinogenesis, both in vivo and in vitro, are still highly controversial, the processes involved in the development of a malignant transformed cell in vitro appear to be similar in nature to those that occur in vivo in animals and in human populations. The continued use of in vitro transformation systems should help to further elucidate the mechanisms involved in carcinogenesis, as well as aid in screening and evaluating agents that can induce, enhance, or suppress skin carcinogenesis in human populations.

This chapter reviews our previous studies on the induction of transformation in vitro and the agents that have been shown to modify the conversion of a normal cell to the malignant state.

METHODS AND RESULTS

Most of the in vitro transformation studies to be discussed here were performed with the C3H/10T1/2 cell system, which was adapted for studies of radiation transformation in vitro in our laboratory. Our studies on radiation transformation in C3H/10T1/2 cells have indicated that the first step in malignant transformation is a high-frequency event in the irradiated cells (4-9). Evidence that such a high-frequency, tumor-initiating event also occurs in chemical carcinogenesis, both in vivo and in vitro, has been recently reviewed (9). We assume that a major consequence of the high-frequency, first step in carcinogenesis is that it confers on cells an altered probability that a subsequent event, which leads directly to malignant transformation, will occur (4-9). Our own studies have shown that this later event in the transformation process occurs during division of a population of cells that have undergone initiation, at a frequency expected for a mutational event (approximately 10^{-6} per cell per generation) (7,8). The frequency of this later, rare event can be greatly altered; some agents, such as tumor promoters, can raise the frequency, and other agents, such as protease inhibitors, can reduce the frequency of the later event.

The initiating event in malignant transformation is heritable and has effects that persist over many cellular generations; it has been observed that tumor-promoting agents (10) and anticarcinogenic agents (3,11) can have modifying effects on the transformation process long after cells have been exposed to a carcinogen. Such modifying agents are capable of having a great effect on the yield of malignantly transformed cells. For tumor-promoting agents, such as 12-O-tetradecanoylphorbol-13-acetate (TPA), the enhancing effect on radiation transformation in vitro is greatest at low doses of radiation, as has been discussed in detail elsewhere (12) and is shown graphically in Figure 1. As can be

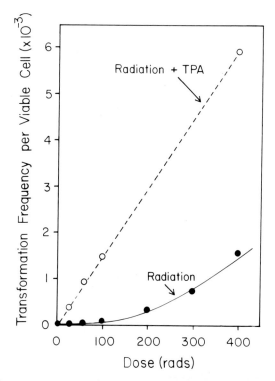

Figure 1. Dose-response curve for radiation transformation in vitro with and without enhancement by 12-O-tetradecanoylphorbol-13-acetate (TPA). Radiation treatment alone results in a quadratic curve, and radiation treatment followed by promotion yields a linear curve. Data are from ref. 12.

observed in Figure 1, the presence of the promoting agent results in a linear curve, and the curve observed for radiation treatment alone is of a quadratic form. Promoting agents have a similar effect on the shape of the dose-response curve in radiation carcinogenesis studies in vivo [for an example of this in vivo effect, see Figure 2 (13)]. Evidence that promoting agents affect the incidence of human cancer in a similar fashion has recently been reviewed (14). As human cancer risks resulting from exposure to carcinogens are estimated on the basis of such dose-response curves, promotional factors must be considered in risk assessment.

Although the mechanism of tumor promotion is still unknown, many theories have been proposed. Recently, there has been much interest in the role of free radicals in tumor promotion (15). Many of the agents shown to modify transformation may do so by affecting free radical reactions (1,2,16). We have recently reported that near-ultraviolet (UV) light can act as a promoter of carcinogen-induced transformation in vitro (17); we have hypothesized that the near-UV light induction of free radicals (18,19) could account for some of UV light's ability to act as a promoter of transformation in vitro.

Many different classes of anticarcinogenic agents suppress the carcinogenic process. We have observed that several different agents can suppress radiation-induced transformation in vitro, although they appear to act in different ways (3). Of the classes of anticarcinogenic agents we have studied, protease inhibitors have proved to be the most effective in suppressing radiation-induced transformation in vitro, as recently reviewed (3,20,21). We have now extended our in vitro studies on protease inhibitors to in vivo studies and observed that these agents can prevent cancer in animals as well (reviewed in ref. 21).

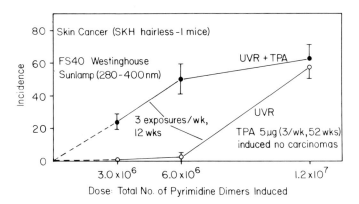

Figure 2. Dose-response curve for ultraviolet light-induced skin cancer in animals, with and without TPA promoter treatments. TPA treatment produces a linear dose-response curve, while the curve is of a quadratic nature for radiation treatment alone. Abbreviations: TPA, 12-O-tetradecanoylphorbol-13-acetate; UVR, ultraviolet radiation. (Reprinted with permission from Fry RJM, Ley RR, in Slaga TJ (ed): Mechanisms of Tumor Promotion, Vol. 2, 1978, pp 73-96. Copyright CRC Press, Inc., Boca Raton, FL.)

DISCUSSION

This discussion focuses on how the results of our own studies relate to human skin carcinogenesis. Radiation is a known potent inducer of human skin cancer, and human skin cancer appears to develop in a manner similar to that observed in animal skin carcinogenesis studies. For example, carcinogens such as ionizing radiation can produce persistent cell populations that have undergone initiation and are capable of producing tumors when exposed to other agents at much later times. Patients who were irradiated early in their lives are extraordinarily sensitive to later psoralen plus near-UV (360-nm) light (PUVA)-induced skin cancer (22). In a study of patients treated with PUVA for psoriasis, those patients with known histories of ionizing radiation exposure (or of previous skin tumors) had a significantly elevated risk of developing skin cancer compared with that of controls (22). These results can be considered an example of two-stage carcinogenesis involving the initiation and promotion stages in the development of human cancer. Presumably, the patients at elevated risk had persistent cells that had undergone initiation, resulting from the previous exposure to radiation, which were promoted by the PUVA therapy. As indicated above, PUVA treatment involves sequential exposures to near-UV light, and near-UV light has been shown in our studies to act in the manner expected for a promoting agent (17). In fact, near-UV light may act as a potent promoting agent for much of human skin cancer. Exposure to solar radiation has been implicated in human skin cancer (23-25). The majority of wavelengths in the solar spectrum are 295 nm and longer, but little is known about the ability of these longer wavelengths to induce malignant transformation. Most of the studies on the ability of various UV light wavelengths to induce transformation in vitro have utilized the UV-C (200-290 nm) or UV-B (290-320 nm) spectral regions (reviewed in ref. 17). UV-A light (320-400 nm) was of particular interest to us as a possible promoter of carcinogenesis, as it is capable of inducing anionic free radicals (18,19). Such anionic free radicals as the superoxide anion radical are known to be induced in cells by tumor-promoting agents (26) and may play an important role in tumor promotion.

Although how cancer is induced is still unknown, recent evidence from several laboratories suggests that the first step in physical and chemical carcinogenesis is a common event that occurs in a large fraction of carcinogen-treated cells (reviewed in ref. 9). We have assumed that this heritable early event in carcinogenesis represents a change in gene expression, as carcinogens are known to induce such changes (27), and there is evidence that radiation produces such gene expression changes at high frequencies (28). It is further assumed that the cellular process induced at high frequency in turn leads to a rare genetic event that gives rise to the malignantly transformed phenotype. Such processes are known to exist. For example, radiation induces the SOS system in *Escherichia coli* as a high-frequency event; this error-prone DNA repair system then gives rise to rare genetic changes (i.e., mutations) (29). To explain the results of our transformation studies, the induced process must persist for a long period of time, which is not the case for SOS functions. Radiation-induced recombination in yeast is a system that is activated for long periods of time; recombinational events continue to occur at elevated levels for many cellular generations after the radiation exposure (30).

Such an induced system could result in a recombinational event that produces the genotype of a malignant cell. For any system induced by radiation, it is assumed that proteases would be involved in the activation process, as proteolytic enzymes are known to play a central role in gene regulation (31). It is of interest that a protease is involved in the induction of SOS functions (32) and that SOS functions are known to be blocked by protease inhibitors (33). Radiation-induced recombination in yeast also can be blocked by certain protease inhibitors, and chymotrypsin inhibitors are the most effective of the protease inhibitors studied (34). In our studies on radiation-induced transformation in vitro, the protease inhibitors that are the most effective at preventing or suppressing radiation transformation are also those that inhibit the enzyme chymotrypsin (11), suggesting a possible association between the process involved in the induction of malignant transformation and that involved in radiation-induced recombination. We assume that radiation is capable of inducing a process at a high frequency that leads to a rare genetic event that results in the malignant genotype; it is assumed that the anticarcinogenic protease inhibitors turn off this activity, which can be thought of as a search for the transformed genotype/phenotype, before the cancer-causing event occurs.

There is some evidence that a high-frequency early event occurs in skin carcinogenesis. For example, the experiments of Fujii and Mizuno (reviewed in ref. 35) showed that a widespread response to an implanted membrane filter occurred in carcinogen-treated epidermal cells such that they did not behave and grow in the fashion expected for normal epidermal cells. In two-stage skin carcinogenesis experiments, Stenbäck et al. (36) observed approximately the same final tumor yield when the skin was treated with different initiating doses of 7,12-dimethylbenz[a]anthracene (DMBA) and then with TPA. One explanation for their results is that all of the available cells underwent initiation, even with DMBA doses as low as 20-50 µg/cm² and that initiation in the mouse skin is characterized by a high-frequency first step (36). Other results also suggest that cancer in animals begins with such a high-frequency event (9).

Agents that modify skin carcinogenesis in animals similarly modify radiation-induced transformation in vitro (see refs. 1 and 2). The anticarcinogenic agents that are the most effective at preventing or suppressing radiation transformation in vitro are certain protease inhibitors, as has been recently reviewed (21). Protease inhibitors are also potent anticarcinogenic agents in mouse skin carcinogenesis studies (37-39). Our studies suggest that protease inhibitors may exert their anticarcinogenic activity through a reduction in c-myc expression and/or inhibition of the activity of a specific protease, as reviewed in ref. 21.

Thus, dermal carcinogenesis appears to have many of the characteristics observed for in vitro transformation induced by physical and chemical carcinogens. It is likely that similar mechanisms operate in the induction of malignancy in these experimental systems.

ACKNOWLEDGMENT

Research investigations performed in our laboratory were supported by National Institutes of Health grants CA-22704, CA-34680, and ES-00002.

OPEN FORUM

Dr. Kenneth Kraemer: Could you elaborate on your findings for Bloom's syndrome?

Dr. Ann Kennedy: We have been studying Bloom's syndrome cells for a while now. We published a paper a few years ago showing that the anticarcinogenic protease inhibitors reduced the levels of sister chromatid exchanges and chromosome aberrations. Many of the agents that affect Bloom's syndrome cells work outside the cell or from a membrane interaction, suggesting that a genetic end point can be affected by an agent that does not reach the nucleus.

Dr. Stuart Yuspa: Dr. Kennedy, as I understand it, you are proposing that the carcinogen induces some kind of epigenetic change, which is somehow sustained for a period of time and then leads to a spontaneous mutation that imparts the neoplastic phenotype on the cell. What is the limiting dose-response component? Second, if there were an activation and prolonged expression of a growth factor directly or indirectly, you might predict that the growth to confluency would occur more quickly in your single-cell experiment than in a controlled single cell. Finally, I would like to challenge the idea that cancer is a disturbance of growth. I do not think that the changes you were calling disturbances in growth—metaplasias and dysplasias—really are. I think they are disturbances in morphogenesis and that they may have a very different basis than a growth factor.

Dr. Kennedy: The dose-response relationship is there in the studies I described with different cell densities. At high doses of radiation you get the same response as with 100 rad of radiation and TPA treatments. Lower doses of radiation lead to a lower response in terms of the transformation yield. There is no reason to suspect that there is not a dose-response relationship for an alteration in gene expression. We know that carcinogens do alter gene expression. There is no question of that. Bob Scott's work suggests that 80% of the cells are altered by a relatively low dose of UV light. So, changes in gene expression, like the first event in transformation, can be a high-frequency, heritable event with a dose response. In our own differentiation studies, there is a very clear dose-response relationship for radiation-induced differentiation in several cell systems, even at low doses. This response is synergistic with TPA treatment. It fulfills many of the characteristics of the dose-response relationship seen in a transformation assay. I do not see any conflict in the idea that an alteration in gene expression is something that can explain the results of transformation experiments.

Dr. Yuspa: I think you would have to test it. I would predict that the saturation dose for a change in gene expression is going to be considerably lower than the saturation dose for focus formation. I think cells can only express so much epigenetically before some structural change in the genome is required— either a deletion of a regulator, an amplification, or a rearrangement. I would predict that, for example, if *myc* expression increases fourfold at a dose of 100 rad, it would probably increase only fourfold at 500 rad, yet the frequency of transformation might be much higher at 500 rad.

Dr. Kennedy: But we can show that TPA alters the response, even in the differentiation systems we are studying. It synergizes the radiation response, just as it does for transformation. At 100 rad, we are not at the saturation level for transformation yields. TPA has to synergize the response brought about by a low dose of radiation such that we end up with a high transformation yield that is like the yield obtained with a high radiation dose.

Dr. Yuspa: But if you went to 500 rad, you could substitute for TPA.

Dr. Leo Sachs: Dr. Kennedy, is your use of a mesenchymal system and the relationship to inhibitors in skin carcinogenesis a model system for carcinogenesis, or are you proposing that developmental, epithelial-mesenchymal interactions are important for epithelial tissue morphogenetic events?

Dr. Kennedy: Admittedly the cell is different from that in which skin carcinogenesis normally arises, but it responds to the same modifying agents and in many respects bears a relationship to what we believe the process of carcinogenesis is in the epithelial cells of the skin. It is a very well behaved system. We can convert cells to the malignant state; these cells then can produce tumors in animals and can kill the animals. There is not a good reproducible epithelial cell system that can be used in the same way as the fibroblast transformation systems at this time.

Dr. Allan Balmain: You mentioned that the radiation induces *myc* expression. In some of your earlier talks, you suggested that *myc* amplification might be induced. What do you think about that?

Dr. Kennedy: Mary Jean Sawey showed that there were alterations in *myc* in 10 of 12 radiation-induced tumors. She has now looked for that same alteration in in vitro transformation systems and not found it. We believe a later change occurs in the development of a cancer cell that allows that cell to form a focus and that that change is not there earlier. One way to look at this is to irradiate cells and allow them to form a monolayer. If you start with one cell on the dish and you get a monolayer and then one focus or more arises from those normal cells (all of which arose from one cell initially), you should be able to tell whether a change occurred later by comparing the cells in a focus with those in the monolayer from which they arose. We have found an internal rearrangement within *myc* when the focus arises, but not earlier. In these experiments, we are not finding changes in *ras*.

Dr. G. Tim Bowden: We have also looked for *myc* amplification rearrangement in radiation-initiated skin tumors. We do not see it in any that we have looked at.

REFERENCES

1. Kennedy AR. Promotion and other interactions between agents in the induction of transformation in vitro in fibroblasts. In Slaga TJ (ed): Mechanisms of Tumor Promotion, Vol. 3. Tumor Promotion and Carcinogenesis In Vitro. Boca Raton, FL: CRC Press, 1984, pp 13-55.
2. Kennedy AR. Role of free radicals in the initiation and promotion of radiation-induced and chemical carcinogen-induced cell transformation. In Breccia A, Rodgers MAJ, Semerano G (eds): Oxygen and Sulfur Radicals in Chemistry and Medicine. Bologna, Italy: Edizioni Scientifiche, 1986, pp 201-209.
3. Kennedy AR. Implications for mechanisms of tumor promotion and its inhibition by various agents from studies of in vitro transformation. In Langenbach R, Barrett JC, Elmore E (eds): Tumor Promoters: Biological Approaches for Mechanistic Studies and Assay Systems. New York: Raven Press, 1988, pp 201-212.
4. Kennedy AR, Fox M, Murphy G, Little JB. Relationship between x-ray exposure and malignant transformation in C3H 10T1/2 cells. Proc Natl Acad Sci USA 77:7262-7266, 1980.
5. Kennedy AR, Little JB. An investigation of the mechanism for the enhancement of radiation transformation in vitro by TPA. Carcinogenesis 1:1039-1047, 1980.
6. Kennedy AR, Little JB. High efficiency, kinetics and numerology of transformation by radiation in vitro. In Burchenal JH, Oettgen HF (eds): Cancer: Achievements, Challenges and Prospects for the 1980s. New York: Grune and Stratton, 1981, pp 491-500.
7. Kennedy AR, Cairns J, Little JB. The timing of the steps in transformation of C3H10T1/2 cells by X-irradiation. Nature 307:85-86, 1984.
8. Kennedy AR, Little JB. Evidence that a second event in x-ray induced oncogenic transformation in vitro occurs during cellular proliferation. Radiat Res 99:228-248, 1984.
9. Kennedy AR. Evidence that the first step leading to carcinogen-induced malignant transformation is a high frequency, common event. In Barrett JC, Tennant RW (eds): Carcinogenesis: A Comprehensive Survey, Vol. 9. Mammalian Cell Transformation: Mechanisms of Carcinogenesis and Assays for Carcinogens. New York: Raven Press, 1985, pp 355-364.
10. Kennedy AR, Murphy G, Little JB. The effect of time and duration of exposure to 12-O-tetradecanoyl-phorbol-13-acetate (TPA) on x-ray transformation of C3H 10T1/2 cells. Cancer Res 40:1915-1920, 1980.
11. Kennedy AR. The conditions for the modification of radiation transformation in vitro by a tumor promoter and protease inhibitors. Carcinogenesis 6:1441-1446, 1985.
12. Kennedy AR, Mondal S, Heidelberger C, Little JB. Enhancement of X-ray transformation by 12-O-tetradecanoyl-phorbol-13-acetate in a cloned line of C3H mouse embryo cells. Cancer Res 38:439-443, 1978.
13. Fry RJM, Ley RR. Ultraviolet radiation carcinogenesis. In Slaga TJ (ed): Mechanisms of Tumor Promotion, Vol. 2. Tumor Promotion and Skin Carcinogenesis. Boca Raton, FL: CRC Press, 1984, pp 73-96.

14. Kennedy AR. Relevance of tumor promotion to carcinogenesis in human populations. In Kaufman DG, Siegfried JM, Steele VE, Nesnow S, Mass MJ (eds): Carcinogenesis: A Comprehensive Survey, Vol. 8. Cancer of the Respiratory Tract: Predisposing Factors. New York: Raven Press, 1985, pp 431-436.
15. Copeland ES. Free radicals in promotion: A chemical pathology study section workshop. Cancer Res 43:5631-5637, 1983.
16. Kennedy AR, Symons MCR. "Water structure" vs. "radical scavenger" theories as explanations for the suppressive effects of DMSO and related compounds on radiation-induced transformation in vitro. Carcinogenesis 8:683-688, 1987.
17. Baturay NZ, Targovnik HS, Reynolds RJ, Kennedy AR. Induction of in vitro transformation by near-UV light and beta-propiolactone. Carcinogenesis 6:465-468, 1985.
18. Webb RB. Lethal and mutagenic effects of near-ultraviolet radiation. In Smith KC (ed): Photochemical and Photobiological Reviews. New York: Plenum Press, 1977, pp 168-261.
19. Peak KG, Foote CS, Peak MS. Protection by DABCO against inactivation of transforming DNA by near-ultraviolet light: Action spectra and implications for involvement of singlet oxygen. Photochem Photobiol 34:45-49, 1981.
20. Kennedy AR. Prevention of radiation-induced transformation in vitro. In Prasad KN (ed): Vitamins, Nutrition and Cancer. Basel: S. Karger AG, 1984, pp 166-179.
21. Kennedy AR, Billings PC. Anticarcinogenic actions of protease inhibitors. In Cerutti P, Nygaard OF, Simic MG (eds): Anticarcinogenesis and Radiation Protection. New York: Plenum Press, 1987, pp 285-295.
22. Stern RS, Thibodeau LA, Kleinerman RA, Parrish JA, Fitzpatrick TB, and 22 participating investigators. Risk of cutaneous carcinoma in patients treated with oral methoxsalen photochemotherapy for psoriasis. N Engl J Med 300:809-813, 1979.
23. Schreiber MM, Shapiro SI, Berry CZ, Dahlen RF, Friedman RP. The incidence of skin cancer in southern Arizona. Arch Dermatol 104:124-127, 1971.
24. Silverstone H, Searle JHA. The epidemiology of skin cancer in Queensland: The influence of phenotype and environment. Br J Cancer 24:235-252, 1970.
25. Setlow RB. The wavelengths in sunlight effective in producing skin cancer: A theoretical analysis. Proc Natl Acad Sci USA 71:3363-3366, 1974.
26. Goldstein BD, Witz G, Amoruso M, Stone DS, Troll W. Stimulation of human polymorphonuclear leukocyte superoxide anion production by tumor promoters. Cancer Lett 11:257-262, 1981.
27. Fahmy MJ, Fahmy OG. Intervening DNA insertions and the alteration of gene expression by carcinogens. Cancer Res 40:3374-3382, 1980.
28. Scott RE, Maercklein PB. An initiator of carcinogenesis selectively and stably inhibits stem cell differentiation: A concept that initiation of carcinogenesis involves multiple phases. Proc Natl Acad Sci USA 82:2995-2999, 1985.
29. Witkin EM. Ultraviolet mutagenesis and inducible DNA repair in Escherichia coli. Bacteriol Rev 40:869-907, 1976.
30. Fabre F, Roman H. Genetic evidence for inducibility of recombination competence in yeast. Proc Natl Acad Sci USA 74:1667-1671, 1977.
31. Gottesman MN. Regulation by proteolysis. In Neidhardt Frederich (ed): Escherichia coli and Salmonella typhimurium. Washington DC: American Society for Microbiology, 1987, pp 1308-1312.
32. Little JW, Edmiston SH, Pacelli LZ, Mount DW. Cleavage of the Escherichia coli lexA protein by the recA protease. Proc Natl Acad Sci USA 77:3225-3229, 1980.

33. Meyn MS, Rossman T, Troll W. A protease inhibitor blocks SOS functions in Escherichia coli: Antipain prevents λ repressor inactivation, ultraviolet mutagenesis, and filamentous growth. Proc Natl Acad Sci USA 74:1152-1156, 1977.

34. Wintersburger U. The selective advantage of cancer cells: A consequence of genome mobilization in the course of the induction of DNA repair processes? (Model studies of yeast). Adv Enzyme Regul 22:311-323, 1984..

35. Süss R, Kinzel V, Scribner JD. Cancer: Experiments and Concepts. New York: Springer-Verlag, 1973, pp 87,88.

36. Stenbäck F, Peto R, Shubik P. Initiation and promotion at different ages and doses in 2200 mice. III. Linear extrapolation from high doses may underestimate low-dose tumour risks. Br J Cancer 44:24-34, 1981.

37. Troll WA, Klassen A, Janoff A. Tumorigenesis in mouse skin: Inhibition by synthetic inhibitors of proteases. Science 169:1211-1213, 1970.

38. Hozumi M, Ogawa M, Sugimura T, Takeuchi T, Umezawa H. Inhibition of tumorigenesis in mouse skin by leupeptin, a protease inhibitor from Actinomycetes. Cancer Res 32:1725-1728, 1972.

39. Slaga TJ, Klein-Szanto AJP, Fischer SM, Weeks CE, Nelson K, Major S. Studies on the mechanism of action of anti-tumor promoting agents: Their specificity in two-stage promotion. Proc Natl Acad Sci USA 77:2251-2254, 1980.

Skin Carcinogenesis: Mechanisms and Human Relevance, pages 113–125

Human Epidermal Keratinocyte Cell Culture and Xenograft Systems: Applications in the Detection of Potential Chemical Carcinogens and the Study of Epidermal Transformation

James G. Rheinwald

Division of Cell Growth and Regulation, Dana-Farber Cancer Institute and Department of Cellular and Molecular Physiology, Harvard Medical School, Boston, Massachusetts 02115

About 70 years ago, the first experimental animal model was developed to identify chemicals that induce squamous cell carcinoma when topically applied to the epidermis (1). This research was initially undertaken to study how workers exposed to petroleum and its products develop skin cancer. Since then, much has been learned about the identities of carcinogenic chemicals and the dose and treatment schedules that induce benign and malignant epidermal lesions on mice (2,3). Over the past 5 years, epidermal cells have been cultured from the skin of mice treated with carcinogens, and the growth and differentiation properties of these cells have been characterized in some detail (4,5). These studies have been very important for identifying epidermal growth regulatory mechanisms, but many of the results cannot be extrapolated directly to humans. Human tissues are generally more refractory to carcinogens than is mouse skin, and induced cancers usually take many years to develop rather than less than a year, as in mice. Acquisition of unlimited replicative potential by cells (immortalization) appears to be an early event in mouse epidermal carcinogenesis. In contrast, this has never been reported to be a property of human cells cultured either from preneoplastic lesions or from histologically normal areas at risk because of previous exposure to carcinogens. Ca^{2+} induces irreversible growth arrest and terminal differentiation in normal mouse epidermal cells (5), and mouse epidermal cells that undergo initiation with carcinogen treatment can be identified in culture by their resistance to Ca^{2+} (6). Normal human epidermal cells are quite resistant to Ca^{2+} for growth in culture (7,8), however. Therefore this phenotype cannot be used to identify or select in culture human cells that may have become initiated by exposure to carcinogens in vivo. Human epidermis is thicker than mouse epidermis is and, therefore, has different permeability characteristics. Thus, there are many reasons to use, whenever possible, experimental systems that permit direct study of chemical carcinogenesis in human epidermis. The challenge, of course, is to find biologically relevant and experimentally feasible models that do not violate ethical constraints on human experimentation.

Identification of the mitogen requirements of normal human epidermal keratinocytes for clonal growth and serial cultivation in vitro (9-12) has permitted detailed comparisons between cells from normal epidermis and those from squamous cell carcinoma, the cancer that arises from epidermal cells. These studies have identified cancer-associated phenotypic markers that are relevant both to humans and to the epidermal cell type (13,14). Cultured human epidermal keratinocytes have also been used as a direct mutagenesis system for assessing the ultimate genotoxicity of polycyclic aromatic hydrocarbons (12). Cultures of normal or malignant epidermal cells can be grafted to the dermis of athymic nude mice, where they differentiate into a histologically normal epidermis (15-19); the in vivo histogenic potential of cultured human cells can therefore be assessed. Native, full-thickness human skin has also been grafted onto nude mice (20,21) and maintained in a histologically normal condition for up to 1 year, suggesting its potential as an experimental in vivo carcinogenesis model for human tissue. This chapter is a brief review of research (primarily from my own laboratory) in these areas, with comments on potential application of the results to the practical problem of predicting the carcinogenic risk of chemicals and evaluating the alterations induced by such carcinogens in human epidermis.

EXPERIMENTAL QUESTIONS

Is There a Feasible In Vivo Experimental System for Studying Chemical Carcinogenesis in the Human Epidermis?

Ethical considerations, of course, preclude direct testing on humans of chemicals suspected of being carcinogenic. However, small pieces of full-thickness human skin can be grafted onto athymic (nude) mice using a simple procedure, and these grafts remain histologically normal for as long as a year or more (20,21, and T. O'Connell and J.G. Rheinwald, unpublished observations). The longevity of such grafts seems limited only by the life span of the nude mouse, which is usually less than a year and a half. Theoretically, histological evaluation of the grafted human skin would be limited by the ability to distinguish the graft from the surrounding mouse skin. In our experience, some grafts appear to take several months to heal in completely; these often prove to eventually have mouse epidermal cells occupying at least part of the area originally occupied by the graft. Fortunately, specific reagents permit the unequivocal identification of human epidermal and dermal cells in tissue sections. Antibodies specific for the epidermal differentiation protein involucrin (22) specifically recognize human epidermis because no immunologically cross-reacting homologue is present in mouse epidermis. We have also found that a commercially available monoclonal antibody, V9 (Boehringer-Mannheim, Indianapolis, IN), specific for the intermediate filament protein vimentin (23), recognizes human but not mouse vimentin in formalin-fixed, paraffin-embedded tissue sections. Thus the cellular elements of human dermis are readily distinguished from those of the adjacent mouse dermis. The fluorescent DNA binding dye Hoechst 33258 also is a useful reagent for distinguishing mouse from human cells because mouse centromeric heterochromatin stains particularly intensely with Hoechst 33258 to give a speckled pattern in mouse nuclei that is not present in human nuclei.

We have found (O'Connell T, Rheinwald JG, unpublished observations) that human dermal fibroblasts and epidermal keratinocytes can be recovered in culture for at least 1 year after full-thickness human skin is grafted to nude mice. The cells have identical growth factor requirements and replicative life spans to cells taken from the same tissue sample but placed directly in culture without grafting. Thus, theoretically, these human skin xenografts should be an excellent model system for topical carcinogenesis studies. Studies have been attempted using this system; Yuspa and colleagues reported a preliminary result nearly 10 years ago that a chemically induced papilloma arose at the edge of such a xenograft (24), but the cells were not evaluated for human or mouse origin. We have performed similar experiments (Allen-Hoffman BL, Rheinwald JG, unpublished observations), topically applying 100 µg dimethylbenz[a]anthracene (DMBA) once a week for 6 weeks. By 2 months after these treatments, a large (1 cm long) papilloma had grown up at the edge of one of the grafts, and the mouse also had eight smaller papillomas on other areas of its own skin. Part of the papilloma was placed in culture to recover the cells, and they were found to be an epidermal growth factor (EGF)-independent, immortal mouse epidermal cell line. Thus it appears that either mouse epidermal cells are much more sensitive to the transforming effect of chemical agents than are human epidermal cells, or progression of chemically altered cells proceeds much more rapidly in mouse skin than in human skin. In any event, direct extension of the animal model of topical epidermal carcinogenesis to human xenografts is probably not feasible. Nevertheless, the ability to recover in culture proliferative human epidermal cells from grafts leaves open the possibility that the effects of relatively short (1- to 2-month) periods of carcinogen application could be assessed by evaluating in culture the cells grown out of such treated grafts rather than waiting for overt tumors to arise. The ability to do this depends upon the knowledge of suitable phenotypic alterations exhibited by malignant or premalignant epidermal cells that can be identified in culture.

Can Premaligant or Malignant Human Epidermal Cells Be Identified in Culture?

Normal human epidermal keratinocytes exhibit very different mitogen requirements than fibroblasts do for growth in culture. Keratinocytes also display a great propensity to undergo an irreversible commitment to terminal differentiation in vitro. Thus they require a special culture medium for growth, and they must be handled carefully if they are to be serially transferred through numerous passages. Normal epidermal cells do not appear to respond directly to serum mitogens for growth but instead depend upon EGF, hydrocortisone (HC), insulin or insulin-like growth factor 1 (IGF-1), and an agent that elevates the intracellular level of cAMP (such as cholera toxin) (10-12). They also require an as yet unidentified and unpurified factor or factors referred to here as keratinocyte growth factor (KGF) that is secreted by normal connective tissue fibroblasts (9) and is also present in the brain and pituitary gland (25). (It is not known whether the fibroblast-secreted and pituitary extract factors are identical.) Because normal epidermal cells do not exhibit such fastidious requirements for replication at high cell density in primary culture, confluent cultures of normal human epidermal cells can be obtained in many different kinds of media from explant outgrowths of minced epidermis (26) or from very-high-density platings of trypsinized epidermal cell suspensions (27,28), as was first reported 20 years ago.

Two different culture systems have been developed for clonal growth and serial cultivation of normal epidermal cells. One, commonly known as the 3T3 feeder layer system (9-12), is particularly well suited for the identification of many differences in growth and differentiation phenotypes exhibited by malignant epidermal cells (i.e., squamous cell carcinoma). The other system (8,25,29), is often referred to as a "defined medium" for epidermal cells, even though it depends on a high concentration of crude bovine pituitary extract for optimal and serial growth. This medium does not support very good growth of most squamous carcinoma cell lines we have examined (unpublished observations) but has permitted the study of the effects of transforming growth factor (TGF)-beta, as described below.

Normal human epidermal cells have a particularly interesting response to the polypeptide hormone EGF (10). In the 3T3 feeder layer system, epidermal cells grow as tightly adherent, epithelioid colonies from single-cell platings. Until about 7 days after plating, the epidermal cells grow at the same rate with or without EGF. Thereafter, colonies grown in the absence of EGF become increasingly tightly packed and multilayered and their growth slows substantially, whereas colonies growing in the presence of EGF are less heavily stratified and the cells are more flattened and spread out. With EGF, cells in large colonies can continue to divide at their maximal rate until the culture becomes confluent by the merging of neighboring colonies. When the cultures of epidermal cells grown with and without EGF are compared, it is found that cells growing without EGF form new colonies after subculture at a greatly reduced frequency compared with cells that were growing with EGF before subculture. It appears that EGF acts by reducing the probability that epidermal cells in crowded conditions will irreversibly depart from the cell cycle, stratify, and become committed to terminal differentiation (10). It has been suggested recently that EGF works on epidermal cells in culture as a migration-enhancing factor (30); thus EGF is likely to be important in vivo in wound healing.

Epidermal cells that lose contact with the plastic culture dish surface and migrate upward to form the stratified layers of the colony no longer replicate. They instead begin to synthesize components of the cornified envelope—the terminal differentiation structure of the epidermal cell. We therefore asked whether loss of attachment to the substratum would be a sufficient signal to induce irreversible commitment to terminal differentiation in normal epidermal cells. We found that if normal epidermal cells are transiently deprived of anchorage by immobilizing them as a single-cell suspension in culture medium made semisolid by the addition of methylcellulose, the cells lose their ability to reinitiate growth when recovered from suspension and replated in surface culture (31). Thus loss of the right type of cell-substratum adhesion is a sufficient signal in culture, and may also be the signal in vivo, to cause epidermal cells to stop proliferating and embark upon their differentiation program.

Normal human epidermal cells cannot divide and form colonies from low-density (less than about 500 cells per cm^2) platings in standard types of culture media, but they are able to do so if cocultivated with a nearly confluent monolayer of previously irradiated or mitomycin-treated connective tissue fibroblasts (9). In this feeder cell system, the epidermal cells attach directly to the culture dish surface and push away the surrounding feeder fibroblasts as the epidermal colonies expand. The cultures become confluent as neighboring epidermal colonies merge, by which time all the feeder fibroblasts have been dislodged and have been removed at culture medium changes.

The feeder fibroblasts appear to secrete both soluble and substratum-associated proteins that are necessary for epidermal cells to begin dividing from single-cell platings (Rheinwald JG, Green H, unpublished observations). Our early attempts at characterizing the fibroblast "feeding" function indicated that the 3T3 feeder cells also altered the nutrient composition of Dulbecco's modified Eagle's medium, making it more favorable for epidermal cell growth. Peehl and Ham (25) found that a modification of Ham's F-12 medium, called MCDB153, is a more optimal nutrient medium for epidermal cells that does not require adjustment by metabolic action of fibroblast feeder cells. In such a medium, crude bovine pituitary extract can be used to replace the growth factors secreted by fibroblast feeder cells, and it helps promote rapid proliferation of epidermal cells from low-density platings.

About 10 years ago, my laboratory began to characterize the growth and differentiation properties of naturally arising human squamous cell carcinomas (SCCs). We wished to identify lesions in the control of growth and/or differentiation that were responsible for the malignant behavior of these cells. We found that epidermal and oral SCCs could be cultured rather routinely (with a 30%-50% success rate) from tumor biopsies taken from these sites (14). We initially cultured the cancer cells in the feeder layer system under conditions that would also permit the growth of normal keratinocytes so that we would not subject the SCC cell populations to selection pressure for reduced growth requirements or enhanced growth potential. For this reason, we did not bias our collection toward the isolation of only the most abnormal cancer cell types. We found that the 18 SCCs we were able to culture all were replicatively immortal and were tumorigenic in nude mice. They were less dependent upon the 3T3 feeder layer than were normal keratinocytes, although they grew more rapidly and with higher colony-forming efficiencies with feeder cells and some grew very poorly without feeder support. All of the lines were absolutely EGF-independent, and all were much more resistant to transient suspension in methylcellulose medium. Thus they could not be triggered to commit to terminal differentiation as readily as could normal keratinocytes (13). Parkinson and colleagues (32) found that normal human epidermal keratinocytes are strongly inhibited in their growth by the phorbol ester tumor promotor 12-O-tetradecanoylphorbol-13-acetate (TPA), whereas our SCC lines were resistant to this agent to the same degree to which we had found they resisted transient anchorage deprivation in semisolid medium.

Shipley and colleagues (33), using Ham's MCDB153 medium, found that normal epidermal cells are strongly inhibited by the polypeptide hormone TGF-beta, whereas one of our SCC lines (SCC-25) was resistant to TGF-beta. Our own study (Rollins B, O'Connell T, Bennett G, Burton L, Stiles C, Rheinwald J, submitted) indicates that a number of our SCC lines are indeed more resistant to TGF-beta inhibition than are normal epidermal cells in MCDB153 medium. However, we have found that normal epidermal cells are greatly protected from TGF-beta by cultivation in the presence of 3T3 fibroblast feeder cells. This greatly reduced sensitivity of normal epidermal cells to inhibition by TGF-beta in the 3T3 feeder layer system and the EGF independence exhibited by normal epidermal cells in MCDB153 demonstrates that both culture systems must be used to evaluate all possible differences in growth phenotypes distinguishing normal from malignant epidermal keratinocytes.

The altered phenotypes exhibited by naturally occurring malignant keratinocytes (human SCC cells), which could be used to select for rare, experimentally induced transformants among a large population of normal keratinocytes in culture include EGF-independent growth, keratinocyte growth factor (KGF)-independent growth, resistance to anchorage deprivation, growth in presence of TPA, growth in presence of TGF-beta, and replicative immortality. The retention of colony-forming ability after several days in an anchorage-deprived state (13) is probably the most powerful selection technique because it can be applied to a large number of cells ($>10^6$) in a small volume of medium and it provides a single-step selection for cells exhibiting this important SCC-associated phenotype. Progressive growth in the absence of EGF or KGF (as provided by the fibroblast feeder layer or pituitary extract) would require several successive passages in selective medium to substantially enrich a cultured population for cells with either of these altered phenotypes, inasmuch as cells that are unable to grow but remain viable would be present for a time in cultures deprived of EGF or KGF. Selection of TPA- or TGF-beta-resistant cells would also require several passages in selective medium because the inhibition caused by TGF-beta is completely reversible in normal cells (33, and Havican K, Rheinwald JG, unpublished observations) and the inhibition caused by TPA is reversible in a considerable fraction of the cells in cultured normal human keratinocytes (32, and Havican K, Rheinwald JG, unpublished observations). The acquisition of replicative immortality is an easily selectable phenotype, requiring serial cultivation beyond the normal life span of a cell strain to identify and select any cell possessing this cancer-related phenotype.

These strategies are necessary for the detection of transformed keratinocytes because altered phenotypes used traditionally for detecting fibroblast transformation are inappropriate in the keratinocyte system. Only a small proportion of the SCC lines we cultured grew in semisolid medium (14, and our unpublished observations). This appeared to be the result of a low, but finite rate of commitment to terminal differentiation even by malignant keratinocytes during anchorage deprivation in semisolid culture medium (13). Growth in low-serum media is inappropriate because normal keratinocytes do not have a high serum requirement. Focus formation is inappropriate because malignant keratinocytes grow as an unstratified monolayer (14) and therefore do not overgrow a dense culture of normal keratinocytes.

Are Human Epidermal Cells Sensitive in Culture to the Same Chemical Carcinogen Initiators as They Are In Vivo?

As discussed above, experimentally transformed human epidermal cells could be identified and selected in culture by their acquisition of less-stringent growth characteristics. The next question that must be answered is whether human epidermal cells in culture are sensitive to and therefore might be transformed by industrial and environmental chemicals thought to be epidermal carcinogens in vivo. An important class of these are polycyclic aromatic hydrocarbons (PAHs). These chemicals are hydrophobic and therefore are able to penetrate the epidermal lipid barrier and gain access to the stem cells in the basal layer of the tissue. Some common PAHs are not reactive with DNA and therefore are not mutagenic or carcinogenic. However, the epidermis expresses mixed-function oxidase enzymes that convert these PAHs to highly mutagenic epoxides (reviewed in ref. 12 and in other chapters of this volume). Because some tissues can metabolize PAHs to nonmutagenic forms as well, we wished to determine whether PAHs were converted to mutagenic forms in human epidermal cells in culture and, therefore, could act as carcinogenic initiators (12).

We chose the nonessential, X-linked gene hypoxanthine-guanine phosphoribosyl transferase (HPRT). Only one allele of this gene is expressed in male and female cells, and the disabling of the gene by any means, whether by point mutation or deletion, results in no growth disadvantage to cells in normal culture medium but does confer resistance to the purine analogue 6-thioguanine (TG). We first selected a TG^r 3T3 clone (3T3M1) to serve as a feeder layer for keratinocytes growing in the presence of this selective agent. We optimized the dose, treatment time, phenotypic expression time, and plating density for selection by using the easily cultivated SCC line SCC-13. A subclone, SCC-13Y, exhibited a 50% colony-forming efficiency and a low spontaneous mutation rate ($<10^{-6}$/cell/generation). Benzo[a]pyrene (BaP) and DMBA induced HPRT$^-$, TG^r mutants at a frequency as high as 10^{-4}. We found that we could get statistically significant quantitative data on PAH activation to mutagenic forms with an experimental protocol that employs about 10^6 treated SCC-13 cells distributed among 10–100 mm culture dishes per experimental point.

This system was then extended to normal human epidermal keratinocytes. By treating cells in their second passage with chemicals and culturing them in the 3T3 feeder layer system, we were able to achieve colony-forming efficiencies of 5% to 35% in the mutant-selection plates and to obtain statistically significant quantitative data using 3 to 5 x 10^6 treated cells selected among 10 to 30 culture dishes per experimental point. Normal keratinocytes exhibited a spontaneous TG^r mutation frequency of ≤ 10^{-6}, whereas HPRT$^-$ mutants were induced by BaP and DMBA at frequencies of 3 to 9 x 10^{-5}. Thus human epidermal cells in culture do metabolize these chemicals to mutagenic and potentially carcinogenic forms. Aside from its practical value for screening potentially harmful agents, this system could be used to attempt to generate premalignant epidermal cells that have undergone initiation and may be identified and selected according to the properties outlined above.

Is There an In Vitro System for Evaluating Premalignant Characteristics of Initiated or Partially Transformed Epidermal Cells?

The formation of a progressively growing tumor by cell suspensions that have been inoculated subcutaneously into nude mice has long been the standard test used for the detection of malignant transformation. Diploid human cells have been found to be refractory to chemically induced transformation in culture, however. Epidermal cells that have been exposed to radiation or chemical carcinogens in vivo frequently form a premalignant lesion, which precedes invasive carcinoma. It follows that human epidermal cells that have been treated in culture with a sufficient dose of an initiating chemical and that may have acquired one or more of the altered growth characteristics of SCC cells might be similar to the cells that form premalignant lesions in vivo. Ca^{2+}-resistant variants (which also prove to be replicatively immortal) can be detected and isolated from mouse skin treated with a single dose of an initiating chemical (6). To assess the similarity between growth variants selected in culture and premalignant cells, however, it is necessary to put the cells back into an in vivo environment that permits their expression of either normal or dysplastic histogenic behavior.

Normal human epidermal cells respond to being placed in contact with connective tissue or granulation tissue in vivo by organizing into a stratified, differentiating tissue nearly identical in appearance to that formed by cells native to human epidermis (17,19). Several transplantation methods have been developed to protect cultured epidermal cells from drying until they are able to form a stratum corneum and isolate the transplanted cells in such a way that they cannot be displaced by ingrowth of the surrounding mouse epidermis. One employs a flanged, covered chamber first described by Yuspa and colleagues (15) and used extensively by Worst et al. (16) and Boukamp et al. (18). Single-cell suspensions of cultured epidermal cells are inoculated into a closed chamber covering the exposed panniculus carnosus, which normally underlies the mouse skin. In this system, normal cultured epidermal cells re-form a histologically normal epidermis, while partially or completely transformed cultured epidermal cells form a tissue exhibiting the expected histopathological abnormalities.

In a system recently described by Morgan et al. (19), an intact confluent cultured cell sheet is implanted. The sheet is removed from the culture vessel surface with Dispase, in the same way cell sheets are prepared for burn therapy (34). A semicircular flap is opened in the mouse skin, and the cell sheet supported by a circle of silicon membrane is placed with its basal surface against the inner side of the mouse dermis. The flap is then closed with surgical staples, leaving the silicon membrane between the panniculus carnosus and the outer surface of the cultured cell sheet. By 7 days after grafting, the epidermal cells have stratified and differentiated normally. Histologically abnormal tissue structures, resembling carcinoma in situ or early invasive SCC are formed by fully malignant cell lines (Lindberg K, Rheinwald J, submitted) and are similar to those reported by Boukamp and colleagues using plastic chambers (18). Furthermore, a clone (SCC-12F2) of one of our SCC lines that we found not to form progressively growing tumors in nude mice (35) does form an abnormal, dysplastic lesion similar to that produced by the fully malignant and tumorigenic SCC lines when grafted by the sheet-implant method. Thus the short-term graft system provides a method for assessing the acquisition of premalignant characteristics by variants selected in culture after treatment with chemical carcinogens.

CONCLUSIONS

Because of differences among species, and even among inbred strains of the same species, with respect to susceptibility to carcinogenesis induced by topically applied chemicals, it is essential to find a human system for studying this phenomenon and acquiring quantitative data on comparative risk of exposure to environmental and industrial chemicals. The purpose of this chapter has been to demonstrate the direct applicability of human epidermal cell culture and xenograft methods as assay systems and experimental models of epidermal carcinogenesis. Although these systems are more technically demanding than are bacterial mutagenesis or mouse skin assays, they are more relevant and therefore should be considered as an alternative strategy for assessing the carcinogenic potential of chemicals on human skin.

OPEN FORUM

Dr. R. K. Boutwell: Is anyone trying to determine what the factor is in the pituitary or in the fibroblasts that gives the keratinocyte cofactor?

Dr. James G. Rheinwald: I spent about one postdoctoral year trying to fractionate that from fibroblast-conditioned medium. It was not possible, at least using old-fashioned liquid chromatography columns. The factors seemed unstable when serum proteins initially present were removed. It is unfortunate that this very important factor has not yet been characterized.

Dr. Boutwell: Is it polypeptide in nature?

Dr. Rheinwald: Yes.

Dr. Boutwell: Then perhaps protease inhibitors are needed to stabilize the peptide during isolation.

Dr. Byron Butterworth: Dr. Rheinwald, you said you were disappointed when the human skin graft did not respond to DMBA. Why did you not simply accept that as the right answer?

Dr. Rheinwald: We know human skin (relative to mouse skin) is very resistant to chemical carcinogenesis, but we wanted to produce initiated cells. Except for the papilloma that formed at the mouse skin margin, which was mouse in origin, we were unable to identify any cells exhibiting altered properties when we cultured them, at least in the few experiments we did. I think with different regimens and larger grafts, they might be found.

Dr. Butterworth: Suppose you had found that the chemical was 1,000-fold more potent for tumor induction in human skin than in mouse skin. You would probably have concluded that that chemical was dangerous to humans. These species comparisons are vital both to understand mechanisms and to provide better risk assessments. I urge you to continue this work.

Dr. Rheinwald: A small basic science laboratory cannot do this. An industrial lab or a large applied research facility would be best suited for this work.

Dr. Butterworth: If your system was functioning and you were confident in it, would you trust it more than the mouse system for human relevance?

Dr. Rheinwald: Yes. It is real human tissue that in long-term xenografts on mice continues to look normal and produces the normal set of differentiation-related proteins. Normal human epidermal cells can be cultured out of it even after a year in the graft.

Dr. Butterworth: Maybe part of the problem was the metabolic activation of the DMBA. Have you ever tried direct-acting mutagens?

Dr. Rheinwald: No.

Question: Earlier you said that mouse skin was either one or several thousand times as sensitive as human skin. Could you expand on the basis for this?

Dr. Rheinwald: I was referring to the rapidity with which papillomas and carcinomas appear on skin after treatment. Some people have spent a large portion of their lives immersing their hands more than once a week in cutting oils, lubricants, croton oil, etc., and it takes much longer than 10 weeks (as is the case for mice) for them to get papillomas. Even people who are in the sun all their lives do not usually develop solar keratoses, squamous cell carcinomas, and basal cell carcinomas until late in their lives.

Question: Do you think that the immune system would have the same response to human skin on mice as to human skin on humans?

Dr. Rheinwald: I think that immune response would be important in the future progression of the lesion. It probably would have minimal impact on the immediate, initiating effects of the carcinogen treatment. Ultimately, the immune system probably would play some role, and it may well be very different in mice and humans.

Dr. Stuart Yuspa: Several years ago, we published a paper describing the human skin system as presented today by Dr. Rheinwald. We initiated with an intraperitoneal injection of urethane and then used TPA as a promoting agent. Tumors developed in what looked like the graft site, but at the periphery. We did not have the markers to prove that the tumors were human in origin. The two subsequent studies—yours and the one from Denmark—show that the tumors that arise are from mice. It is likely that in our initial report we also produced host tumors.

Dr. Rheinwald: You could find out if metabolism of a procarcinogen took place in the skin by excising the treated area, recovering the cells in culture, and selecting for thioguanine-resistant mutants, which should have been induced by an activated form of the chemical. We did not do this in our limited study.

REFERENCES

1. Yamagiwa K, Ichikawa K. Experimental study of the pathogenesis of carcinoma. J Cancer Res 3:1-29, 1918.
2. Berenblum I, Shubik P. A new quantitative approach to the study of chemical carcinogenesis in the mouse skin. Br J Cancer 1:379-382, 1947.
3. Slaga TJ, Fischer SM, Nelson K, Gleason GL. Studies on the mechanism of skin tumor promotion: Evidence for several stages in promotion. Proc Natl Acad Sci USA 77:3659-3663, 1980.
4. Yuspa SH, Hawley-Nelson P, Koehler B, Stanley RJ. A survey of transformation markers in differentiating epidermal cell lines in culture. Cancer Res 40:4694-4703, 1980.
5. Hennings H, Michael D, Cheng C, Steinert P, Holbrook K, Yuspa SH. Calcium regulation of growth and differentiation of mouse epidermal cells in culture. Cell 19: 245-254, 1980.
6. Yuspa SH, Morgan DL. Mouse skin cells resistant to terminal differentiation associated with initiation of carcinogenesis. Nature 293:72-74, 1981.
7. Boyce ST, Ham RG. Calcium-regulated differentiation of normal human epidermal keratinocytes in chemically defined clonal culture and serum-free serial culture. J Invest Dermatol 81 (Suppl 1):33s-40s, 1983.
8. Wille JJ Jr, Pittelkow MR, Shipley GD, Scott RE. Integrated control of growth and differentiation of normal human prokeratinocytes cultured in serum-free medium: Clonal analyses, growth kinetics, and cell cycle studies. J Cell Physiol 121:31-44, 1984.
9. Rheinwald JG, Green H. Serial cultivation of strains of human epidermal keratinocytes: The formation of keratinizing colonies from single cells. Cell 6:331-344, 1975.
10. Rheinwald JG, Green H. Epidermal growth factor and the multiplication of cultured human epidermal keratinocytes. Nature 265:421-424, 1977.
11. Green H. Cyclic AMP in relation to proliferation of the epidermal cell: A new view. Cell 15:801-811, 1978.
12. Allen-Hoffman BL, Rheinwald JG. Polycyclic aromatic hydrocarbon mutagenesis of human epidermal keratinocytes in culture. Proc Natl Acad Sci USA 81:7802-7806, 1984.

13. Rheinwald JG, Beckett MA. Defective terminal differentiation in culture as a consistent and selectable character of malignant human keratinocytes. Cell 22:629-632, 1980.

14. Rheinwald JG, Beckett MA. Tumorigenic keratinocyte lines requiring anchorage and fibroblast support cultured from human squamous cell carcinomas. Cancer Res 41:1657-1663, 1981.

15. Yuspa SH, Morgan DL, Walker RJ, Bates RR. The growth of fetal mouse skin in cell culture and transplantation to F_1 mice. J Invest Dermatol 55:379-389, 1970.

16. Worst PKM, Valentine EA, Fusenig NE. Formation of epidermis after reimplantation of pure primary epidermal cell cultures from perinatal mouse skin. JNCI 53:1061-1064, 1974.

17. Banks-Schlegel S, Green H. Formation of epidermis by serially cultivated human epidermal cells transplanted as an epithelium to athymic mice. Transplantation 29:308-313, 1980.

18. Boukamp P, Rupniak HT, Fusenig NE. Environmental modulation of the expression of differentiation and malignancy in six human squamous cell carcinoma cell lines. Cancer Res 45:5582-5592, 1985.

19. Morgan JR, Barrandon Y, Green H, Mulligan RC. Expression of an exogenous growth hormone gene by transplantable human epidermal cells. Science 237:1476-1479, 1987.

20. Reed ND, Manning DD. Long-term maintenance of normal human skin on congenitally athymic (nude) mice. Proc Soc Exp Biol Med 143:350-353, 1973.

21. Manning DD, Krueger GG. Use of cyanoacrylate cement in skin grafting congenitally athymic (nude) mice. Transplantation 18:380-383, 1974.

22. Rice R, Green H. Presence in human epidermal cells of a soluble protein precursor of the cross-linked envelope: Activation of the cross-linking by calcium ions. Cell 18:681-694, 1979.

23. Osborn M, Debus E, Weber K. Monoclonal antibodies specific for vimentin. Eur J Cell Biol 34:137-143, 1984.

24. Yuspa S, Viguera C, Nims R. Maintenance of human skin on nude mice for studies of chemical carcinogenesis. Cancer Lett 6:301-310, 1979.

25. Peehl D, Ham RG. Clonal growth of human keratinocytes with small amounts of dialyzed serum. In Vitro 16:526-540, 1980.

26. Flaxman BA, Lutzner M, Van Scott EJ. Cell maturation and tissue organization in epithelial outgrowths from skin and buccal mucosa in vitro. J Invest Dermatol 49:322-332, 1967.

27. Karasek M. In vitro culture of human skin epithelial cells. J Invest Dermatol 47:533-540, 1966.

28. Briggaman R, Abele S, Harris S, Wheeler C. Preparation and characterization of a viable suspension of postembryonic human epidermal cells. J Invest Dermatol 48:159-168, 1967.

29. Tsao MC, Walthall BJ, Ham RG. Clonal growth of normal human epidermal keratinocytes in a defined medium. J Cell Physiol 110:219-229, 1982.

30. Barrandon Y, Green H. Cell migration is essential for sustained growth of keratinocyte colonies: The roles of transforming growth factor-alpha and epidermal growth factor. Cell 50:1131-1137, 1987.

31. Rheinwald JG. The role of terminal differentiation in the finite culture lifetime of the human epidermal keratinocyte. Int Rev Cytol 10:25-33, 1979.

32. Parkinson EK, Grabham P, Emmerson A. A subpopulation of cultured human keratinocytes which is resistant to the induction of terminal differentiation-

related changes by phorbol, 12-myristate, 13-acetate: Evidence for an increase in the resistant population following transformation. Carcinogenesis 4:857-861, 1983.

33. Shipley GD, Pittelkow MR, Wille JJ Jr, Scott RE, Moses HL. Reversible inhibition of normal human prokeratinocyte proliferation by type beta transforming growth factor-growth inhibitor in serum-free medium. Cancer Res 46:2068-2071, 1986.

34. Gallico GG III, O'Connor NE, Compton CC, Kehinde O, Green H. Permanent coverage of large burn wounds with autologous cultured human epithelium. N Engl J Med 311:448-451, 1984.

35. Rheinwald JG, Germain E, Beckett MA. Expression of keratins and envelope proteins in normal and malignant human keratinocytes and mesothelial cells. In Harris CC, Autrup HN (eds): Human Carcinogenesis. New York: Academic Press, 1983, pp 85-96.

Skin Carcinogenesis: Mechanisms and Human Relevance, pages 127–135

Consequences of Exposure to Initiating Levels of Carcinogens In Vitro and In Vivo: Altered Differentiation and Growth, Mutations, and Transformation

Stuart H. Yuspa, Anne E. Kilkenny, Dennis R. Roop, James E. Strickland, Robert Tucker, Henry Hennings, and Susan Jaken

Laboratory of Cellular Carcinogenesis and Tumor Promotion, National Cancer Institute, Bethesda, Maryland 20892 (S.H.Y., A.E.K., D.R.R., J.E.S., H.H.), Johns Hopkins Oncology Center, Baltimore, Maryland 21205 (R.T.), and Alton Jones Cell Science Center, Lake Placid, New York 12946 (S.J.)

From studies using chemical agents to induce cancer on mouse skin, three operationally distinct stages have been defined: initiation, promotion, and malignant conversion. Initiation is accomplished rapidly, is irreversible, and is commonly caused by mutagens. A point mutation in a single gene, the Ha-*ras* gene, is sufficient to produce an initiated epidermal cell (1), although alterations involving other, as yet undefined genes, are certain to be initiating events as well. Promotion must occur after initiation and requires repeated frequent exposure to agents that are generally not mutagenic, although mutagenic agents such as ultraviolet light may have promoting properties. Promotion is reversible if terminated prior to the appearance of tumors. Promoters influence the homeostasis of the target tissue to produce an environment conducive to the selective clonal outgrowth of initiated cells (2). The clinical result of initiation and promotion in mouse skin is the formation of multiple squamous papillomas, each representing a clone of a million or more initiated cells. Carcinomas result when a papilloma cell incurs additional genetic changes that must complement the initiating genetic alterations (3). Because of its genetic basis, malignant conversion occurs at a low frequency spontaneously, but it can be induced by mutagens or by the introduction of mutated genes into benign tumor cells. Thus, at least two structural genetic alterations in the same cell are required to produce a cancer cell, and the probability of achieving these is low because the risk is the product of the frequency of each individual event. By producing a million-fold increase in the number of cells expressing the initiating mutation, tumor promoters act as the principal determinant of the probability of producing a cancer cell.

Cancer is considered a disease in which rapid, unregulated proliferation causes the unbridled expansion of tumor cells to a clinically relevant end point. This concept is supported by the discovery of oncogenes that cause rapid proliferation in appropriate target cells and are commonly related to growth factors or growth factor receptors. However, the transformation-sensitive target cells for oncogenes generally have been simple cell types (fibroblasts) or cells that are already abnormal by virtue of a previous treatment or extended cultivation in vitro. In vivo, cancers develop more commonly in epithelial cells, particularly lining epithelia such as those of the skin, bronchus, gastrointestinal tract, pancreatic duct, mammary duct, or urogenital tract. These epithelia are complex in structure, and many have a stringently regulated program of differentiation that can counteract aberrant proliferative activity. This suggests that the carcinogenesis process in epithelia requires an alteration in the program of terminal differentiation in addition to aberrant growth control. The development of a differentiation abnormality must constitute a rate-limiting step in cancer development in lining epithelia.

Aberrant differentiation of a fundamental type may occur early in carcinogenesis. Patients carrying the autosomal dominant gene for multiple polyposis have a genetic predisposition to develop intestinal tract cancer and demonstrate an abnormal differentiation pattern in their nonneoplastic colonic mucosa (4). A similar lesion has been documented during the induction of colon cancer in mice and rats by chemical carcinogens (5). In experimental skin carcinogenesis, papillomas contain cells that proliferate in the strata that is confined to differentiating cells in normal skin, suggesting that initiation is associated with an altered response to signals for terminal differentiation (6,7). Similarly, the earliest changes noted during chemical induction of rat mammary tumors is an inhibition of the normal differentiation of terminal end buds into alveolar buds (8).

THE PHENOTYPE OF INITIATION

The use of epidermal cell culture systems in association with biochemical and molecular techniques has contributed to a cellular and molecular understanding of some of the changes that underlie the biology of tumor development in skin (9). In 1980, it was first reported that extracellular Ca^{2+} regulates the differentiation of normal keratinocytes in vitro (10). Subsequently, a number of other studies from a variety of laboratories have confirmed and extended the initial observations to suggest that Ca^{2+} acts as a signal to trigger other changes that permit differentiation to proceed (9). Additional changes include modification of the cell membrane and receptors (11), intracellular ion distribution (12), and the expression of differentiation-specific genes (13).

When epidermal cells are grown in medium with a Ca^{2+} concentration (Ca_o) below 0.1 mM, they are phenotypically similar to basal epidermal cells. Elevation of Ca_o above 0.1 mM leads to vertical stratification and a rapid change in morphology and biochemistry that is irreversible after 48 to 72 h. Within 3 to 7 days, stratifying cells form mature squames, which ultimately slough from the culture dish. This model was used to examine modifications in differentiation associated with carcinogen exposure. When cultured epidermal basal cells were exposed to initiating carcinogens, cellular foci evolved that were resistant to the Ca^{2+} signal, and although stratified, cells in these foci continued to proliferate under conditions of high Ca^{2+} (14). Since similar cellular foci were derived from mouse skin initiated in vivo and subsequently selected in culture by an increased Ca_o (15), it is presumed that these cells represent initiated cells. Additional experimental studies strengthened this presumption. The number of foci increased with exposure to more-potent initiating agents and with increasing doses of initiators (16,17). Furthermore, the focus-forming potential of skin exposed to initiating agents persisted at least 10 weeks after initiation, as would be expected for a process associated with a mutation (16). The characteristics of carcinogen-induced foci—some cells stratify and produce fully mature squames while others proliferate in high-Ca^{2+} medium—are similar to the differentiation pattern of papillomas in vivo. Also, cells isolated from benign and malignant skin tumors display a similar phenotype in vitro.

To confirm the initiated state, we isolated cells from chemically induced papillomas and cultured them in vitro (18,19). As demonstrated for initiated cells, papilloma cells proliferate in high-Ca^{2+} medium, but a population also expresses the differentiated phenotype. When initiated cells or papilloma cells were removed from culture and grafted to nude mice as a reconstituted skin, some cell lines produced papillomas, while others produced carcinomas, and a few even produced normal skin.

A number of studies in vivo and in vitro have suggested that activation of the Ha-*ras* gene by point mutation is sufficient to initiate carcinogenesis in mouse epidermis (1,20-23). When an activated Ha-*ras* oncogene is introduced into normal keratinocytes, recipient cells are resistant to Ca^{2+}-induced differentiation. Under high-Ca^{2+} culture conditions, cells with an activated Ha-*ras* oncogene remain in a late basal cell stage of differentiation (24). The cultured cells express basal cell markers but have a reduced capacity to proliferate. They do not express the suprabasal keratins (13), which are among the earliest markers of the differentiated phenotype. This finding strongly links a defect in the response to Ca^{2+} as a differentiation signal with the initiation of skin carcinogenesis.

THE REGULATION OF NORMAL EPIDERMAL DIFFERENTIATION

To address how initiation alters the control of epidermal differentiation, it is necessary to define the factors that regulate normal differentiation. The discovery that extracellular Ca^{2+} regulates many aspects of epidermal differentiation in vitro provided a model for further exploration. Furthermore, analysis of Ca^{2+} content in epidermis in vivo indicates that a Ca^{2+} gradient exists in which total and free Ca^{2+} are low in the basal cell and first suprabasal cell layers relative to serum and dermal content (25,26). Ca^{2+} in the granular cell layer is extraordinarily high. Nevertheless, the existence of this gradient in the epidermis supports the potential importance of Ca_o as a physiological regulator of epidermal differentiation in vivo.

Important insights into the precise metabolic pathways involved in epidermal differentiation were provided by reports that the tumor promoter 12-O-tetradecanoylphorbol-13-acetate (TPA) could induce epidermal differentiation in vivo and in keratinocytes cultured in 0.05 mM Ca^{2+} medium (27-29). Because the biological activities associated with TPA responses are mediated through the activation of protein kinase C, this enzyme appears to play a role in the differentiation response. This concept was linked to the Ca^{2+} pathway, as the pattern of changes in epidermal protein synthesis and protein phosphorylation that occur within 1 or 2 h after exposure to either Ca^{2+} or TPA were found to be similar (30). Additional studies showed that exogenous bacterial phospholipase C and exogenous diacylglycerol could mimic the action of TPA in epidermal differentiation (31). Together, these results suggest a pathway regulating epidermal differentiation that involves exposure to increasing concentrations of extracellular Ca^{2+} activating an endogenous phospholipase C, a Ca^{2+}-requiring enzyme.

Phospholipase C activation is associated with the rapid metabolism of cellular phosphatidylinositol (PI), yielding two intracellular second messengers, diacylglycerol and inositol triphosphate (IP3) (32). Diacylglycerol is the endogenous activator of protein kinase C, and IP3 mobilizes intracellular Ca^{2+} (Ca_i) from bound stores. In epidermal cell cultures prelabeled with [^{3}H]inositol in 0.05 mM Ca^{2+} medium, the addition of Ca^{2+} to 1 mM increased inositol phosphates, the water-soluble metabolites of phosphatidylinositol, within 2 min (33). There was a corresponding decrease in radiolabeled phosphoinositide, suggesting that these were the source of the increased IPs. After 3 h in 1 mM Ca^{2+} medium, each of the IPs remained elevated, at 130%–140% of control levels. Two Ca^{2+} ionophores, A23187 and ionomycin, also increased IP levels in cells maintained in 0.05 mM Ca^{2+}, suggesting that a rise in Ca_i is important in the increased turnover of phosphatidylinositol. Phorbol esters stimulated phosphatidylcholine metabolism but not phosphatidylinositol turnover. In concert with ionomycin, phorbol esters become more potent inducers of differentiation (Table 1), suggesting that protein kinase C activation, elevation of Ca_i, and PI turnover were important components of the signal for epidermal differentiation.

To confirm that Ca_i was elevated in response to a change in Ca_o, we employed digital image technology by loading cells with a calcium-sensitive probe, Fura-2, and measuring a change in intracellular fluorescence (34). When the Ca_o was increased from 0.05 mM to 1.2 mM, a four- to fivefold increase in Ca_i occurred within a few minutes and was sustained for at least 30 min. The magnitude of this response was greatest in the presence of serum, but individual cells showed substantial heterogeneity in both time course and magnitude of response. In contrast, serum-free conditions reduced the Ca_i increase to two- to threefold, but the response was nevertheless sustained and the cells responded homogeneously. Such results suggest that exogenous factors found in serum could influence the differentiation response in individual cells. Because both Ca_i and PI metabolism are increased simultaneously by a change in Ca_o and both are sustained and tightly linked to the differentiation response, a rise in Ca_i is likely to be an intracellular signal responsible for the induction of terminal differentiation in keratinocytes.

Table 1. Combined Effects of TPA and Ionomycin on Epidermal Differentiation*

Treatment	% Cornified envelopes	
	Experiment 1	Experiment 2
TPA, ng/ml (0.05 mM Ca²⁺)		
0	0.7	0.1
1	0.7	1.8
10	1.8	3.5
100	2.8	—
TPA, ng/ml (ionomycin) (0.05 mM Ca²⁺)		
0	1.3	0.5
1	4.3	4.6
10	2.9	—
100	3.5	—
1.4 mM Ca²⁺	—	2.3

*Primary mouse keratinocytes were grown for 1 week in 0.05 mM Ca^{2+} medium. At the commencement of treatment, dishes were rinsed once with phosphate-buffered saline, and fresh medium with indicated test agents was added. Data are from individual culture dishes in which total cell number ranged from 5 to 7×10^6 cells/dish. No significant change in cell number among the groups was observed. Cornified envelopes were measured 24 h after treatment. The ionomycin concentration was 13 μM in experiment 1 and 6.5 μM in experiment 2. A (–) indicates that the group was omitted. Abbreviation: TPA, 12-O-tetradecanoylphorbol-13-acetate.

MECHANISM OF ALTERED DIFFERENTIATION IN INITIATED CELLS

It could be postulated that initiation of carcinogenesis in mouse epidermis is associated with a change in Ca^{2+} transport or in the Ca^{2+} requirements of enzymes involved in PI metabolism. We investigated these possibilities utilizing papilloma cell lines and normal cultured keratinocytes into which we have introduced the v-Ha-*ras* gene. PI metabolism was stimulated in papillomas and v-Ha-*ras* cell lines switched from 0.05 mM to 1.0 mM Ca^{2+}. However, the generation of IP3 was extremely low in some papilloma cell lines relative to normal cells. Papilloma cells in 0.05 mM Ca^{2+} had a twofold greater Ca_i than normal cells. When these cells were switched to 1.0 mM Ca^{2+}, Ca_i rapidly increased 5- to 10-fold, but this increase was sustained for only several minutes, after which Ca_i remained about twofold greater than starting values. Papilloma cells responded more homogeneously than normal cells, and they were less influenced by serum factors. Together, these results suggest that Ca^{2+} homeostasis and the link to PI metabolism are fundamentally altered in initiated keratinocytes, but the precise cause of this defect is not clear.

Defining a defect in Ca^{2+} homeostasis in the initiation of epidermal carcinogenesis provides a target for chemoprevention. Using ionomycin to cause a sustained increase in Ca_i, the differentiation of papilloma cells and v-Ha-*ras* keratinocytes can be induced in vitro. Preliminary data also indicate that the limited application of ionomycin to mouse skin treated with initiating agents prior to the commencement of tumor promotion can reduce the tumor yield (data not shown). Thus, these studies on the basic mechanisms involved in the early stages of neoplastic development may lead to new strategies for the prevention of tumor formation.

OPEN FORUM

Dr. Helen Gensler: Have you tried the activated form of vitamin D3 in your system, since this has been shown to be an antipromoter and to regulate skin cancer-binding protein in vivo?

Dr. Stuart Yuspa: We tried it some years ago and were not impressed with its activity. At that time, we did not have specific or sensitive markers to study differentiation. Several groups have shown that vitamin D3 induces differentiation in this model, but we have not retried it.

Dr. Thomas O'Brien: One of the important properties of initiated cells is that after promoter treatment there is a selective clonal expansion of those cells relative to the other cells in the epidermis. Dr. Yuspa, using your foci model, have you initiated in vivo and then promoted for a short time, and does that increase the yield of in vitro cells that are resistant to differentiation?

Dr. Yuspa: We tried those experiments several years ago, and they were unsuccessful. Recently, Miller et al. repeated them and found an increase in the size (but not the number) of the colonies that evolved after TPA treatment. That study was published in *Cancer Research*.

Question: How do the intracellular calcium levels in epithelial and nonepithelial cells compare? For example, if you put fibroblasts into the same test tube and you change the level of extracellular calcium, is there a different response between an epithelial cell with the potential to keratinize and a nonepithelial cell that does not have this potential?

Dr. Yuspa: We have preliminary data showing that fibroblasts do respond differently from keratinocytes. The classic studies have been done with fibroblast cell lines like 3T3. I do not know whether they respond to extracellular calcium, but they do respond to certain other stimuli with an increase in intracellular calcium. It is very transient—a minute or two. We are seeing elevations for at least 30 min, and we suspect it may be longer since there is no indication of a decrease in the profiles. This appears to be a unique type of response. We do not have data on other epithelial cells. It may be unique to epidermal cells but we do not know that.

Dr. Allan Balmain: Dr. Yuspa, you have shown very nicely that the papilloma cell lines that you get from in vivo-induced papillomas have the activated Ha-*ras* gene. We know that virtually all the papillomas in vivo have that mutation. If you initiate in vitro with the same carcinogen and select using the calcium switch, what proportion of the calcium-resistant clones have that mutation?

Dr. Yuspa: I do not know. We have not examined that many cell lines derived in vitro for the mutation. We have looked for the mutation in some lines, but most of these were initiated with MNNG (N-methyl-N'-nitro-N-nitrosoguanidine). These do not have the codon 61 mutation. The only DMBA (7,12-dimethylbenz[a]anthracene) line from our in vitro assay that we have studied is 308, which was initiated in vivo by DMBA and selected in vitro. This has the codon 61 mutation.

Dr. Balmain: It would be interesting to know that because the frequency of initiation in vitro is high. If you throw DMBA onto the cultures and then select in high calcium, the frequency of these clones is quite high. I wonder what the frequency of that specific mutation is, or if there is a group of genes that can allow that type of selection in vitro.

Dr. Yuspa: I am not sure the frequency is as high as you imply. In fact, it may not be much higher than in vivo. You have to make some assumptions to answer that question. One assumption is that every focus is clonal. Second, you must assume that when you initiate in vivo, you are only initiating basal cells, so that the number of cells at risk is not the entire section of skin that receives the carcinogen, but only perhaps one-fourth of that. Then you try to guess at the number of cells at risk. For example, if there are 107 cells at risk and you get 10 papillomas per animal, the frequency is 1 in 106. Our focus assay starts with about 3 million cells in a dish, all of which presumably have the basal cell phenotype and are thus at risk. With an average of two to four foci per dish, we are not that far off from the in vivo frequency if all those assumptions are correct.

Dr. Balmain: When you add TGF-beta to the papilloma cells, it stops DNA synthesis and prevents the cells from dividing. Does it have any effects on morphology or on differentiation? Calcium, for example, stops the growth of ras-initiated cells but also seems to flatten them out.

Dr. Yuspa: It does not visibly affect their morphology. Without using specific markers, I cannot say for sure that it does not influence their differentiation state. We have one experiment in which we looked at K1 expression—the 67-kDa keratin. We did not see K1 expressed, but that was not really a controlled study. We have no evidence that it induces differentiation. It simply seems to stop the cells from growing.

Dr. J. Michael Holland: Do you have any information on the form of the calcium in either the control or initiated cell line? Is it ionic, protein bound, or associated in some way with a cytosolic constituent?

Dr. Yuspa: The technique we are using only measures free calcium, not bound calcium.

REFERENCES

1. Balmain A. Transforming ras oncogenes and multistage carcinogenesis. Br J Cancer 51:1-7, 1985.
2. Yuspa SH. Tumor promotion. In Fortner JG, Rhoads JE (eds): Accomplishments in Cancer Research. Philadelphia: JB Lippincott Co., 1987, pp 169-182.
3. Hennings H, Shores R, Wenk M, Spangler EF, Tarone R, Yuspa SH. Malignant

134 / Yuspa et al.

conversion of mouse skin tumours is increased by tumour initiators and unaffected by tumour promoters. Nature 204:67-69, 1983.

4. Deschner EE, Lipkin M. Proliferative patterns in colonic mucosa in familial polyposis. Cancer Res 35:413-418, 1975.

5. Deschner EE. Early proliferation defects induced by six weekly injections of 1,2-dimethylhydrazine in epithelial cells of mouse distal colon. Zeitschrift fur Krebsforschung 91:205-216, 1978.

6. Yuspa SH. Alterations in epidermal differentiation in skin carcinogenesis. In Pullman B, T'so POP, Schneider ED (eds): Interrelationship among Aging, Cancer and Differentiation. Dordrecht, Holland: D. Reidel Publishing Company, 1985, pp 67-81.

7. Yuspa SH, Hennings H, Lichti U. Initiator and promoter induced specific changes in epidermal function and biological potential. Journal of Supramolecular Structure and Cell Biochemistry 17:245-257, 1981.

8. Russo J, Tay LK, Ciocca DR, Russo IH. Molecular and cellular basis of the mammary gland susceptibility to carcinogenesis. Environ Health Perspect 49:185-199, 1983.

9. Yuspa SH. Methods for the use of epidermal cell culture to study chemical carcinogenesis. In Skerrow D, Skerrow C (eds): Methods in Skin Research. Sussex: John Wiley and Sons, 1985, pp 213-249.

10. Hennings H, Michael D, Cheng C, Steinert P, Holbrook K, Yuspa SH. Calcium regulation of growth and differentiation of mouse epidermal cells in culture. Cell 19:245-254, 1980.

11. Strickland JE, Jetten AM, Kawamura H, Yuspa SH. Interaction of epidermal growth factor with basal and differentiating epidermal cells of mice resistant and sensitive to carcinogenesis. Carcinogenesis 5:735-740, 1984.

12. Hennings H, Holbrook K, Yuspa SH. Factors influencing calcium-induced terminal differentiation in cultured mouse epidermal cells. J Cell Physiol 116:265-281, 1983.

13. Roop DR, Huitfeldt H, Kilkenny A, Yuspa SH. Regulated expression of differentiation-associated keratins in cultured epidermal cells detected by monospecific antibodies to unique peptides of mouse epidermal keratins. Differentiation 35:143-150, 1987.

14. Kulesz-Martin M, Koehler B, Hennings H, Yuspa SH. Quantitative assay for carcinogen altered differentiation in mouse epidermal cells. Carcinogenesis 1:995-1006, 1980.

15. Yuspa SH, Morgan DL. Mouse skin cells resistant to terminal differentiation associated with initiation of carcinogenesis. Nature 293:72-74, 1981.

16. Kawamura H, Strickland JE, Yuspa SH. Association of resistance to terminal differentiation with initiation of carcinogenesis in adult mouse epidermal cells. Cancer Res 45:2748-2752, 1985.

17. Kilkenny AE, Morgan D, Spangler EF, Yuspa SH. Correlation of initiating potency of skin carcinogens with potency to induce resistance to terminal differentiation in cultured mouse keratinocytes. Cancer Res 45:2219-2225, 1985.

18. Yuspa SH, Morgan DL, Lichti U, Spangler EF, Michael D, Kilkenny A, Hennings H. Cultivation and characterization of cells derived from mouse skin papillomas induced by an initiation-promotion protocol. Carcinogenesis 7:949-958, 1986.

19. Strickland JE, Greenhalgh DA, Koceva-Chyla A, Hennings H, Restrepo C, Balaschak M, Yuspa SH. Development of murine epidermal cell lines which contain an activated rasH oncogene and form papillomas in skin grafts on athymic nude mouse hosts. Cancer Res 48:165-169, 1988.

20. Bizub D, Wood AW, Skalka AM. Mutagenesis of the Ha-*ras* oncogene in mouse skin tumors induced by polycyclic aromatic hydrocarbons. Proc Natl Acad Sci USA 83:6048-6052, 1986.

21. Quintanilla M, Brown K, Ramsden M, Balmain A. Carcinogen specific mutation and amplification of Ha-*ras* during mouse skin carcinogenesis. Nature 322:78-80, 1986.

22. Brown K, Quintanilla M, Ramsden M, Kerr IB, Young S, Balmain A. v-*ras* Genes from Harvey and BALB murine sarcoma viruses can act as initiators of two-stage mouse skin carcinogenesis. Cell 46:447-456, 1986.

23. Roop DR, Lowy DR, Tambourin PE, Strickland J, Harper JR, Balaschak M, Spangler EF, Yuspa SH. An activated Harvey ras oncogene produces benign tumours on mouse epidermal tissue. Nature 323:822-824, 1986.

24. Yuspa SH, Kilkenny AE, Stanley J, Lichti U. Keratinocytes blocked in phorbol ester-responsive early stage of terminal differentiation by sarcoma viruses. Nature 314:459-462, 1985.

25. Menon GK, Grayson S, Elias PM. Ionic calcium reservoirs in mammalian epidermis: Ultrastructural localization by ion-capture cytochemistry. J Invest Dermatol 74:508-512, 1985.

26. Malmqvist KG, Carlsson LE, Forslind B, Roomans GM, Akselsson KR. Proton and electron microprobe analysis of human skin. Instrumentation and Methods in Physics Research [Sec. B] 3:611-617, 1984.

27. Yuspa SH, Ben T, Hennings H, Lichti U. Phorbol ester tumor promoters induce epidermal transglutaminase activity. Biochem Biophys Res Commun 97:700-708, 1980.

28. Yuspa SH, Ben T, Hennings H. The induction of epidermal transglutaminase and terminal differentiation by tumor promoters in cultured epidermal cells. Carcinogenesis 4:1413-1418, 1983.

29. Reiners JJ, Slaga TJ. Effects of tumor promoters on the rate and commitment to terminal differentiation of subpopulations of murine keratinocytes. Cell 32:247-255, 1983.

30. Wirth PJ, Yuspa SH, Thorgeirsson SS, Hennings H. Induction of common patterns of polypeptide synthesis and phosphorylation by calcium and 12-O-tetradecanoylphorbol-13-acetate in mouse epidermal cell culture. Cancer Res 47:2831-2838, 1987.

31. Jeng AY, Lichti U, Strickland JE, Blumberg PM. Similar effects of phospholipase C and phorbol ester tumor promoters on primary mouse epidermal cells. Cancer Res 45:5714-5721, 1985.

32. Berridge MJ. Inositol triphosphate and diacylglycerol as second messengers. Biochem J 220:345-360, 1984.

33. Jaken S, Yuspa SH. Early signals for keratinocyte differentiation: Role of Ca^{2+}-mediated inositol lipid metabolism in normal and neoplastic epidermal cells. Carcinogenesis 9:1033-1038, 1988.

34. Williams DA, Fogarty KE, Tsien RY, Fay FS. Calcium gradients in single smooth muscle cells revealed by the digital imaging microscope using Fura-2. Nature 318:558-561, 1985.

Skin Carcinogenesis: Mechanisms and Human Relevance, pages 137–145

Initiation of Skin Carcinogenesis Can Occur by Induction of Carcinogen-Specific Point Mutations in the Harvey-*ras* Gene

B. Bailleul,* K. Brown, M. Ramsden,† F. Fee, and A. Balmain

Beatson Institute for Cancer Research, Bearsden, Glasgow G61 1BD, U.K.

Evaluation of the risk to humans of exposure to environmental chemicals is severely hampered by lack of knowledge of the mechanisms by which such chemicals induce specific biological responses. The most severe of these responses is neoplasia, and while a great deal of information has been accumulated on the metabolism and DNA-binding properties of tumor-inducing chemicals, the nature of the resulting mutations and their effects on critical target genes has remained obscure.

Animal model systems are invaluable in the study of these questions. The ability to control the dose, route of exposure, and duration of treatment with specific chemical agents vastly increases the probability of reaching meaningful conclusions with regard to the mechanisms involved. The use of inbred rodent strains furthermore eliminates problems associated with variations in the degree of metabolic activation or genetic susceptibility to tumor development.

Of the animal model systems used in carcinogenesis studies, mouse skin has provided most of the currently accepted biological principles. The concepts of initiation, promotion, and progression were developed using this model system, and a wealth of information has been accumulated over the past 40-50 years (1). We have chosen to use this system to investigate the molecular events associated with the different stages of carcinogenesis. Most of the work to be described will be related to mechanisms of initiation, but it should be noted that different classes of chemicals can induce the subsequent events in promotion and progression. There is therefore enormous potential to exploit the available knowledge of tumor biology to determine at the molecular level how chemical agents act.

* On leave from U.124 INSERM, Institut de Recherches sur le Cancer, 59045 Lille Cedex, France

† Present address: Fermentation Development Department, Glaxochem Ltd., Ulverston, Cumbria, U.K.

PROTO-ONCOGENES AS TARGETS FOR INITIATING AGENTS

For many years the critical targets for the mutagenic action of chemical carcinogens were unknown. The discovery of proto-oncogenes has raised the possibility that these genes, which play important roles in the control of cell growth and differentiation (2), could be activated by environmental chemicals or radiation. This possibility was supported by the demonstration of multiple activating mechanisms for these genes, including single point mutations, gene amplification, translocations, or deletions (3). All of these genetic changes can be induced by various types of mutagens (4).

RAS GENE ACTIVATION IN CHEMICALLY INDUCED TUMORS

Our initial experiments on the role of oncogenes in mouse skin carcinogenesis showed that a member of the *ras* family of proto-oncogenes was reproducibly activated in both papillomas and carcinomas initiated with 9,10-dimethyl-1,2-benzanthracene (DMBA) (5-7). This family, of which the three members known as Harvey (Ha)-, Kirsten (Ki)-, and N-*ras* have been the most intensively studied, is found to be activated in a substantial proportion (10%–40%) of human tumors (8). The Ha-*ras* gene has been most frequently activated in squamous carcinomas and melanomas, whereas the Ki-*ras* is activated in a wide spectrum of malignancies of different types. N-*ras* is found predominantly in tumors of hematopoietic cells. It is noteworthy that the gene found to be mutated in chemically induced papillomas and carcinomas of mouse skin (5-7) and the rat mammary gland (9) was the Ha-*ras* gene, while mainly the N-*ras* gene was mutated in thymic lymphomas (10). This supports the relevance of animal models for human carcinogenesis, since the type of gene activated is similar in tumors of the same general type in different species.

STRUCTURE AND TRANSCRIPTIONAL CONTROL OF THE MOUSE HA-*RAS* GENE

In view of the apparent importance of the mouse cellular Ha-*ras* gene in skin carcinogenesis, we undertook a study of the structure and transcriptional control of this gene in normal cells. This study was essential for two reasons. First, the normal sequence of the gene would provide the necessary basis for comparison of the mutated forms found in the tumors. Second, some tumors of either animal or human origin do not have altered forms of the Ha-*ras* structural gene, but rather show increased expression of the normal proto-oncogene product (11). Structural elements that control the transcription of this gene could therefore be important alternative targets for chemical mutagenesis.

A genomic clone of the normal mouse Ha-*ras* gene was obtained by screening a genomic library prepared using a λ Charon 30 phage vector. The single clone isolated (λN1-*ras*) was restriction mapped, and the Ha-*ras* hybridizing regions were sequenced. Full details of the sequence will be published elsewhere (12). Figure 1 shows the sequenced regions of the gene and indicates that the clone λN1-*ras* contains the first two coding exons of the Ha-*ras* gene, but lacks exons 3 and 4. Even by repeated screening of this and other genomic libraries, we have consistently failed to isolate the 3' end of the mouse Ha-*ras* gene, despite the fact that both rat (13) and human (14) genes have been cloned and sequenced. We conclude that there is a sequence within the mouse 3' end that precludes isolation by propagation in phage or plasmid vectors.

The presence in λN1-*ras* of coding exons 1 and 2 together with 20 kb of 5' flanking sequence enabled us to investigate the transcriptional control of this gene in some detail. A combination of nucleotide sequencing, primer extension analysis, and S1 mapping was used to show that initiation of transcription starts at the three sites shown in Figure 1. No differences in the relative intensities of these three start sites and no additional start sites were found when tumor cells were compared with normal cells (12). In addition, the use of probes from the 5' end of the gene showed that the structural gene was intact in over 70 chemically induced tumors that were tested. We therefore find no evidence that truncation of the *ras* gene plays any role in its activation, as has previously been postulated (15).

The upstream region containing the transcription start sites (exon-1) is highly conserved between mouse and human and contains several potential SP1 binding sites. Similar elements have been noted in the promoter regions of several "housekeeping" genes (16). The promoter activity of this sequence was directly tested by fusion to a promoterless chloramphenicol-acetyl-transferase gene (CAT) followed by transfection into 208F fibroblast cells and an assay for CAT enzyme activity. The results showed that the exon-1 region does indeed have promoter activity comparable to that previously detected in the human gene (17,18). Interestingly, the activity was substantially increased by the

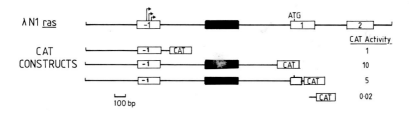

Figure 1. The structure and promoter activity of the mouse Ha-*ras* gene 5' flanking sequence. Primer extension analysis and S1 mapping show three transcription start sites (↑) in exon-1. The shaded box represents a sequence within the first intron that is highly conserved between mouse and human DNA. The open boxes represent either coding (1 and 2) or noncoding (-1) exons. The CAT enzyme activities obtained with three constructs have been compared. The first one showed significant enzyme activity compared to the promoterless gene. The inclusion of the first intron increased promoter activity by 5- to 10-fold.

inclusion of the first intron in the fusion construct (Fig. 1), suggesting that a previously undetected enhancer element may be present within this intron (12). A possible candidate for this enhancer element is a highly conserved sequence of about 300 bp found in the first intron (12).

In conclusion, analysis of the overall structure and transcriptional control of the Ha-*ras* gene in normal and tumor cells suggests that the only differences detectable to date are single point mutations within the coding exons, which confer dominant transforming activity. It remains possible that additional mutations may be found within the putative enhancer region in the first intron, which could lead to elevated expression in some tumors.

ANALYSIS OF CARCINOGEN-SPECIFIC MUTATIONS IN THE HA-RAS GENE

Initiation in mouse skin carcinogenesis can be accomplished by a single treatment with any one of a variety of carcinogens—benzo[*a*]pyrene (BP), 7,12-dimethylbenz[*a*]anthracene, methylcholanthrene (MCA), N,N^1-dimethylnitrosourea, N-methyl-N´-nitro-N-nitrosoguanidine (MNNG), 4-nitroquinoline 1-oxide, β-propiolactone, and *bis*(chloromethyl) ether. The list of initiators includes both direct-acting alkylating agents such as MNNG and polycyclic aromatic hydrocarbons or aromatic amine derivatives requiring metabolic activation. Chemicals of these two classes are known to induce different types of point mutations by forming specific promutagenic lesions with the target DNA. MNNG can methylate the 0^6 position of the guanosine residue, which causes GC→AT transitions by miscoding during the next round of DNA replication (19). Polycyclic hydrocarbons form bulky adducts with both guanosine and adenosine residues, with the formation predominantly of transversion mutations after error-prone repair (20). Heterocyclic aromatic amines such as 4-nitroquinoline 1-oxide are known to bind to purine bases (21, 22), forming bulky adducts, which induce largely GC→AT transitions. We have therefore investigated the types of oncogene mutations that can be found in tumors initiated with these two classes of mutagens. The rationale for this approach is that if the oncogene mutations that can be detected had the correct carcinogen specificity, that would provide strong evidence that the mutations occur at the time of initiation by direct interaction between the carcinogen and the oncogene DNA. Alternatively, if the mutations found are nonspecific or random, it would be more likely that they arise at a later stage, possibly during the proliferative phase induced by tumor promoters—those that bind protein kinase C: 12-O-tetradecanoylphorbol-13-acetate (TPA) and dihydroteleocidin; and others: phenol, anthralin, chrysarobin, and skin wounding. Additional experiments were therefore carried out using promoters of different classes to determine whether tumors promoted with TPA, which acts by binding to protein kinase C (23), have a different spectrum of mutations from those promoted by non-TPA-type agents (chrysarobin) (24).

The techniques used to investigate the pattern of mutations included DNA transfection into NIH/3T3 cells, nucleotide sequencing, analysis of induced

Table 1. Ha-*ras* Gene Activation in Mouse Skin Tumors

Tumor	Carcinogen	Promoter	No. analyzed	Ha-*ras* activation	Mutation
Papilloma	DMBA	TPA	42	39	$A^{182} \rightarrow T$
				1	Codon 61
Papilloma	DMBA	Chrysarobin	5	5	$A^{182} \rightarrow T$
Carcinoma	DMBA	TPA	13	10	$A^{182} \rightarrow T$
				1	$G^{35} \rightarrow T$
Carcinoma	DMBA	DMBA	8	4	$A^{182} \rightarrow T$
Papilloma	MCA	TPA	5	2	$A^{182} \rightarrow T$
Carcinoma	MCA	TPA	7	4	Codon 13
Papilloma	BP	TPA	2	1	$G^{35} \rightarrow T$
Carcinoma	BP	TPA	3	1	$G^{35} \rightarrow T$
Papilloma	MNNG	TPA	14	11	$G^{35} \rightarrow A$
Carcinoma	MNNG	TPA	9	1	$G^{35} \rightarrow A$

Abbreviations used: DMBA, 7,12-dimethylbenz[a]anthracene; MCA, methylcholanthrene; BP, benzo[a]pyrene; MNNG, *N*-methyl-*N'*-nitro-*N*-nitrosoguanidine.

restriction fragment length polymorphisms (RFLPs) (5-7), and oligonucleotide hybridization (25). Some of the results obtained are shown in Table 1.

Two main conclusions can be drawn from the results shown. The first is that the type of Ha-*ras* mutation seen is dependent upon the initiating agent used. An AT→TA transversion mutation is seen in a very high proportion of tumors initiated with DMBA. This mutation is seen only rarely in MCA-initiated tumors and not at all in tumors initiated with BP or MNNG. In contrast, variation of the promoting agent had no effect on the mutations seen. These results therefore support the conclusion that the *ras* mutations are induced at an early stage of carcinogenesis (6) and probably at the time of initiation (7,9).

Further evidence in favor of this interpretation comes from analysis of the MNNG-induced tumors. A substantial proportion of these exhibited the GC→AT transition predicted on the basis of the known mechanisms of action of this carcinogen (19). This transition mutation has not been detected in any tumors initiated with the polycyclic hydrocarbons.

A further conclusion from Table 1 is that there appears to be a discrepancy in the mutational pattern shown by the papillomas and carcinomas initiated with MNNG. While the GC→AT transition was frequently seen in the papillomas, it was rare in the carcinomas. It would therefore appear that the majority of carcinomas in this case do not arise by progression from the "typical" papilloma with the GC→AT transition. Those papillomas that do not have this mutation may constitute a subpopulation with a very high probability of malignant conversion. Alternatively, some of the carcinomas may arise de novo, without passing through an obvious papilloma stage. The existence of carcinomas with these properties has been postulated previously (26,27). These results constitute the first molecular evidence for the existence of multiple pathways leading to papillomas and carcinomas. An important future goal is to determine the nature of the lesion in those tumors that do not have the typical GC→AT transition, since this knowledge may provide valuable clues as to the events important for malignant progression.

RELEVANCE TO HUMAN CANCER

The majority of human cancers are carcinomas, which are known from epidemiological studies to arise by a multistep mechanism. Many of these are caused by exposure to chemicals present in the environment. It therefore seems highly likely that animal models for the multistage development of chemically induced carcinomas will be relevant to human carcinogenesis, but there is as yet no proof of this assumption. Initial comparisons based on molecular evidence are nevertheless encouraging. The *ras* genes are activated by similar point mutations in both human and animal tumors (28). The broad tissue specificity in the activation of particular *ras* family members in human tumors is also reflected in the equivalent types of animal tumors. Although mutations in premalignant tumors were first found in mouse skin papillomas, a similar situation exists in human colon tumors in which certain premalignant polyps also contain mutated *ras* genes. It is therefore possible that while mouse skin carcinogenesis may not be an exact replica of human skin tumor development, the basic principles emerging from studies of this kind are probably relevant to human carcinomas of different tissues.

ACKNOWLEDGMENTS

B.B. was supported by European Medical Research Councils and European Science Foundation (1987) and by the Association pour la Recherche sur le Cancer (ARC, 1988). The Beatson Institute is supported by the Cancer Research Campaign.

OPEN FORUM

Dr. Hiroshi Yamasaki: In your study, the percentage of Ha-*ras* mutations at the 61st codon was quite similar in papillomas and carcinomas. I think it is important to take papillomas before any carcinomas appear, because what is being compared is the prevalence of papillomas that may become carcinomas. At which stage did you assess papillomas? We have done extensive work with transplacental initiation with DMBA and postnatal promotion with TPA. We saw the same mutation you have found. The transplacental initiation was carried out on gestation day 15, and the back skin was painted with TPA. When skin tumors were analyzed for the presence of a A to T transmission of the 61st codon of Ha-*ras*, only 50% had positive papillomas. But all the carcinomas had this mutation. We suspect that this mutation may serve as a selective pressure for papillomas.

Dr. Allan Balmain: Those statistics appear to be the opposite of what we found by doing the initiation-promotion with the adult mice. There, 90% to 95% of the papillomas and a smaller percentage of the carcinomas have the mutation. In terms of what stage of papillomas we have looked at, we have taken papillomas at about 10 weeks and those that are still present at the end of the experiment. We find no difference. There is a uniformly high percentage in these particular experiments.

Dr. Claudio M. Aldaz: Dr. Balmain, you presented a table showing Ha-*ras* activation in different human and animal neoplasias. That table did not list human skin squamous cell carcinoma. Apparently Ha-*ras* activation has not been shown there. Do you think that the *ras* role is played in human skin tumors by a different oncogene, similar to what may happen in the rat mammary system and human breast tumors (in the rat system apparently *ras* activation is important but human breast tumors show mainly activation of the *neu* oncogene)?

Dr. Balmain: To my knowledge, no one has published a comprehensive survey of human squamous cell tumors. Steven White in our laboratory has been looking at human skin tumors, concentrating on basal cell carcinomas. To date, he has found one basal cell carcinoma that has an activated *ras* gene with a codon 12 mutation. He is presently working on some squamous cell carcinomas. We do not have any definitive results yet. Mammary carcinomas have very low frequencies of activated *ras* genes, while most other human tumors have an average of 10% to 20%. In the colon, the frequency is 40%.

Dr. Rheinwald: In their early studies, Bob Weinberg and Geoff Cooper both looked for DNA sequences in four of my squamous carcinoma cell lines that would confer focus-forming ability in 3T3 cells. They did not find any. I think there will always be some cases of every histological type of cancer that have mutationally activated *ras* genes; some tumor types may tend to have it at a higher frequency. Squamous cell carcinoma does not appear to have *ras* activation at a very high frequency, nor does it have any other gene that confers focus-forming ability to fibroblasts.

Dr. Stuart Yuspa: I have heard rumors that there is a fairly high incidence of erbB-2 activation or high expression of EGF receptor in human squamous cell cancers, but I have not seen it published. Dr. Balmain, have you found that carcinomas that do not have the *ras* mutation contain a transforming gene as detected by transfection into 3T3 cells?

Dr. Balmain: We have looked for the *ras* mutation mainly by polymorphism analysis and oligohybridization. In some cases, we have also done transfections. A proportion of the carcinomas do not appear to have any transforming gene. This is an important point because there may be one or more genes that are not detectable by transfection assays but that are more potent inducers of carcinomas than of papillomas.

Dr. G. Tim Bowden: You mentioned that carcinoma cells are refractory to TGF-beta. We have shown recently that carcinoma cells in culture when treated with TGF-beta show an enhanced level of transin, suggesting that maybe there is an autocrine mechanism by which the carcinoma cells stimulate themselves to produce transin.

Dr. Balmain: Did you find any effects on growth rates?

Dr. Bowden: We have not looked at that yet.

Dr. Yuspa: We have looked at the effects of TGF-beta on growth of papilloma cell lines in vitro, and we have found that their growth is inhibited. The clonal growth of several cell lines that have an activated *ras* gene with a codon 61 mutation and produce papillomas when grafted to nude mouse skin sites were inhibited. We have not examined carcinoma cells, but any scheme describing differential response to TGF-beta in tumor promotion must address these results on benign tumor cells.

REFERENCES

1.   Hecker E, Fusenig NE, Kunz W, Marks F, Thielman HW, eds. Cocarcinogenesis and Biological Effects of Tumour Promoters. New York: Raven Press, 1982.
2.   Bishop JM. Cellular oncogenes and retroviruses. Annu Rev Biochem 52:301-354, 1983.
3.   Weinberg RA. The action of oncogenes in the cytoplasm and nucleus. Science 230:770-776, 1985.
4.   Klein G, Klein E. Oncogene activation and tumor progression. Carcinogenesis 5:429-435, 1984.
5.   Balmain A, Pragnell IB. Mouse skin carcinomas induced in vivo by chemical carcinogens have a transforming Harvey-*ras* oncogene. Nature 303:72-74, 1983.
6.   Balmain A, Ramsden M, Bowden GT, Smith J. Activation of the mouse cellular Harvey-*ras* gene in chemically induced benign skin papillomas. Nature 307:658-660, 1984.
7.   Quintanilla M, Brown K, Ramsden M, Balmain A. Carcinogen-specific mutation and amplification of Ha-*ras* during mouse skin carcinogenesis. Nature 322:78-80, 1986.
8.   Bos JL. The *ras* gene family and human carcinogenesis. Mutat Res 195:255-268, 1988.
9.   Zarbl H, Sukumar S, Arthur AV, Martin-Zanca D, Barbacid M. Direct mutagenesis of Ha-*ras*1 oncogene by N-nitroso-N-methylurea during initiation of mammary carcinogenesis in rats. Nature 315:382-386, 1985.
10.   Guerrero I, Pellicer A. Mutational activation of oncogenes in animal model systems of carcinogenesis. Mutat Res 185:293-308, 1987.
11.   Slamon DJ, Cline MJ. Expression of cellular oncogenes during embryonic and fetal development of the mouse. Proc Natl Acad Sci USA 81:7141-7145, 1984.
12.   Brown K, Bailleul B, Ramsden M, Fee F, Krumlauf R, Balmain A. Isolation and characterisation of the 5' flanking region of the murine Harvey-*ras* gene. Molecular Carcinogenesis (in press) 1988.
13.   Damante G, Filetti S, Rapoport B. Nucleotide sequence and characterization of the 5' flanking region of the rat Ha-*ras* protooncogene. Proc Natl Acad Sci USA 84:774-778, 1987.

14. Capon DJ, Chen EY, Levinson AD, Seeburg PH, Goeddel DV. Complete nucleotide sequence of the T24 human bladder carcinoma oncogene and its normal homologue. Nature 302:33-37, 1983.

15. Cichutek K, Duesberg PH. Harvey *ras* gene transform without mutant codons, apparently activated by truncation of a 5' exon (exon -1). Proc Natl Acad Sci USA 83:2340-2344, 1986.

16. Dynan WS, Tjian R. Control of eukaryotic messenger RNA synthesis by sequence-specific DNA-binding proteins. Nature 316:774-778, 1985.

17. Ishii S, Merlino GT, Pastan I. Promoter region of the human Harvey-*ras* proto-oncogene: Similarity to the EGF receptor proto-oncogene promoter. Science 230:1378-1381, 1985.

18. Spandidos DA, Riggio M. Promoter and enhancer activity at the 5' end of normal and T24 Ha-*ras* 1 genes. FEBS Lett 203:169-174, 1986.

19. Eadie JS, Conrad M, Toorchen D, Topal MD. Mechanism of mutagenesis by 06-methylguanine. Nature 308:201-203, 1984.

20. Eisenstadt E, Warren AJ, Porter J, Atkins D, Miller JH. Carcinogenic epoxides of benzo[*a*]pyrene and cyclopenta[*cd*]pyrene induce base substitutions via transversions. Proc Natl Acad Sci USA 79:1945-1949, 1982.

21. Bailleul B, Galiegue S, Loucheux-Lefebvre MH. Adducts from the reaction of O,O-diacetyl or O-acetyl derivatives of the carcinogen 4-hydroxyaminoquinoline 1-oxide with purine nucleosides. Cancer Res 41:4559-4565, 1981.

22. Galiegue-Zouitina S, Bailleul B, Ginot TM, Perly B, Vigny P, Loucheux-Lefebvre MH. N2-Guanyl and N6-adenyl arylation of chicken erythrocyte DNA by the ultimate carcinogen of 4-nitroquinoline 1-oxide. Cancer Res 46:1858-1863, 1986.

23. Castagna M, Takai T, Kaibuchi K, Sano K, Kikkawa U, Nishizuka T. Direct activation of calcium-activated phospholipid-dependent protein kinase by tumor-promoting phorbol esters. J Biol Chem 257:7847-7851, 1982.

24. DiGiovanni J, Boutwell RK. Tumor promoting activity of 1,8-dihydroxy-3-methyl-9-anthrone (chysarobin) in female SENCAR mice. Carcinogenesis 4:281-284, 1983.

25. Verlaan-de Vries M, Bogaard ME, van den Elst H, van Boom JH, van der Eb AJ, Bos JL. A dot-blot screening procedure for mutated ras oncogenes using synthetic oligodeoxynucleotides. Gene 50:313-320, 1986.

26. Scribner JD, Scribner NK, McKnight B, Mottet NK. Evidence for a new model of tumor progression from carcinogenesis and tumor promotion studies with 7-bromomethylbenz[*a*]anthracene. Cancer Res 43:2034-2041, 1983.

27. Reddy AL, Caldwell M, Fialkow PJ. Sequential studies of skin tumorigenesis in phosphoglycerate kinase mosaic mice: Effect of resumption of promotion on regressed papillomas. Cancer Res 47:1947-1951, 1987.

28. Barbacid M. *Ras* genes. Annu Rev Biochem 56:779-827, 1987.

Skin Carcinogenesis: Mechanisms and Human Relevance, pages 147–164
© 1989 Alan R. Liss, Inc.

Differential Gene Expression in Skin Tumors Initiated by Ionizing Radiation or Chemical Carcinogens

G. Tim Bowden, Deborah Jaffe, Peter Krieg, Keith Bonham, and Larry Ostrowski*

Department of Radiation Oncology (G.T.B., K.B., L.O.), University of Arizona Health Sciences Center, Tucson, Arizona 85724; Department of Radiation Oncology (D.J.), University of Chicago Medical School, Chicago, Illinois, 60637; and Institute for Virus Research (P.K.), German Cancer Research Center, 6900 Heidelberg, West Germany

During the process of either chemical or radiation carcinogenesis, the progression of target cells through a premalignant to a malignant state is accompanied by a variety of morphological and biochemical changes. Some of these phenotypic changes may result from qualitative changes in the encoded gene products or changes in the levels of expression of cellular genes. One class of cellular genes that is altered during carcinogenesis and is thought to play a functional role in tumor progression is that of cellular proto-oncogenes (1-3). In addition there is a class of cellular tumor-suppressor genes whose inactivation may be required for expression of the tumorigenic phenotype because the genes' active expression may override the transforming action of highly expressed oncoproteins (4). The activation of the cellular proto-oncogenes can be either qualitative or quantitative. In general, the activation of proto-oncogenes that encode proteins located in the cytoplasm or at the plasma membrane involves structural alterations in the encoded proteins. In contrast, the proto-oncogenes that encode proteins located at the nucleus are activated by mechanisms that enhance the expression of the proto-oncogene products.

Over the last 5 years a number of laboratories have studied proto-oncogene activation (5-11) and the overexpression of tumor-associated genes (12-17) during tumor progression, using the multistage model of mouse skin carcinogenesis. The detection of transforming genes in both experimental animal and human tumors has in part been made possible by the development of the DNA-mediated gene-transfer technique. The transfection of genomic DNA isolated

---

* Present address: Department of Radiation Oncology, University of Arizona Health Sciences Center, Tucson, Arizona 85724

from tumors into NIH3T3 recipient cells, producing transformed foci, has made possible the identification of activated oncogenes in tumors. The activated oncogenes detected by this gene-transfer technique include the *ras* family of oncogenes (18,19) and a number of other oncogenes including *met, neu, raf, erb*B, B-*lym*, and *dbl* (20-25). Two laboratories (6,8) have described the activation of the cellular Harvey-*ras* gene in both benign and malignant mouse skin tumors that have been initiated with the chemical carcinogen 7,12-dimethylbenz[*a*]anthracene (DMBA). Besides looking for the activation of dominant transforming genes in chemically induced mouse skin tumors, we have used differential screening of cDNA libraries to isolate a number of cellular sequences that are overexpressed during mouse skin tumor progression (12-17). These sequences include the six "*mal*" sequences (12) and the transin gene, which encodes a secreted metalloproteinase (13).

Information related to molecular mechanisms of skin carcinogenesis could lead to the development of molecular markers of skin tumor progression as well as provide the rationale for strategies of intervention in human skin cancer. In addition, these molecular markers involving the activation or inactivation of cellular genes including proto-oncogenes and tumor-suppressor genes could be useful in assessing the risk for potential human skin carcinogens.

METHODS

Tumor Induction

The mouse skin tumors used in this study were produced according to procedures published previously (26-28). Ionizing radiation-induced skin tumors were initiated in SENCAR or Charles River CD-1 mice with a single dose of 4 MeV photons and then promoted twice a week for 60 weeks with 8 nmol 12-O-tetradecanoylphorbol-13-acetate (TPA) per treatment. Chemical carcinogen-initiated skin tumors used in the reported studies were initiated with DMBA or N-methyl-N'-nitro-N-nitrosoguanidine (MNNG), and the tumors were promoted with TPA as described previously (28).

Transfection Assays

The DNA transfection assays were performed as described by Wigler et al. (29). Briefly, freshly propagated NIH3T3 or Rat2 fibroblasts were grown in Dulbecco's modified Eagle's medium supplemented with 10% fetal calf serum and antibiotics. As controls, each transfection assay included cultures treated with calcium phosphate alone (mocks), DNA from untreated NIH3T3 cells (negative control), and DNA from a human T24 bladder carcinoma cell line (30). Foci were picked, and transformed cells of interest were grown and used as sources of DNA for second- and third-round transfection experiments.

DNA and RNA Isolation

Total tissue DNA and RNA were extracted from mouse skin tumors and epidermis by a procedure previously described (31).

Isolation of Plasmid DNA and Preparation of Labeled Probes

Plasmids were isolated from chloramphenicol-amplified cultures and purified by column chromatography (32). Purified plasmid DNA was ^{32}P labeled by nick translation (33).

Southern and Northern Analyses

DNAs from normal epidermis, tumors, and transfectants were digested with restriction enzymes using the conditions recommended by the supplier. The digested DNAs (10 μg) were separated by electrophoresis through horizontal agarose slab gels and transferred to nitrocellulose filters (34). Nick-translated ^{32}P-labeled probes with specific activities of 3–10 x 10^7 cpm/μg were hybridized to the nitrocellulose filters in 50% formamide, 5 x Denhardt's solution, 150 mM NaCl plus 15 mM sodium citrate (SSC), 0.1% sodium dodecyl sulfate (SDS), and 100 mg/ml denatured salmon-sperm DNA at 43°C for 18-24 h (35). Filters were washed three times, for 10 min each, in 2.0 x SSC, 0.1% SDS at room temperature. The final wash stringency was 0.2 x SSC, 0.3% SDS at 65°C. Autoradiography was performed with Kodak XAR film and intensifying screens.

DNA Sequencing

DNA sequence was determined using either the Maxam-Gilbert technique (36) or M13 dideoxy technique with ^{35}S dATP and buffer gradient gels (37).

RESULTS

Detection of Dominant Transforming Genes in Radiation-Induced Mouse Skin Tumors

Recently, we showed that ionizing radiation can act as an initiator of both squamous cell (26,27) and basal cell carcinomas (27) in the mouse skin when followed by promotion with TPA. It was of considerable interest to compare the dominant transforming genes present in these radiation-initiated skin tumors with the ones found in mouse skin tumors initiated with chemical carcinogens. Previously, in collaboration with Dr. Balmain, we showed that both benign and malignant mouse skin tumors initiated with the polycyclic hydrocarbon DMBA and promoted with TPA contained an activated Harvey-*ras* oncogene (6).

Subsequently, Balmain's laboratory demonstrated that greater than 90% of the DMBA-initiated tumors had an activating A→T transversion mutation at the second nucleotide of codon 61 of the Harvey-*ras* gene (7). In addition, we have recently obtained preliminary data to indicate that the majority of both benign and malignant mouse skin tumors initiated with urethane have an activating A→T transversion mutation, also in the 61st codon of the cellular Harvey-*ras* gene (16).

To examine the role of oncogene activation in the radiation-induced mouse skin tumors and address the issue of carcinogen specificity, tumor DNAs were examined for the presence of dominant transforming activity using the NIH3T3 and Rat2 transfection focus-formation assays. Eighty-two percent of all of the skin tumor DNAs studied were positive in the NIH3T3 assay. Dominant transforming activity was observed in all tumor types (papilloma, basal cell carcinoma, and squamous cell carcinoma [SCC]) initiated by ionizing radiation but not in normal or treated (x-radiation- and TPA-treated) epidermis. To study the potential transforming genes transferred from the tumors to the recipient NIH3T3 cells, DNAs from the NIH3T3 transfectant cell lines were analyzed by Southern blot technique for the presence of activated forms of the three cellular *ras* genes, Harvey (Ha), Kirsten (Ki), and N. If restriction sites closely linked to the transferred gene were destroyed by restriction digestion before transfection, then DNA prepared from transformed foci would contain novel restriction fragments hybridizing to the gene probes of interest. Novel restriction fragments were not observed in any of the NIH3T3 transfectant DNAs examined, nor were any of the endogenous fragments amplified. Secondary Rat2 transfectant DNAs were also probed with the same three *ras* genes to determine whether the Rat2 transfectants contained any mouse *ras* sequences, presumably transferred from the mouse tumor. This can be done because the restriction patterns for the mouse and rat *ras* genes are quite different. It was found that the Rat2 transfectants contained only the endogenous rat *ras* sequences. These data indicated that the putative transforming genes were not members of the *ras* gene family.

The majority of oncogenes detected in the NIH3T3 focus assay have been shown to be genetically altered versions of one of three closely related *ras* genes. However, oncogenes unrelated to *ras* (B-*lym*, *erb*B, *met*, *neu*, *raf*) have also been detected by DNA transfection assays. Southern blots of primary and secondary NIH3T3 transfectants were screened for the presence of amplified or rearranged B-*lym*, *erb*B, *met*, *neu*, and *raf*. Amplification and rearrangements were not detected with any of the probes used in any of the transfectant cell lines studied.

Further characterization of the dominant transforming genes in the radiation-induced mouse skin tumors was carried out by studying the effects of restriction enzyme cleavages on the dominant transforming activity in transfectant DNAs. The characterization of potential dominant transforming genes in genomic DNA has been assisted by studies of the sensitivity of the gene to inactivation by restriction endonucleases (18,38). Restriction enzyme endonuclease mapping was performed on primary and secondary NIH3T3 transfectant

DNAs containing dominant transforming activity. The results of the mapping of four transfectants derived from four different SCCs with four different enzymes indicated three different mapping patterns.

Expression of the Differentially Expressed *mal* Genes in Benign and Malignant Mouse Skin Tumors

To investigate molecular mechanisms involved in the process of skin carcinogenesis, it is useful to identify and characterize genes whose expression is altered during tumor development. To achieve this goal using the mouse skin multistage model, we have recently isolated a number of sequences (*mal*-1 to *mal*-6) that were overexpressed at different stages during skin tumor progression (12,15-17). These sequences (cDNAs) were isolated using the technique of differential screening of cDNA libraries that were made from poly(A)+ RNA isolated from SCCs induced by DMBA initiation and TPA promotion. The libraries were screened using cDNA probes made from RNA isolated from normal epidermis and SCCs.

To investigate a potential role of the *mal* sequences in the process of skin carcinogenesis, we asked whether there was a correlation between the stage of tumor development and the level of expression of the different *mal* genes. Both benign and malignant skin tumors were induced in mice by initiation with either DMBA or MNNG and promotion with TPA. Northern blot analysis (Fig. 1) was performed with total-tissue RNA isolated from mouse epidermis, benign papillomas, a benign keratoacanthoma, and malignant squamous cell carcinomas using *mal* cDNA clones as probes. As a control in all northern blot analyses, the RNA bound to the filters was hybridized either simultaneously or in a second round of hybridization with a probe for 7S cytoplasmic RNA, which is present in the same abundance in normal and in tumor tissues (39). With one exception (*mal*-4), the transcripts corresponding to the *mal* cDNA clones were already overexpressed in the papilloma stage, and we did not observe a further increase of expression of these sequences during progression from the papilloma to the SCC. There were no detectable differences in the expression of *mal*-1-related sequences in tumor promoter-dependent papillomas (Fig. 1h,i) as compared with tumor promoter-independent papillomas (Fig. 1f,g). In contrast, *mal*-2 expression was slightly enhanced in tumor promoter-dependent tumors (Fig. 1f-i). A keratoacanthoma, another benign tumor sometimes arising during skin carcinogenesis, showed only a weak expression of *mal*-1 and -2 (Fig. 1a). In all malignant SCCs we observed high levels of steady-state transcripts for *mal*-1- and -2-related sequences. There were only small differences in the expression levels in several individual carcinomas induced by the two-stage protocols with either DMBA/TPA (Fig. 1c-e) or MNNG/TPA (Fig. 1b).

In contrast to these findings, the patterns of the *mal*-3-related transcripts changed during tumor development in the mouse skin. In normal epidermis, low steady-state levels of three transcripts were detected (i.e., 1.3, 2.3, and 2.9 kb)

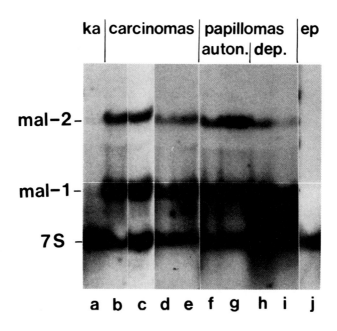

Figure 1. Expression of *mal*-1 and *mal*-2 in different mouse skin tumors. Ten micrograms of total RNA from normal epidermis or tumors was applied to each lane, size fractionated in 1.4% agarose/2.2 M formaldehyde gels, blotted onto nitrocellulose paper, and hybridized to a mixed probe of nick-translated plasmid DNA p*mal*-1, p*mal*-2, and pA6. Tumor induction, preparation of tumor and epidermal tissues, and RNA isolation and hybridization were performed as described in "Methods." (a) RNA from a keratoacanthoma; (b) RNA from a squamous cell carcinoma induced by *N*-methyl-*N'*-nitro-*N*-nitrosoguanidine (MNNG) and 12-*O*-tetradecanoylphorbol-13-acetate (TPA); (c-e) induced by 7,12-dimethylbenz[*a*]anthracene and TPA; (f,g) RNA from tumor promoter-independent papillomas; (h,i) from tumor promoter-dependent papillomas; and (j) RNA from normal epidermis. Abbreviations: Ka, keratoacanthomas; auton., autonomous; dep., dependent; ep, epidermis.

(Fig. 2a). In benign papillomas the 1.3- and 2.3-kb transcripts were overexpressed, whereas the largest, 2.9-kb, transcript was not detectable (Fig. 2b). In malignant SCCs, this largest transcript related to *mal*-3 was always overexpressed, whereas the 2.3-kb transcript either disappeared or was expressed at a lower level (Fig. 2c,d). In all benign tumors tested so far, we only detected an overexpression of the 1.3- and 2.3-kb transcripts. Thus, overexpression of the

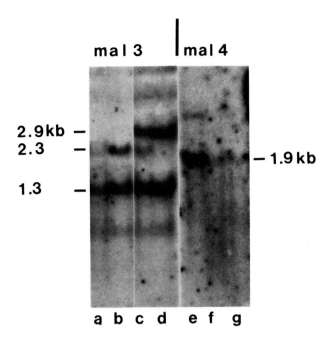

Figure 2. Expression of *mal*-3 and *mal*-4 in different mouse skin tumors. Northern blots were performed as described in the legend to Figure 1. (a-d) Hybridized with p*mal*-3; (e-g) hybridized with p*mal*-4; (a,g) RNA from normal epidermis; (b,f) RNA from papillomas; (c-e) RNA from squamous cell carcinomas.

2.9-kb transcript may be related to the malignant state. In a similar manner, overexpression of *mal*-4-related sequences appeared also to be specific for the malignant state. Northern analysis of RNA using *mal*-4 cDNA as a probe showed a slight overexpression of *mal*-4-related transcripts in benign papillomas as compared with normal epidermis (Fig. 2f,g). In malignant SCCs, however, these *mal*-4-related sequences were in high abundance (Fig. 2e). As estimated by densitometry of the autoradiograms, the factor of elevated transcript levels in carcinomas as compared with papillomas and normal epidermis was greater than 10.

In addition to studying the expression pattern of the *mal* sequences, we have been actively sequencing p*mal* cDNA inserts and full-length cDNAs for the *mal* sequences, which we obtained from a λgt10 cDNA library made from poly(A)+ RNA from carcinomas or tumorigenic epidermal cell lines. Sequencing of the p*mal*-4 clone and a full-length cDNA for *mal*-4 has revealed a high degree of similarity between *mal*-4 and mouse β-actin cDNA (Ostrowski and Bowden, unpublished observations). It is not clear whether we have cloned a normal or mutated β-actin. A mutated human β-actin has been implicated in the chemically induced malignant transformation of human fibroblasts in culture (40).

Differential Expression of the Transin Gene During Late Stages of Mouse Skin Tumor Progression

In addition to studying the expression pattern of the *mal* genes during skin tumor progression, we have investigated the expression of a gene called transin during mouse skin tumor progression. Transin RNA is a 1.9-kb RNA transcript induced by oncogenes and epidermal growth factor in rat embryo fibroblast cell lines. Recently we showed that an RNA species complementary to a rat transin cDNA is present in mouse skin SCCs induced by a classic initiation-promotion protocol but is not found to be expressed in either benign papillomas or in normal epidermis (13). In the same paper we reported that the transin RNA encodes for a secreted protease that, after activation, degrades α-casein. Of interest is the recent report indicating that there is a high degree of similarity between rabbit stromelysin, a secreted metalloproteinase that degrades proteoglycans found in the basement membrane, and the amino acid sequence predicted from rat transin cDNA (13). The inappropriate expression of the transin gene may, therefore, be causally involved in one or more steps of tumor progression from a benign papilloma to an invasive, malignant, and eventually metastatic squamous cell carcinoma.

We undertook research to investigate the expression pattern of the transin gene during the progression of benign papillomas to nonmetastatic SCCs to metastatic SCCs. We first developed a mouse cDNA transin probe by screening a cDNA library made from poly(A)+ RNA isolated from an SCC (DMBA- plus

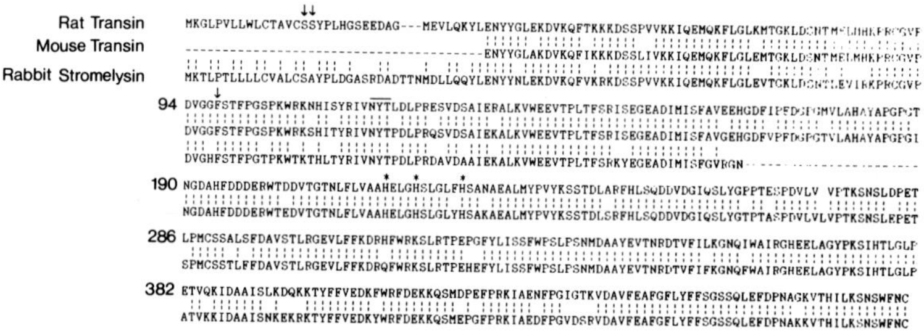

Figure 3. Amino acid sequences of members of the metalloproteinase family. The predicted amino acid sequences of rat transin-1, mouse transin, and rabbit stromelysin are compared. Gaps have been introduced to give the maximum homologies. Amino acids identical to those found in rat transin-1 are marked with a dot. The arrows indicate possible cleavage sites between the leader sequence and protransin and protransin and the activated form of transin. The overlined amino acids represent a potential site for N-linked glycosylation. The starred residues are potential zinc-binding sites.

TPA-induced), using the rat transin-1 cDNA as a probe. One putative mouse transin cDNA clone called TR11A was isolated and sequenced.

The predicted amino acid sequence for TR11A, rat transin-1, and the determined amino acid sequence of the amino terminus of rabbit stromelysin are presented in Figure 3. TR11A showed a 90% amino acid sequence similarity to rat transin-1, which may be a rat homologue of stromelysin (41). In Figure 3 several conserved features between the sequences have been indicated. The arrow at residue 98 indicates a possible cleavage site between the protransin and the activated form of transin. A potentially conserved glycosylation site is present at residues 125-127 of transin, and a conserved region containing three histidine residues that could be involved in the binding of a zinc atom is present between residues 216 and 226. These data indicated that a mouse homologue of rat transin-1 had been isolated, although functional comparative studies on the isolated mouse and rat proteins need to be performed.

It has recently been shown that it is possible to induce metastasizing SCCs with a carcinogen regimen involving repeated treatments of the mouse skin with MNNG or BaP (42). These SCCs were found to metastasize primarily to the lung

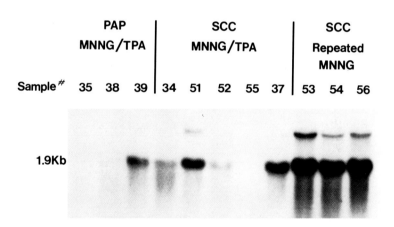

Figure 4. Northern blot analysis of transin transcripts in various tumors induced by two-stage and complete carcinogenesis protocols. Ten micrograms of total tumor RNA was separated on a 1.4% agarose formaldehyde gel, blotted onto nitrocellulose paper, and probed with a ^{32}P nick-translated mouse transin cDNA. The blot was posthybridized with a ^{32}P nick-translated probe for 7S ribosomal RNA to verify that the amounts of total RNA loaded were equivalent. The tumor induction protocols included (1) initiation treatment with N-methyl-N'-nitro-N-nitrosoguanidine (MNNG) followed by tumor promotion with 12-O-tetradecanoylphorbol-13-acetate (TPA) and (2) repeated MNNG treatments of the skin. Abbreviations: PAP, papillomas; SCC, squamous cell carcinomas.

or lymph nodes. The induction of SCCs by a two-stage protocol of initiation and promotion leads to tumors with a much lower probability of demonstrating metastasis (42). To study the expression pattern of the mouse transin gene in late stages of mouse skin tumor progression, total RNA was isolated from benign papillomas induced by MNNG initiation and TPA promotion, SCCs induced by MNNG and TPA, and SCCs induced by repeated MNNG treatments. These RNAs were run on northern gels, blotted, and probed with a nick-translated mouse transin cDNA probe. In addition, the blots were reprobed with a 7S specific probe to control for the amount of RNA loaded onto the gels and blotted. The results of this probing are presented in Figure 4.

Three benign papilloma RNAs were investigated on this northern blot, and one of the three showed a measurable level of transin transcripts, perhaps identifying this as a papilloma with an increased probability of conversion. The levels of transin transcripts seen in the SCCs induced by MNNG initiation and TPA promotion were more variable but were consistent with our previous results (13) and examination of more than 20 SCCs induced by various protocols (data not shown). With one exception (SCC 55 in Fig. 2), the level of transin transcripts

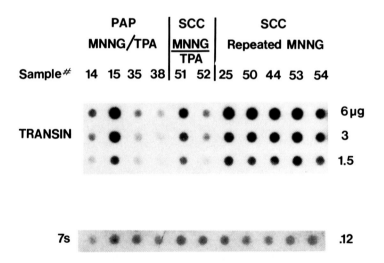

Figure 5. Dot blot analysis of transin transcripts in various tumors induced by two-stage and complete carcinogenesis protocols. Six, 3, 1.5, or 0.12 µg of total RNA from various tumors [papillomas (PAP) and squamous cell carcinomas (SCC)] was dotted onto nitro-cellulose paper, fixed by heating, and then probed with ^{32}P nick-translated mouse transin or 7S ribosomal cDNA probes. The tumor-induction protocols included (1) initiation treatment with N-methyl-N'-nitro-N-nitrosoguanidine (MNNG) followed by tumor promotion with 12-O-tetradecanoylphorbol-13-acetate (TPA) and (2) repeated MNNG treatments of the skin.

was always higher in SCCs than in normal epidermis. A very strong 1.9-kb hybridizing transcript was seen in the RNA from three SCCs induced by repeated MNNG treatment. The level of transin transcripts in SCCs induced by repeated MNNG treatment was always higher than the somewhat variable expression levels in SCCs induced by MNNG initiation and TPA promotion.

Additional tumor RNAs, some of which were partially degraded, were analyzed by dot blot analysis (Fig. 5). For comparison, some of the samples used in Figure 4 were included on this filter. All five of the RNAs from tumors induced with repeated MNNG exposure showed strong autoradiographic signals indicative of high levels of transin transcripts. Of the four RNA samples from benign papillomas (induced by MNNG and TPA), one sample showed a strong autoradiographic signal. Therefore, by northern and dot blot analyses, the levels of transin transcripts were consistently higher in SCCs induced by repeated MNNG treatment than that found in either benign papillomas or SCCs induced by MNNG initiation and TPA promotion.

We looked for potential rearrangements and amplification of the mouse transin gene that might explain the gene's overexpression in certain tumor

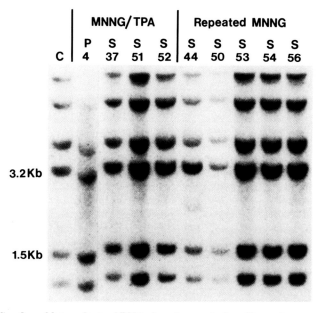

Figure 6. Southern blot analysis of DNAs from tumors induced by various carcinogenesis protocols. Ten micrograms of high-molecular-weight, genomic DNA was digested with the restriction enzyme *Pst* I, separated on an 0.8% agarose gel, blotted onto nitrocellulose paper, and probed with a ^{32}P nick-translated mouse transin cDNA probe. Abbreviations: C, control epidermis; S, SCC; P, papilloma; MNNG, *N*-methyl-*N'*-nitro-*N*-nitrosoguanidine; TPA, 12-*O*-tetradecanoylphorbol-13-acetate.

samples. Therefore, high-molecular-weight genomic DNAs from various tissues, including epidermis, papillomas, and SCCs induced by different protocols, were cut with *Pst*-I, run on a Southern gel, blotted, and probed with a nick-translated mouse transin cDNA probe (TR11A). The major hybridizing fragments seen were: 12, 6.7, 4.1, 3.2, 1.5, and 1.2 kb (Fig. 6). There were no real differences in either the band intensities or in the restriction-fragment patterns. Therefore, we have no evidence for either rearrangement or amplification of the mouse transin gene in any of the tumor DNAs studied.

DISCUSSION

Experimental results from a number of laboratories (6,8) have demonstrated the activation of the Harvey-*ras* proto-oncogene in polycyclic aromatic hydrocarbon-initiated mouse skin papillomas and SCCs. These data have suggested that the activation of the cellular Harvey-*ras* gene is an early event associated with the initiation of mouse skin tumors by certain polycyclic aromatic hydrocarbons. The detection of initiator-specific mutations in mouse skin tumors (7) and the recent demonstration that an activated *ras* gene can initiate mouse skin tumors (43) lend support to the idea that at least in some carcinogenesis systems, initiation may involve direct mutation of a *ras* proto-oncogene.

In comparing chemical to ionizing radiation initiation of mouse skin tumors, we have found that ionizing radiation-initiated tumors contained non-*ras*, dominant transforming genes. The nature of the activated oncogene in the mouse skin system appeared to be dependent upon the initiating agent used and independent of the tumor promoter applied. Our data also suggest that the targets for oncogenic activation are different for chemical initiators versus ionizing radiation. Support for our findings has recently been presented by Borek et al. (38). Their work has shown that in vitro malignant transformation of mammalian cells (hamster embryo and mouse C3H/10T1/2) by a single direct exposure to x-radiation resulted in the activation of oncogenic sequences with detectable transforming activity. The oncogenes activated did not represent activated forms of the *ras* gene family, which have been implicated in chemically transformed C3H/10T1/2 cells. These activated oncogenes were also none of a series of non-*ras* oncogenes that have been detected by the NIH3T3 focus assay. In vivo studies of chemical versus radiation carcinogenesis have also shown that different transforming genes are activated depending on the nature of the carcinogen (chemical versus radiation) (44).

The cloning, characterization, and identification of gene sequences that are differentially expressed during tumor progression could lead to the discovery of gene products that play functional roles in skin tumor progression or in maintenance of various progressive phenotypes. Previous studies resulted in the discovery of sequences that were overexpressed during mouse skin tumor progression (12,15-17). These sequences were called the *mal* sequences. Molecular characterization of these sequences showed that they were not similar to 20 known retroviral oncogenes or to mouse keratin genes. Overexpression of one of these *mal* sequences (*mal*-4) was a marker for the malignant state, because this sequence was not overexpressed in benign tumors but transcriptional activation occurred during the progression from benign papilloma to malignant SCC. In contrast to the *mal*-4 expression pattern, overexpression of *mal*-1- and *mal*-2-related transcripts was specific for neoplasia in that they were activated in both papillomas and SCC. A change in the transcript pattern of the *mal*-3-related sequences was observed during the progression of a benign to a malignant tumor. It is not known whether the multiple transcripts were different precursor molecules reflecting a change in RNA processing or whether they were different mature mRNA species. Southern analysis of the genomic organization detected at least four copies of the *mal*-3-related sequences (15). These data suggest that a gene family of *mal*-3 sequences exists. Nevertheless, in all benign tumors tested, only two transcripts (1.3- and 2.3-kb) were present and overexpressed, and the 2.9-kb transcript was overexpressed only in malignant tumors. Therefore, the overexpression of the 2.9-kb transcript related to *mal*-3 may be used as a genetic marker to distinguish between the benign and malignant state of tumor progression in mouse skin.

Besides studying the expression pattern of the *mal* sequences during mouse skin tumor progression, we have also studied the expression of the transin gene during late stages of tumor progression. We have shown that the steady-state levels of transin transcripts in DMBA/TPA-induced SCCs were considerably higher than in benign papillomas (13). In these initial studies we used a rat transin-1 probe. Subsequently, we cloned a mouse cDNA that turned out to have considerable sequence similarity with the rat transin-1 cDNA as well as with rabbit stromelysin. The high degree of similarity between either rat or mouse transin and rabbit stromelysin suggested a potential role for the overexpression of the transin gene in invasion and metastasis. It has been shown that rabbit stromelysin degrades many of the protein components of extracellular matrices including proteoglycans, fibronectin, laminin, soluble type IV collagen, and elastin (45). All of these proteins are components of the basement membrane that must be degraded by invasive as well as metastatic tumor cells.

The metastatic phenotype results most likely from a complex series of steps involving the expression of multiple gene products. It is highly likely that the increased metastatic potential of some tumors is due to the increased expression of certain necessary but not sufficient gene products that confer a selective advantage on these cells. Since the transin gene could be one of these genes involved in metastasis, we have studied the expression pattern of this gene in SCCs with different potentials for metastasis. Our consistent finding that the levels of transin transcripts in SCCs induced by repeated MNNG were always higher than levels seen in SCCs with a lower probability of metastasis suggests that the higher levels of transin product enhance the probability that the tumor cells penetrate the continuous basement membranes, which separate tissue compartments and surround blood vessels and muscle.

A similar observation was made by Garbisa et al. (46). These workers found that transfection of cultured cells with an activated *ras* oncogene induced metastatic tumors and these metastatic tumors secreted higher levels of type IV collagenolytic protease than nonmetastatic tumors. Garbisa et al. suggested that their data supported a biochemical linkage between expression of type IV collagenase activity and the metastatic phenotype. A consideration of the carcinogenic protocol and latency period needed to induce metastatic tumors in the skin indicated that acquisition of this phenotype is a late event that requires large cumulative doses of a genotoxic complete carcinogen such as MNNG or benzo[a]pyrene (BaP). Despite prolonged genotoxic damage, none of the tumors demonstrated either amplification or rearrangement of the transin gene on Southern analysis. A comparison of genomic alterations with the measured levels of transin transcripts indicated that other mechanisms for enhanced expression of the transin gene must exist.

Ultimately, it is necessary to know whether the overexpression of the transin gene or the *mal* genes play functional roles in skin tumor progression. To test the hypothesized functional roles for these genes in tumor progression it will be necessary to overexpress the gene in specific epidermal precursor cells using appropriate plasmid or defective retroviral vectors and to then look for phenotypic alterations. This approach assumes that the overexpression of a specific gene is necessary and sufficient for some phenotypic alteration. The alternative that the overexpression is necessary but not sufficient can only be tested by blocking specifically the expression of that gene and then looking for the loss of a specific phenotype. These experimental approaches are being pursued in our laboratory to determine whether the transin gene or the *mal* genes play functional roles in mouse skin tumor formation.

ACKNOWLEDGMENTS

The work described in this book chapter was supported in part by National Institutes of Health grants CA-40584, CA-42239, and CA-23074. We thank Ms. Sally Anderson for her expert secretarial assistance.

OPEN FORUM

Dr. Stuart Yuspa: In your 3T3 transfections using DNA from tumors produced by ionizing radiation, did the foci that formed look like the typical transformed 3T3 foci that you would see with *ras* or did they have a different appearance?

Dr. G. Tim Bowden: Their appearance was very similar to the T24-induced foci. Qualitatively, I could not distinguish them.

Dr. Yuspa: We have produced cell lines using several different protocols, and DNA from several of these lines produce 3T3 foci that are unusual.

Dr. Thomas O'Brien: You stated that the *mal* genes and the transin gene are overexpressed in tumors relative to epidermis. I assume you mean untreated epidermis. Did you look for regulation by TPA or other promoters?

Dr. Bowden: The epidermis was untreated. At least three of the *mal* genes and transin are regulated transiently by TPA and RPA (12-*O*-retinoyl-phorbol-13-acetate). We have also looked at EPP (ethyl phenylpropiolate) at doses that give equivalent hyperplasia to the dose of TPA and RPA. It turns out that transin and *mal*-4 are not regulated by EPP, whereas *mal*-1 and -2 are. There is a transient increase in the steady-state levels of transcripts of *mal*-1 and -2. We suggest that the induction of expression of *mal*-4 and transin may be tumor-promoter-specific. Lynn Matrisian has done sequencing of the 5' regulatory region of the rat transin gene, and the same enhancer elements are present that have been described by Michael Karin—the TPA-responsive element (TRE)-enhancer and TPA-responsive elements. I have attempted to look at the 5' regulatory region that has been published for β-actin, and I have not seen these TRE elements yet; however, there are certain sequences within the 5' regulatory region of β-actin that look like enhancer elements found in SV 40. We have not yet done any genomic cloning of *mal*-1 and -2.

Dr. O'Brien: Is it possible that the transin that the tumors make is a mutant transin? Could it have a different catalytic specificity than a transin made in a normal tissue?

Dr. Bowden: Another colleague from Strasbourg, Richard Breathnach, has recently cloned a truncated version of transin that has lost the N terminus and appears to be only the catalytic domain. I have not thought about expression of mutated transin during skin tumor progression.

Dr. F. J. Burns: I am curious about the tumors that you see in the SENCAR mouse with TPA alone. What type of activation pattern do those tumors have?

Dr. Bowden: We have not looked at papillomas induced with TPA alone. Generally, when we do transfections with papillomas induced by radiation and TPA, we see dominant transforming activity in a first round; the efficiencies always go down in subsequent rounds of transfection in 3T3 cells, and we have not been able to passage that activity in a tertiary round into Rat2 cells. I do not know what this means. However, for most malignant tumors that have been initiated and promoted, the dominant transforming activity can be transferred through two rounds of transfection in mouse 3T3 cells and transferred into Rat2 cells.

Dr. Hiroshi Yamasaki: You had transin expression in carcinomas, while in papillomas there was almost no transin expression. If carcinoma is progressing through papillomas, I thought there would be some percentage of papillomas that would be positive in transin or *mal*-4 gene overexpression. Have you ever seen this?

Dr. Bowden: It does occur, but in a very small percentage (maybe in 1 of 20) of the benign papillomas we have looked at.

Dr. A. J. P. Klein-Szanto: Do the transin and β-actin reflect any biological differences in the behavior of those cells? For example, is there proven increase in collagenolytic activity, locomotive capacity, or invasive potential in these cells?

Dr. Bowden: We do not know the answer to that. That may be the function of these genes. Certainly the mutant β-actin does not polymerize as well and may be responsible for disrupting the cytoskeleton network. In the case of transin, antibodies are now available for the encoded protein. We have not looked at the expression level in terms of protein at this point.

Dr. Klein-Szanto: Is the encoded protein equivalent to collagenase IV?

Dr. Bowden: Stromelysin has type IV collagenase activity as well as activity against laminin and fibronectin. However, apparently it is not the same as type IV collagenase. Stromelysin has a high degree of DNA sequence similarity to another metalloprotease called protease activator gene, recently cloned by Connie Brinkerhoffer. That particular activator gene may play an important role in a cascade of activation of different metalloproteases.

Dr. Kenneth Kraemer: I have a question about the Harvey-*ras* A to T transversion that you found with urethane and DMBA. Do you know if the urethane or the DMBA binds to the adenine?

Dr. Bowden: I do not know. In the case of mouse skin, not much is known about the urethane-DNA adducts. In liver, in the case of DNA, it is a 7-oxyethylguanine derivative, which probably would not be miscoding. There are also RNA adducts (ethenoadducts of adenosine and cytosine), but I do not know the relevance of those.

Dr. Kraemer: If the adenine adduct were the crucial one, this might be further evidence toward the A role, where polymerases put in an A opposite a noninstructional lesion. That could explain the UV photoproducts that we found where the TT dimers were not mutagenic. That could also explain AT to TA transversions.

REFERENCES

1. Bishop JM. Cellular oncogenes and retroviruses. Ann Rev Biochem 52:301-354, 1983.
2. Land H, Parada LF, Weinberg RA. Cellular oncogenes and multistep carcinogenesis. Science 222:711-717, 1983.
3. Bowden GT. A National Institutes of Health Workshop report: Chemical carcinogenesis and the oncogenes. Cancer Res 45:914-918, 1985.
4. Klein G. The approaching era of the tumor suppressor genes. Science 238:1539-1545, 1987.
5. Balmain A, Pragnell IB. Mouse skin carcinomas induced in vivo by chemical carcinogens have a transforming Harvey-*ras* oncogene. Nature 303:72-74, 1985.
6. Balmain A, Ramsden M, Bowden GT, Smith J. Activation of the mouse cellular Harvey-*ras* gene in chemically induced benign skin papillomas. Nature 307:658-660, 1984.
7. Quintanilla M, Brown K, Ramsden M, Balmain A. Carcinogen-specific mutation and amplification of Ha-*ras* during mouse skin carcinogenesis. Nature 322:78-80, 1986.
8. Bizub D, Wood AW, Skalka AM. Mutagenesis of the Ha-*ras* oncogene in mouse skin tumors induced by polycyclic aromatic hydrocarbons. Proc Natl Acad Sci USA 83:6048-6052, 1986.
9. Toftgard R, Roop DR, Yuspa SH. Proto-oncogene expression during two-stage carcinogenesis in mouse skin. Carcinogenesis 6:655-657, 1985.
10. Pelling JC, Ernst SM, Strawhecker JM, Johnson JA, Nairn RS, Slaga TJ. Elevated

expression of Ha-*ras* is an early event in two-stage skin carcinogenesis in SENCAR mice. Carcinogenesis 7:1599-1602, 1986.

11. Gibson D, Jaffe D, Barnhart K, Bowden GT. Detection of activated oncogenes in urethane and cisplatin induced mouse skin tumors (abstract). Proceedings of the American Association of Cancer Research 27:76, 1986.

12. Melber K, Krieg P, Furstenberger G, Marks F. Molecular cloning of sequences activated during multi-stage carcinogenesis in mouse skin. Carcinogenesis 7:317-322, 1986.

13. Matrisian LM, Bowden GT, Krieg P, Furstenberger G, Briand JP, Leroy P, Breathnach R. The mRNA coding for the secreted protease transin is expressed more abundantly in malignant than in benign tumors. Proc Natl Acad Sci USA 83:9413-9417, 1986.

14. Krieg P, Finch J, Furstenberger G, Melber K, Matrisian L, Bowden GT. Tumor promoters induce a transient expression of tumor-associated genes in both basal and differentiated cells of the mouse epidermis. Carcinogenesis 9:95-100, 1988.

15. Krieg P, Melber K, Furstenberger G, Bowden GT. In vivo and in vitro expression pattern of genes activated during multistage carcinogenesis in the mouse skin. UCLA Symposium on Molecular and Cellular Biology 58:267-274, 1987.

16. Bowden GT, Furstenberger G, Krieg P, Matrisian LM, Breathnach R. Gene activation during multistep skin carcinogenesis. In Hausen H, Schlenhofer JR (eds): Accomplishments in Oncology, Vol. 2. Philadelphia: J.B. Lippincott, 1987, pp 106-116.

17. Bowden GT, Jaffe DR, Krieg P. Gene activation during multistage carcinogenesis in mouse skin. In Colburn NH (ed): Genes and Signal Transduction in Multistage Carcinogenesis. New York: Marcel Dekker, 1987.

18. Cooper GM. Cellular transforming genes. Science 217:801-806, 1982.

19. Land M, Parada LF, Weinberg RA. Cellular oncogenes and multistep carcinogenesis. Science 222:771-778, 1983.

20. Cooper CS, Park M, Blair DG, Tainsky MA, Huebner K, Croce CM, Vande Woude GF. Molecular cloning of a new transforming gene from a chemically transformed human cell line. Nature 311:29-33, 1984.

21. Schechter AL, Stern DF, Vaidyanathan L, Decker SJ, Prebin JA, Green MI, Weinberg RA. The *neu* oncogene: An erb-B-related gene encoding an 185,000 M_r tumor antigen. Nature 312:513-516, 1984.

22. Fukui M, Yamamoto T, Kawai S, Maruo K, Toyshima K. Detection of a *raf*-related and two other transforming DNA sequences in human tumors maintained in nude mice. Proc Natl Acad Sci USA 82:5954-5958, 1985.

23. Fung YKT, Lewis WG, Crittenden LB, Kung HJ. Activation of the cellular oncogene c-*erb*B by LTR insertion: Molecular basis for induction of erythroblastosis by avian leukosis virus. Cell 33:357-368, 1983.

24. Diamond A, Cooper GM, Ritz J, Lane MA. Identification and molecular cloning of the human B-*lym* transforming gene activated in Burkitt's lymphomas. Nature 305:112-116, 1983.

25. Eva A, Aaronson SA. Isolation of a new human oncogene from a diffuse B-cell lymphoma. Nature 316:273-275, 1985.

26. Jaffe DR, Bowden GT. Ionizing radiation as an initiator in the mouse two-stage model of skin tumor formation. Radiat Res 106:156-165, 1986.

27. Jaffe D, Bowden GT. Ionizing radiation as an initiator: Effects of proliferation and promotion time on tumor incidence in mice. Cancer Res 47:6692-6696, 1987.

28. Jaffe DR, Williamson JF, Bowden GT. Ionizing radiation enhances malignant

progression of mouse skin. Carcinogenesis 8:1753-1755, 1987.

29. Wigler M, Pellicer A, Silverstein S, Axel R. Biochemical transfer of single copy eucaryotic genes using total cellular DNA as donor. Cell 14:725-731, 1978.

30. Reddy EP, Reynolds PK, Santos E, Barbacid M. A point mutation is responsible for the acquisition of transforming properties by the T24 bladder carcinogen oncogene. Nature 300:149-152, 1982.

31. Krieg P, Amtmann E, Sauer G. The simultaneous extraction of high-molecular-weight DNA and of RNA from solid tumors. Anal Biochem 134:288-294, 1983.

32. Suominen AI, Karp MT, Mantsala T. Fractionation of DNA with Sephacryl S-1000. Biochem Int 8:209-215, 1984.

33. Rigby PWJ, Dieckman M, Rhodes C, Berg P. Labeling deoxyribonucleic acid to high specific activity by nick-translation with DNA polymerase I. J Mol Biol 113:237-251, 1977.

34. Southern EM. Detection of specific sequences among DNA fragments separated by gel electrophoresis. J Mol Biol 98:503-517, 1975.

35. Maniatis T, Fritsch EF, Sambrook J. Molecular Cloning: A Laboratory Manual. Cold Spring Harbor, NY: Cold Spring Harbor Laboratory, 1987, pp 382-387.

36. Maxam AM, Gilbert W. Sequencing end-labeled DNA with base-specific chemical cleavages. Methods Enzymol 65:499-560, 1980.

37. Sanger F, Coulson AR, Barrell GB, Smith AJ, Roe BA. Cloning in single-stranded bacteriophage as an aid to rapid DNA sequencing. J Mol Biol 143:161-178, 1980.

38. Borek C, Ong A, Mason H. Distinctive transforming genes in x-ray transformed mammalian cells. Proc Natl Acad Sci USA 84:794-798, 1987.

39. Balmain A, Krumlauf R, Vass JK, Birnie GD. Cloning and characterization of the abundant cytoplasmic 7S RNA from mouse cells. Nucleic Acids Res 10:4259-4277, 1982.

40. Leavitt J, Ng S-Y, Varma M, Latter G, Burbeck S, Gunning P, Kedes L. Expression of transfected mutant β-actin genes: Transitions toward the stable tumorigenic state. Mol Cell Biol 7:2467-2476, 1987.

41. Whitham SE, Murphy G, Angel P, Rahmsdorf NJ, Smith BJ, Lyons A, Harris TJR, Reynolds JJ, Herrlich P, Docherty AJP. Comparison of human stromelysin and collagenase by cloning and sequence analysis. Biochem J 240:913-916, 1986.

42. Patskan GJ, Klein-Szanto AJP, Phillips JL, Slaga TJ. Metastasis from squamous cell carcinomas of SENCAR mouse skin produced by complete carcinogenesis. Cancer Lett 34:121-127, 1987.

43. Brown K, Quintanilla M, Ramsden M, Ken IB, Young S, Balmain A. V-ras genes from Harvey and Balb murine sarcoma viruses can act as initiators of two-stage mouse skin carcinogenesis. Cell 46:447-456, 1986.

44. Guerrero I, Villasante A, Corces V, Pellicer A. Activation of a c-K-ras oncogene by somatic mutation in mouse lymphomas induced by gamma radiation. Science 225:1159-1162, 1984.

45. Chen JR, Murphy G, Werb Z. Stromelysin: A connective tissue-degrading metalloendopeptidase secreted by stimulated rabbit synovial fibroblasts in parallel with collagenase. J Biol Chem 260:12367-12376, 1985.

46. Garbisa S, Pozzatti R, Muschel RJ, Saffiotti U, Ballin M, Goldfarb RN, Khoury G, Liotta LA. Secretion of type IV collagenolytic protease and metastatic phenotype: Induction by transfection with c-Ha-ras but not c-Ha-ras plus Ad2-Ela. Cancer Res 47:1523-1528, 1987.

BIOCHEMICAL ASPECTS

Skin Carcinogenesis: Mechanisms and Human Relevance, pages 167–199
© 1989 Alan R. Liss, Inc.

Metabolism of Polycyclic Aromatic Hydrocarbons and Phorbol Esters by Mouse Skin: Relevance to Mechanism of Action and Trans-Species/Strain Carcinogenesis

John DiGiovanni

Department of Carcinogenesis, Science Park, The University of Texas M. D. Anderson Cancer Center, Smithville, Texas 78957

Carcinogenic polycyclic aromatic hydrocarbons (PAHs) require metabolic activation to highly reactive intermediates for their cytotoxic, mutagenic, and carcinogenic activities (1-6). These reactive intermediates are capable of interacting covalently with a wide variety of cellular macromolecules (1-5). The interaction with DNA, a target for activated hydrocarbon intermediates, has received considerable attention in recent years, and DNA is currently considered the critical cellular macromolecule involved in the initiation of chemical carcinogenesis (1-6).

PAHs are metabolized to a wide variety of organic solvent-soluble metabolites, including epoxides, dihydrodiols, quinones, and phenols (and their sulfate esters), as well as to water-soluble glutathione (GSH) and glucuronide conjugates (7-29 and reviewed in 30). More recently, it has been demonstrated that a number of the products of initial oxidation (i.e., phenols and diols) can be reoxidized and recycled through these pathways (31-34). Figure 1 shows a general scheme for the metabolic processing of any chemical carcinogen and is discussed in this chapter as it illustrates the metabolic pathway of a PAH. Of particular interest is the formation of the diol-epoxides. Studies of the ubiquitous PAH, benzo[*a*]pyrene (BaP), for example, have shown that it is activated to mutagenic and carcinogenic derivatives by a two-step mechanism leading to the formation of a "bay-region" diol-epoxide (33, 35; reviewed in 2, 5, 36, 37) and that the various isomers of this diol-epoxide bind covalently to different extents at various positions on the DNA bases, particularly on guanine residues (38). Growing evidence indicates that other PAHs are activated in a similar way (reviewed in 2, 37-39). Figure 2 highlights this two-step oxidation pathway, showing the chemical structure of the major BaP–DNA adduct formed in a variety of tissues that are targets for PAH carcinogens.

Many factors are known to affect the conversion of PAHs to reactive intermediates such as the epoxides and diol-epoxides discussed above. The ultimate toxic, mutagenic, and carcinogenic potential of a given PAH depends on

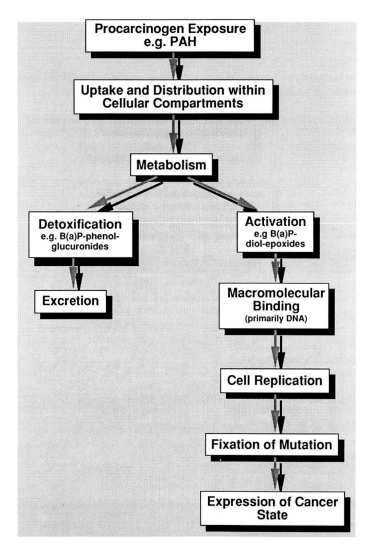

Figure 1. Scheme for the biotransformation and bioactivation of a carcinogenic chemical, for example, polycyclic aromatic hydrocarbons, in mouse skin. Abbreviation: BaP, benzo[*a*]pyrene.

a delicate balance between the rate of formation of these critical intermediates (activation) and the rate of removal by detoxifying reactions. Modifying factors known to affect the balance between activation and detoxification include the

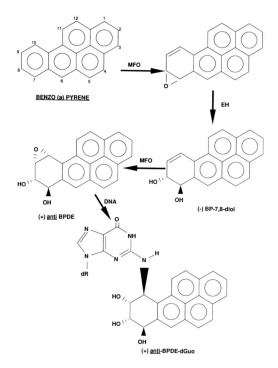

Figure 2. Two-step oxidation pathway leading to the metabolic activation and DNA binding of BaP. The major BaP–DNA adduct in most target tissues is shown, (+)-*anti*-BPDE-*trans*-dGuo. Abbreviations: MFO, cytochrome P-450-mediated mixed-function oxidation; EH, epoxide hydratase; BPDE, benzo[a]pyrene-diol-epoxide.

organism's age, gender, species, strain, tissue, diet, temperature, and previous or concurrent exposure to other drugs or environmental chemicals and the time of day, season, and route of administration.

METABOLISM AND METABOLIC ACTIVATION OF PAH IN MOUSE SKIN

Mouse skin, a widely studied target tissue for PAH carcinogens, serves not only as a model system for carcinogenesis studies in general but also as a potential model for carcinogenesis studies in humans. The epidermal target cells contain a variety of enzymes capable of metabolizing PAHs and other carcinogens and detoxifying them. The major ones catalyzing phase I reactions are monooxygenases (cytochrome P-450), peroxidases (cyclooxygenase), and hydrolases (epoxide hydrolase); those catalyzing phase II reactions are glucuronyltransferases, sulfotransferases, and glutathione-S-transferases. The mouse epidermal aryl hydrocarbon hydroxylase enzyme system (AHH, EC 1.14.14.2) is highly active and inducible by a variety of PAH substrates (40-44). In early studies (40), the highest AHH enzyme activity was found in the superficial layer of the dermis; more detailed studies (41,42) revealed, however, that the epidermal layer contains the highest AHH activity in mouse skin.

Although the cytochrome P-450-dependent monooxygenase system (i.e., AHH) is responsible for the metabolic activation of PAHs in a variety of target tissues, recent studies have implicated enzymes involved in prostaglandin biosynthesis in carcinogen metabolism (45-49). Mouse epidermis contains significant amounts of the enzymes involved in arachidonic acid metabolism (e.g., cyclooxygenase and lipoxygenase) (50-58), but several lines of evidence suggest that these pathways play only a lesser role in the production of DNA-binding intermediates from parent PAHs such as BaP.

First, Figure 3 shows the high-performance liquid chromatography (HPLC) profiles of [^{14}C]BaP metabolites produced in epidermal homogenates from control or DB[a,c]A-pretreated mice. These profiles are remarkably similar in that the major metabolites are the 9- and 3-hydroxy and the 7,8-diol of BaP. We previously noted a similar effect with 7,12-dimethylbenz[a]anthracene (DMBA) as the substrate, using epidermal homogenates from a variety of inducer-pretreated animals (59). These data are consistent with the notion that, compared with other forms of cytochrome P-450, the relative content of MC-P-450 (the form that is induced by 3-methylcholanthrene [MC]) may be high in the skin of uninduced mice as compared with tissues such as the liver (60).

Further support for the hypothesis that cytochrome P-450-mediated pathways are primarily responsible for the metabolic activation of PAHs in mouse epidermis comes from unpublished studies in our laboratory in which we used antisera directed against the MC-inducible form of cytochrome P-450 (i.e., MC-P-450). These data are summarized in Table 1. The antibody, which was obtained from Dr. Harry Gelboin (National Cancer Institute, Bethesda, MD), specifically inhibits this MC-inducible form of cytochrome P-450 (61). As shown in the table, anti-MC-P-450 antibody inhibited the covalent binding of BaP to the same extent whether homogenates were obtained from control or inducer-pretreated mice. In addition, only two major adducts were formed in the DNA coincubated with the homogenates and antibody (data not shown). These adducts, which were formed in about equal proportions, cochromatographed with marker adducts of 9-OH-BaP-4,5-oxide-deoxyguanosine (dGuo) and (+)-7α,8β-dihydroxy-9β,10β-epoxy-7,8,9,10-tetrahydrobenzo[a]pyrene-deoxyguanosine ([+]-$anti$-BPDE-dGuo). The presence of the antibody decreased the formation of both DNA adducts. These data, in conjunction with the data shown in Figure 3, support the notion that a constitutive form of cytochrome P-450 in skin is similar to that induced by MC in rat liver (i.e., MC-P-450). These data may also help support the explanation that mouse epidermis is so sensitive to PAH carcinogens because it constitutively expresses a form of cytochrome P-450 that is highly active in converting BaP to the (–)-7,8-diol and ultimately to the (+)-$anti$-BPDE (reviewed in ref. 2).

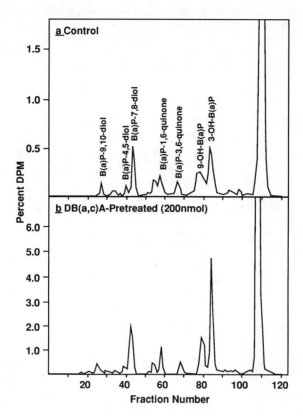

Figure 3. Pattern of [^{14}C]BaP metabolites generated in vitro using epidermal homogenates from control (acetone) or DB[a,c]A-pretreated (200 nmol per mouse) SENCAR mice. The retention times of various synthetic standard compounds are depicted above peak fractions in which they elute in this system. Further details of the methodology can be found in refs. 59 and 67. Abbreviation: DB(a,c)A, dibenz[a,c]anthracene.

Other data in the literature that support this hypothesis concern the effect of antioxidants such as butylated hydroxyanisole (BHA) and butylated hydroxytoluene (BHT) on PAH metabolism in mouse epidermis. These compounds, which are known to inhibit peroxidase-dependent metabolism of PAHs (46,57,62), were examined for their effects on PAH metabolism in mouse epidermis. Interestingly, BHA and BHT had little effect on oxidative metabolism or DNA binding of DMBA when catalyzed by epidermal homogenates in vitro (63,64). Moreover, BHT did not inhibit but rather enhanced the metabolism of BaP catalyzed by epidermal homogenates (65). In addition, BHT had no effect on the epidermal homogenate-mediated binding of BaP to calf thymus DNA (65).

Table 1. Covalent Binding of [³H]BaP to Calf Thymus DNA In Vitro Catalyzed by Epidermal Homogenates: Effect of Anti-Methylcholanthrene (MC)-P-450 Antibody*

Homogenate	Anti-MC-P-450	Total binding (dpm/mg)	% Inhibition of binding
Control	–	12,614	—
Control	+	3,371	73
MC-pretreated	–	86,446	—
MC-pretreated	+	17,415	80

*The assay system for epidermal homogenate-mediated binding of [³H]PAH to DNA used epidermal material from female SENCAR mice that had been pretreated with either acetone (control) or MC (200 nmol/mouse) 18 h before the mice were killed (epidermal scrapings from 5 skins/ml buffer). The standard reaction mixture contained the following components in a final volume of 3 ml: 50 μmol sodium phosphate, pH 7.4; 100 μmol EDTA; 0.5 mg NADPH; 2 mg calf thymus DNA; 0.2 ml epidermal homogenate (4–6 mg of protein), and 36 nmol [³H]PAH (500 Ci/mol). Control tubes contained 0.5 mg/ml nonspecific antibody, whereas antibody tubes contained 0.5 mg/ml of anti-MC-P-450 antibody 1-7-1 p2 (61). Each value is an average from two experiments. Further details, including the procedures for isolating DNA and quantitating hydrocarbon binding, may be found in ref. 63.

To gain further insight into the overall metabolism of PAHs, we used cultured keratinocytes from newborn SENCAR mice (66,67). The use of intact epidermal cells allows determination of the contribution of conjugative (phase II) as well as oxidative (phase I) enzymes to the overall metabolism of PAHs. Figure 4 illustrates the profile of ethyl acetate:acetone (2:1)-extractable metabolites within epidermal cells (panel *a*), those excreted into the medium (panel *b*), and those present in the medium as glucuronide conjugates. The most important observations from these studies were that mouse epidermal cells from newborn mice grown in primary culture produced large amounts of BaP-7,8-diol and retained this metabolite within the cell, major water-soluble metabolites (about 50% of the total water-soluble metabolites) were present as glucuronides, and no sulfate esters of PAH metabolites have ever been detected in cultures of mouse epidermal cells exposed to PAHs. The remaining water-soluble metabolites are probably GSH-conjugates and polyhydroxylated derivatives, but they remain to be identified.

As noted earlier, many factors may affect the metabolism of PAH carcinogens. Since the epidermis does not consist of a single cell type but of a gradient of cells at different stages of terminal differentiation (68), we examined the relationship between the differentiation state and the metabolism of several PAHs (DiGiovanni J, Gill RD, Nettikumara AN, unpublished data) using cultured epidermal cells from adult SENCAR mice. Techniques for establishing and maintaining pure cultures of adult mouse epidermal keratinocytes were recently described (69-71), and the growth of these cultures was characterized reasonably well. An important feature of the culture system is that one can control the proliferative and differentiative capacities of the keratinocytes by altering free-

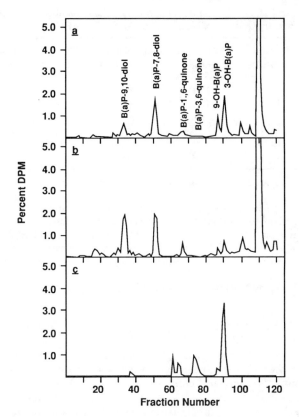

Figure 4. High-performance liquid chromatography profiles of intracellular and extra-cellular metabolites of [³H]BaP produced by primary cultures of neonatal mouse epidermal keratinocytes from SENCAR mice after 24 h of exposure to the hydrocarbon (1 µg/ml). Panel a: ethyl acetate/acetone-soluble metabolites found intracellularly. Panel b: ethyl acetate/acetone-soluble metabolites found extracellularly. Panel c: β-glucuronidase-releasable metabolites found extracellularly. The profile of panel c was obtained by subtracting the ethyl acetate/acetone-soluble metabolites found in the extracellular medium from those found when the medium was treated first with β-glucuronidase before extraction. Retention times of various synthetic standard compounds are depicted as names above the peak fractions in panel a, in which they elute in this system. Reproduced from DiGiovanni et al. Cancer Res 42:2579-2586, 1982, used with permission.

calcium concentrations in the culture medium. In low-calcium medium (0.05-0.10 mM), the cells are in a proliferative state and maintain basal cell morphology, whereas increasing the total free-calcium concentration to 1.4 mM signals the cells to undergo terminal differentiation (70). The calcium concentration and hence differentiation state of the cells also dramatically affect their metabolic

Table 2. Effect of Calcium Concentration on Polycyclic Aromatic Hydrocarbon (PAH) Metabolism in Primary Cultures of Neonatal and Adult Mouse Epidermal Keratinocytes*

Cell type	Calcium concentration	Hydro-carbon	Water-soluble metabolites†	Glucu-ronides‡	Unchanged hydrocarbon§
Adult	High	BaP	57	20	27
	Low	BaP	23	10	82
Adult	High	DMBA	54	—	10
	Low	DMBA	22	—	53
Neonatal	High	BaP	61	23	25
	Low	BaP	33	15	70

*Cultures were prepared as described (70) and exposed to hydrocarbon (0.25 µg/ml) for 24 h.
†Determined by extraction of the medium with ethyl acetate:acetone (2:1) and expressed as a percentage of the total radioactivity recovered in the medium.
‡Expressed as a percentage of the total radioactivity recovered in the medium.
§Expressed as a percentage of the total ethyl acetate:acetone-extractable radioactivity recovered in the medium (and determined from high-performance liquid chromatography profiles).
Abbreviations: BaP, benzo[a]pyrene; DMBA, 7,2-dimethylbenz[a]anthracene.

capacity. In this regard, adult mouse epidermal keratinocytes (MEK) exposed to either [3H]BaP or [3H]DMBA for 24 h showed a dramatic quantitative difference in metabolism of these two substrates depending on whether the cells were maintained in low Ca^{2+} or switched to a normal Ca^{2+} medium. Cultures of adult MEK in normal Ca^{2+} medium consistently converted both PAHs to water-soluble, nonextractable (with ethyl acetate:acetone, 2:1) metabolites at considerably faster rates. The results of these experiments are summarized in Table 2. Also included in this table are the results of an experiment using primary cultures of neonatal MEK. Similar results were obtained with neonatal MEK cultured in low as compared with normal Ca^{2+} media.

Figure 5 shows the HPLC profiles of the BaP metabolites obtained from adult MEK exposed to [3H]BaP for 24 h and after extraction of the media samples with ethyl acetate:acetone (2:1). It is readily apparent that, in cultures of differentiated MEK, [3H]BaP underwent much more extensive overall metabolism compared with the low-Ca^{2+} cultures. The major medium metabolite after a 24-h incubation with [3H]BaP in normal Ca^{2+} cultures was the major tetraol (i.e., r-7,t-8,9,c-10) derived from (+)-*anti*-BPDE (72).

The BaP–DNA adducts formed in mouse epidermal cells (from neonates or adults) and mouse epidermis have been characterized by several research groups including our own (73-80 and J. DiGiovanni, unpublished). Figure 6 shows the HPLC profiles of BaP–DNA adducts formed in mouse epidermis in vivo and in adult MEK switched to a normal Ca^{2+} medium as described in Table 2. The cultures were exposed to 0.25 µg/ml of [3H]BaP for 24 h and treated 48 h after switching to normal Ca^{2+} medium. The DNA adduct profile shown in panel

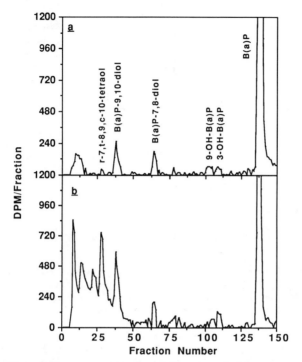

Figure 5. High-performance liquid chromatography profiles of extracellular metabolites of [³H]BaP produced by primary cultures of adult mouse epidermal keratinocytes from SENCAR mice after 24 h exposure to the hydrocarbon (0.25 µg/ml). Panel a: ethyl acetate:acetone (2:1)-soluble metabolites from cultures maintained in low-Ca²⁺ medium. Panel b: ethyl acetate:acetone (2:1)-soluble metabolites from cultures exposed to the hydrocarbon 48 h after switching to normal Ca²⁺ medium.

b is nearly identical to that found after topical application of [³H]BaP to mouse epidermis (panel a). The major observations from these data were that a number of DNA adducts were formed in mouse epidermal cells after exposure to BaP; the major adduct peak in both DNA samples (peak IV) cochromatographed with the major DNA adduct formed after reaction of (±)-*anti*-BPDE or the pure (+) enantiomer of *anti*-BPDE with dGuo (77), and this adduct, well characterized in several laboratories as (+)-*anti*-BPDE-*trans*-dGuo (reviewed in ref. 2), represented about 65% of the total adducts eluted in both chromatograms shown in Figure 6; and many other adducts were routinely detected in DNA from epidermal cells exposed to [³H]BaP. Tentative identifications of these adducts have been made (77) and are presented in the legend for Figure 6. Although the major DNA adduct derived from BaP (i.e., [+]-*anti*-BPDE-*trans*-dGuo) seems to be important for many of the biological effects of this PAH (including tumor initiation on mouse skin, reviewed in refs. 2 and 5), the other adducts may also

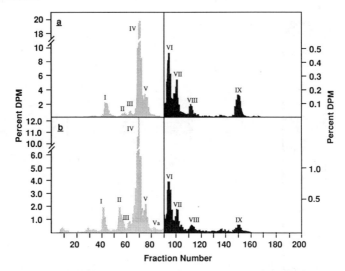

Figure 6. High-performance liquid chromatography profiles of BaP–DNA adducts formed in SENCAR mouse epidermis 24 h after topical application of 200 nmol [³H]BaP (panel a) or 24 h after exposure of adult mouse epidermal keratinocytes from SENCAR mice to 0.25 μg/ml [³H]BaP. Samples containing ~100,000 dpm in 20–50 μl were injected into the column, and immediately after injection 0.5-min fractions were collected directly into scintillation vials and analyzed for radioactivity. The radioactivity in each fraction was expressed as a percentage of the total radioactivity eluted from the column (i.e., % dpm); ▨, uses left-hand scale of % dpm; ■, uses right-hand scale of % dpm. Peak I, 9-OH-4,5-oxide-dGuo; Peak II, unknown; Peak III, (–)-*anti*-BPDE-dGuo; Peak IV, (+)-*anti*-BPDE-dGuo; Peak V, *syn*-BPDE-dGuo; Peak VI, (+)-*anti*-BPDE-dAdo; Peak VII, (–)-*anti*-BPDE-dAdo; Peak VIII, (+)-*anti*-BPDE-dAdo; Peak IX, *syn*-BPDE-DNA. Abbreviations: dGuo, deoxyguanoxine; BPDE, benzo[a]pyrene-diol-epoxide; dAdo, deoxyadenosine.

contribute to the biologic effects of this hydrocarbon. In particular, several adenine adducts are formed from the (+)-*anti*-BPDE in addition to adducts formed from the diastereomeric *syn*-BPDE. Further work is warranted to establish the biologic effects of the different types of DNA adducts formed in mouse epidermal cells as well as other target tissues.

QUALITATIVE COMPARISON OF METABOLISM AND METABOLIC ACTIVATION OF PAHs IN HUMAN COMPARED WITH MOUSE EPIDERMIS

A number of investigative efforts have been aimed at understanding how human skin, and in particular human epidermal cells, metabolize PAHs (80-87). Human epidermis contains a highly active mixed-function oxidase system for metabolizing xenobiotics such as PAHs (88-90). PAH metabolism has been examined in human skin organ cultures (80), human hair follicles (84-86), and epidermal cells in culture (81-83,87). Most of these studies confirmed that human epidermal cells convert BaP to metabolites similar to those observed when using mouse epidermal cells. For example, keratinocyte primary cultures from human skin (83) released BaP-9,10-diol and BaP-7,8-diol into the culture media similar to the way primary cultures of mouse epidermal cells did, as shown in Figure 4. Although large interindividual variations in metabolism of BaP were noted in at least one study (81) in which primary cultures from different human donors were used, relatively modest interindividual differences (two- to threefold) were reported in the metabolism of BaP by primary cultures of human epidermal cells (82,83). Interestingly, however, one of these research groups (83) observed large interindividual differences in the extent and nature of the BaP–DNA adducts formed in different primary cultures of human epidermal cells. Whether this was primarily the result of interindividual differences in metabolism or DNA repair or both remains to be determined. The major adduct in DNA isolated from human epidermal cells exposed to [³H]BaP was (+)-*anti*-BDPE-*trans*-dGuo (83). Although differences exist in the basal level and inducibility of AHH among mouse strains (reviewed in refs. 91-93), no marked differences were observed among different strains in metabolism and DNA adduct formation in epidermis (59,94-101). Therefore, although further studies are needed, the data suggest that the human population may have much greater interindividual variability than do mice in the metabolism of PAHs by epidermis and other epithelial tissues (107-110).

Another apparent difference between human and mouse epidermis relates to conjugation pathways. A major pathway for conjugating primary oxidation products in rodent cells, especially mouse epidermal cells, appears to involve glucuronidation (30,65,66,106). To date, glucuronide conjugates have been found as only minor water-soluble metabolites produced by human epidermal cells in culture (81).

Finally, human epidermal cells activated BaP to mutagenic metabolites for V79 cells in cell-mediated assays (81). Although other human cells and tissues (e.g., human bronchus) have been used in similar cell-mediated assays, they had lower capacities for activating carcinogens than rodent cells (107,108). When human epidermal cells were compared with rodent embryo cells, however, they were found to be more active in converting BaP to mutagenic intermediates. In addition, when compared with MEK, human epidermal cells seemed to behave quite similarly in a V79 cell-mediated assay (81,109). Allen-Hoffman and Rheinwald (110) developed an assay for detecting hypoxanthine phosphoribosyl-transferase-deficient mutants of human epidermal cells exposed to PAH. In this assay, when both DMBA and BaP were metabolized to mutagens, they gave rise to mutation frequencies as much as 50-fold higher than the spontaneous frequency. Thus, the human epidermal cell lines used in these studies were clearly competent to metabolically activate PAH carcinogens to mutagenic intermediates.

The conclusions to be drawn, based on our present knowledge of the metabolism and metabolic activation of PAHs by human and mouse epidermal cells, is that there are differences as well as similarities. Table 3 contains a

Table 3. Qualitative Comparison of the Metabolic Activation of Benzo[a]pyrene in Mouse and Human Epidermal Keratinocytes in Culture

Parameter studied	Comparative response in mouse and human	References
Oxidative metabolism	Similar: Major organic extractable metabolites are non-k-region diol, phenols, and tetraols. BaP is rapidly metabolized by both cell types.	67,81,82
DNA adduct formation	Similar: Major DNA adduct is (+)-anti-BPDE-trans-dGuo	82,83, and J DiGiovanni, unpublished
Conjugate formation	Different: Glucuronides are major water-soluble conjugates formed by mouse epidermal keratinocytes. Little or no glucuronides detected in cultures of human epidermal keratinocytes.	67,81
Cell-mediated mutagenesis	Similar: Both human and mouse epidermal cells activate BaP to mutagenic metabolites for V79 cells.	81,109

Abbreviations: (+)-anti-BPDE-dGuo, (+)-7α,8β-dihydroxy-9β,10β-epoxy-7,8,9,10-tetrahydrobenzo[a]pyrene.

summary of some of the literature and observations discussed above. Judged on a qualitative scale, metabolic events associated with tumor initiation seem to be similar in both human and mouse epidermal cells. What is not clear from the literature is how to relate a quantitative parameter such as specific DNA adduct levels to a biologic end point such as tumor formation in the two species. Perhaps an assay system like the one developed by Allen-Hoffman and Rheinwald (110) will allow such quantitative comparisons in terms of mutation induction at a specific genetic locus. Still, we need other model systems capable of measuring cellular transformation under conditions more like those in vivo.

One system that may allow such quantitative comparisons with human cells under in vivo-like conditions is xenotransplantation of human tracheobronchial epithelium (111-114), which can also be adapted to other epithelial tissues and to species comparisons of specific tissues. In this model, cells of the respiratory tract are enzymatically removed and inoculated into de-epithelialized rat tracheas. These are sealed at both ends and transplanted subcutaneously into nude mice; after 4 weeks, a normal mucociliary epithelium covers the tracheal luminal surface (113). Tracheal transplants containing cells of human origin have been treated with beeswax pellets containing 100 to 200 µg DMBA (113). After 4 to 8 weeks this treatment produces squamous metaplasias without atypias as well as some mild to moderate dysplastic lesions of the human respiratory tract epithelium (113). These data indicated that the xenotransplanted human epithelial cells remain metabolically competent and are capable of responding to a particular PAH, in this case DMBA.

The other system involves transplantation of carcinogen-treated cells into a granulation bed chamber in an immunosuppressed host. Studies from several laboratories showed that isolated epidermal cells, either fresh or cultured, may be reimplanted into appropriate host animals. Yuspa et al. (115) developed a silicone chamber that produces a protected area in the panniculus carnosus. Embryonal keratinocyte cultures transferred into these chambers form a hyperplastic epidermis with normal appendages and hair follicles.

A modification of this method was reported by Worst et al. (116). They implanted a smaller silicone chamber into a highly vascularized granulation tissue formed by the implantation of a glass disk into the subcutaneous tissue. These investigators were able to obtain an organotypic reorganization of normal and malignant mouse epidermal cultures after transplantation to syngeneic or allogeneic recipients (116-118). In recent studies (119) in which a modification of the technique of Mackenzie and Hill (120) was used, single-cell suspensions were placed in a granulation tissue formed with a glass-disk technique, and a small plastic chamber was used to cover and protect the implant. In this system, the skin of the host is closed on top of the chamber, completely covering the implant. This method protects the implant from infection and dessication, which are two problems of the other systems described. The model system developed by Conti et al. (119) may allow a direct comparison of the biologic behavior of epidermal cells from various species under conditions of the same or similar DNA adduct levels.

RELATIONSHIP OF METABOLIC ACTIVATION, DNA BINDING, AND DNA REPAIR IN MOUSE EPIDERMAL CELLS

Several investigations have focused on the ability of genotoxic agents to induce a DNA repair response in skin (121-126). Ultraviolet (UV) light was shown to induce DNA repair in normal human skin, although irradiation of the skin of patients with xeroderma pigmentosum induced little, if any, repair synthesis (127,128). This disease, a genetic disorder characterized by a deficiency in DNA excision repair and a heightened sensitivity to UV irradiation, results in multiple skin cancers during the first few years of life (129). UV-induced DNA repair has also been demonstrated in primary cultures of neonatal mouse epidermal cells (130-133) and in mouse skin in vivo (130,133,134). Hennings and associates (135,136) measured guanine-specific DNA repair in the DNA of nonreplicating cells in mixed epidermal-fibroblast cultures treated with either β-propiolactone (BPL) or N-methyl-N'-nitro-N-nitrosoguanidine (MNNG). Little additional work has been done, however, on chemically induced DNA repair in skin of rodents or humans, especially with regard to PAH-induced DNA damage. Chemically induced unscheduled DNA synthesis (UDS) has been measured autoradiographically in mouse skin in vivo (137). The technique involved clamping the skin, which, although quite drastic, was capable of measuring a UDS response to methylnitrosourea (MNU) and 4-nitroquinoline-

1-oxide (4-NQO). Previous work from our laboratory indicated that mouse epidermal cells in vivo were capable of actively removing hydrocarbon DNA adducts (77,138), whereas Nakayama et al. (76) reported removal of (±)-anti-BPDE–DNA adducts in cultured neonatal MEK. We have developed a UDS assay that can sensitively measure chemically induced DNA damage, including damage induced by PAHs, in primary cultures of adult MEK (139).

The data in Table 4 show that a variety of skin carcinogens induce dose-dependent UDS responses in this system. We found that the detection of UDS induced by direct-acting carcinogens was possible over a relatively wide range of culture conditions; only by using a medium that allowed for extensive terminal differentiation of the cultures was it possible, however, to detect UDS induced by both direct- and indirect-acting carcinogens in primary adult MEK. Under established assay conditions, the cells reached confluency 36 to 40 h after seeding in low-Ca^{2+} medium and gave a dense cobblestone appearance (139). Introduction of normal Ca^{2+} medium rapidly initiated terminal differentiation, and squamous differentiation was visible within 12 h. The level of S-phase cells decreased and, by 48 h in normal Ca^{2+} medium, was reduced to levels that were similar to those observed in vivo (< 5%) (140). This low level of replicating cells allowed quantitation of UDS by autoradiography. The 24-h treatment and labeling time also permitted adequate metabolic activation of indirect carcinogens and a good UDS response for the cells in repair. This overall approach, which involved manipulating experimental conditions to achieve acceptable levels of cells in S phase, eliminated the need to use chemical inhibitors of DNA replicative synthesis. Although such chemicals have been widely used to suppress DNA synthesis in UDS studies, they have been shown to have variable effects on DNA repair. In human epidermal cells, for example, the widely used (and cytotoxic) hydroxyurea has been shown to stimulate DNA repair (141), whereas aphidicolin causes a slight but significant (15%) inhibition of DNA repair.

Although rodent cells are generally believed to be less efficient at DNA repair than human cells (137,142), Bowden and coworkers (130-132) demonstrated that mouse epidermal cells (neonatal) in culture and mouse epidermal cells in vivo were capable of excising, at a low rate, pyrimidine dimers induced by exposure to UV irradiation. In addition, these workers were able to detect nonsemiconservative DNA synthesis after exposure to UV irradiation in both their cell-culture (131) and whole-animal studies (131). Hennings and coworkers (135,136) were unable to measure β-propiolactone- or MNNG-induced DNA repair at nontoxic doses in mixed fibroblast-epidermal cell cultures using [³H]thymidine (Tdr) incorporation. However, as stated earlier, these same investigators were able to measure guanine-specific repair using [³H]dGuo at nontoxic MNNG doses. More recently, UDS was demonstrated in mouse epidermis following exposure to a variety of agents including β-irradiation (143), UV light (133,134), and MNNG, 4-NQO, and 4-hydroxyaminoquinoline-1-oxide (139). All these studies, as well as our previous (77,138) and current data using primary cultures of MEK from adult SENCAR mice (139), demonstrated that mouse epidermal cells are capable of repairing both physically and chemically induced DNA damage. Among possible reasons for the difference between our

Table 4. Induction of Unscheduled DNA Synthesis in Primary Cultures of Adult Mouse Epidermal Keratinocytes by Various Skin Carcinogens*

Compound	Dose (μg/ml)	Net nuclear grains†	% Cells in repair‡
Acetone	–	–3.0 ± 0.6	3 ± 1
MNNG	0.1	9.7 ± 5.2§	64 ± 2
	0.5	24.5 ± 0.0§	92 ± 2
	1.0	41.7 ± 21.4§	100 ± 0
	2.0	57.5 ± 17.6§	100 ± 0
	3.0	70.8 ± 4.2§	100 ± 0
DMBA	0.005	10.1 ± 0.2§	74 ± 3
	0.010	10.4 ± 1.0§	82 ± 8
	0.025	15.3 ± 1.6§	88 ± 11
	0.05	20.0 ± 0.3§	90 ± 2
	0.125	38.5 ± 2.7§	100 ± 0
	0.25	42.3 ± 2.1§	100 ± 0
	0.5	40.0 ± 0.8§	100 ± 0
(±)anti-BPDE	0.005	–2.5 ± 0.5	14 ± 9
	0.010	0.2 ± 0.0§	16 ± 0
	0.025	1.2 ± 0.0§	16 ± 0
	0.050	14.9 ± 0.4§	78 ± 0
	0.125	19.5 ± 0.9§	95 ± 1
	0.25	41.6 ± 0.2§	100 ± 0
	0.5	46.9 ± 0.0§	100 ± 0
	1.0	39.3 ± 0.4§	100 ± 0

*Keratinocytes were isolated and cultured as described (70). Test compounds (in acetone) and [^{3}H]Tdr (10 μCi/ml) were added 48 h after switching to normal Ca^{2+} medium, and cultures were incubated for 24 h.

†Net nuclear grains are nuclear grains minus background grains. Fifty cells were scored per cover slip and values represent an average of two slides. Values represent the mean ± SE (slide-to-slide variation).

‡An individual cell with ≥ 5 net nuclear grains was considered in repair.

§Greater than the average of the control slides by the unpaired t-test for the equality of two means at a significance level of $P \leq 0.05$ (see ref. 139 for further details).

Abbreviations: MNNG, N-methyl-N′-nitro-N-nitrosoguanidine; DMBA, 7,12-dimethyl-benz[a]anthracene; BPDE, 7α,8β-dihydroxy-9β,10β-epoxy-7,8,9,10-tetrahydrobenzo[a]pyrene; Tdr, thymidine.

findings and those of Hennings and coworkers (135,136) could be that we used MEK from adult rather than newborn mice or that mixed epidermal-fibroblast cultures were used in the latter studies. However, Hosomi and Kuroki (124) also recently demonstrated UDS in primary cultures of mouse epidermal cells from newborn C3H/He and SENCAR mice following exposure to UV light; in that study, the extent of UV light-induced UDS was nearly the same in both human and mouse epidermal cells. MEK derived from newborn mice appeared, therefore, to undergo UDS (using [³H]Tdr), as did the adult MEK used in our study. Such other differences as culture conditions may explain the apparent discrepancies between our data and those of Hennings and coworkers (135,136), and these remain to be explored. In addition, species comparisons of DNA repair responses may be more appropriately performed in target epithelial cells rather than fibroblasts, which were used in earlier studies (142).

Several studies also have suggested that the differentiation state of epidermal cells may play a role in their ability to undergo a DNA repair response. In this regard, Bowden et al. (131) suggested that epidermal basal cells but not epidermal cells committed to the differentiation pathway were capable of repairing UV light-induced DNA damage. In addition, Liu et al. (144) reported that the repair of UV light-induced DNA damage in human epidermal basal cells was much greater than that in differentiated cells from the same skin preparation. Nakayama et al. (76), in contrast, reported that differentiating populations of newborn epidermal keratinocytes in culture efficiently removed DNA adducts formed from BaP. Our data also indicated that cultures of mouse epidermal cells, which were highly differentiated, displayed significant DNA repair capacity when exposed to a variety of chemical carcinogens. Thus, although we did not directly compare UDS in basal and differentiated cell populations, it seems probable that some differentiated cells in mouse epidermis are capable of exhibiting a DNA-repair response after exposure to chemical carcinogens. We are currently investigating this possibility.

In summary, a sensitive assay for measuring chemically induced DNA repair in primary cultures of adult MEK has been established. In this assay, which can detect both direct- and indirect-acting chemicals, the MEK seem to retain the tissue specificity of mouse epidermis in vivo for metabolic activation. The assay should be useful in evaluating the genotoxic potential of various chemicals for skin epidermal cells. In addition, this assay system may be useful for clarifying the relationships between biologic potency, DNA repair, and tumor initiation. Finally, the assay may be useful for comparing epidermal cells from various species.

Preliminary experiments (Table 5) were conducted to examine the relationship between biologic potency, DNA adduct formation, and DNA repair in adult MEK using this UDS assay system. For these experiments, we compared the diastereomeric diol-epoxides of BPDE for their ability to bind to DNA and induce a UDS response. The data in Table 5 show that (±)-syn-BPDE bound to epidermal DNA much less extensively than (±)-anti-BPDE at comparable doses. However, the UDS response was very similar despite the dramatic differences in DNA adduct levels. These data are interesting in light of the remarkable lack of tumor-initiating activity of the (±)-syn-BPDE for mouse skin (145,146). In addition, the data are consistent with the report of Pelling and Slaga (147), whose data suggested that the DNA adducts formed from (±)-syn-BDPE after topical application to mouse skin were removed more rapidly than those from (±)-anti-BPDE. The data in Table 5 suggest that (±)-syn-BPDE adducts may induce a greater DNA repair response in MEK. Further work along these lines is in progress.

Table 5. Relationship Between DNA Adduct Formation and Induction of Unscheduled DNA Synthesis (UDS) in Mouse Epidermal Keratinocytes (MEK)*

Compound (μg/ml)	Net nuclear grains	pmol Bound/mg keratinocyte DNA	Net nuclear grains per pmol bound to DNA
(±)-*anti*-BPDE			
0.050	23.54 ± 0.93	59.98	0.393
0.125	28.46 ± 1.02	88.79	0.321
0.250	41.62 ± 0.26	203.73	0.204
(±)-*syn*-BPDE			
0.050	14.18 ± 1.34	9.64	1.47
0.125	27.98 ± 0.34	21.34	1.31
0.250	35.22 ± 1.50	42.78	0.82

*UDS values were determined as described in Table 4 and ref. 139. DNA adduct levels were determined by treating cultures of epidermal keratinocytes with [³H]-*anti*- or [³H]-*syn*-BPDE at the concentrations indicated. All cultures and treatment conditions were similar to those used for the UDS experiments. Three hours after treatment, cells were harvested, and DNA was isolated for quantitation.
Abbreviations: (±)-*anti*-BPDE, (±)-7α,8β-dihydroxy-9β,10β-epoxy-7,8,9,10-tetrahydrobenzo[a]pyrene; (±)-*syn*-BPDE, 7α,8β-dihydroxy-9α,10α-epoxy-7,8,9,10-tetrahydrobenzo[a]pyrene.

METABOLISM OF TUMOR PROMOTERS IN MOUSE SKIN AND ITS RELATIONSHIP TO BIOLOGIC ACTIVITY

Investigators in several laboratories have shown clearly that 12-*O*-tetradecanoylphorbol-13-acetate (TPA) does not require metabolic activation for its promoting action in mouse skin (148-150). The major metabolic pathways for TPA in mouse skin involve formation of monoesters and the parent alcohol, phorbol, as shown in Figure 7 (148,150). Table 6 contains a summary of information in the literature showing marked species and strain differences in response to two-stage epidermal carcinogenesis when phorbol esters were used as promoters. As the data in Table 6 show, the responsiveness to initiation-promotion in general followed the responsiveness to phorbol ester-induced sustained epidermal hyperplasia (reviewed in ref. 151). The postulation has been, therefore, that species and strain differences in epidermal carcinogenesis are primarily determined by differences in response to the promoter (reviewed in 151). One possible reason for these species and strain differences could reside in genetic differences in the metabolism of phorbol esters. Reiners et al. (109,152) suggested that, "since the skins of CD-1 mice and Syrian hamsters are similar in their ability to clear and metabolize TPA, it is unlikely that differences in metabolism can account for differences in response to TPA promotion." Barrett and coworkers (153) also provided convincing evidence that species differences in responsive-

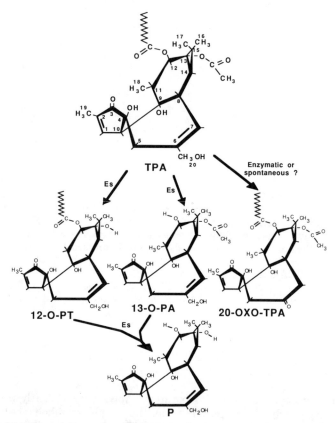

Figure 7. Major metabolic pathways for 12-*O*-tetradecanoylphorbol-13-acetate (TPA) in mouse skin. Abbreviations: Es, esterase; 12-*O*-PT, 12-*O*-phorbol tetradecanoate; 13-*O*-PA, 13-*O*-phorbol acetate· P, phorbol.

ness to phorbol esters are not related to the ability or inability to deacylate TPA. It seems unlikely, therefore, that differences in the pharmacokinetics of TPA in mouse skin can explain the species differences in response to TPA promotion.

Differences between species and strains are usually not apparent until TPA has been applied repeatedly (i.e., during sustained hyperplasia) (154). Interestingly, when mouse skin is treated with TPA before epidermal homogenates are isolated, metabolism is enhanced (149). The possibility exists, therefore, that some aspect of the absorption, distribution, metabolism, or elimination of TPA from the skin changes after multiple but not single treatments in the various mouse stocks and strains. Furthermore, Shoyab et al. (155) reported that a tissue

Table 6. Species and Strain Comparison of Response to Two-Stage Epidermal Carcinogenesis and Epidermal Hyperplasia Using TPA*

Species/ strain	Hyperplasia after multiple treatments	Responsiveness to two-stage epidermal carcinogenesis
Hamster	+	+/−
Rat	++	+/−
Mouse		
SENCAR	+++++	+++++
DBA/2	++++	++++
CD-1	+++	+++
C3H	+++	+++
BALB/c	++	++
C57BL/6	+	+/−

*Data reviewed in ref. 151.

esterase capable of metabolizing TPA rapidly might explain genetic differences in responsiveness to phorbol esters. The enzyme is apparently present in the skin of hamsters (a species relatively resistant to TPA) and virtually absent from the skin of mice, but the extent to which it is induced or elevated after high doses of or repetitive treatments with TPA on mouse skin is unknown.

Finally, Segal et al. (156) reported the formation of a reduction product at the C-5 carbonyl group of TPA in mouse skin, phorbol-5-ol myristate acetate. The extent to which this and other potential metabolites (157) are formed in mouse skin and play a role in genetically determined sensitivity to phorbol ester promotion remains to be determined.

To explore further the role of metabolism in mediating genetic differences in response to phorbol ester promoters, we examined the metabolism of TPA in skin of DBA/2 and C57BL/6 mice (DiGiovanni J, Naito Y, unpublished). DBA/2 and C57BL/6 mice represent extremes in sensitivity and resistance, respectively, to phorbol ester skin tumor promotion (158). In determining the clearance and metabolite profiles in skin after both single and multiple treatments with this tumor promoter, we found that although TPA clearance was faster and overall metabolism greater in mouse skin after multiple treatments, no significant differences were seen between DBA/2 and C57BL/6 mice that could account for differences in promotion sensitivity (Fig. 8).

We also examined the nature of the TPA metabolites formed in the skin of these two inbred strains and found detectable quantities of both monoesters as well as the parent alcohol, phorbol, over a 24-h time course after a single [³H]TPA application. When [³H]TPA was given as the last of four applications, a similar metabolite distribution (Figure 9) was observed, although larger amounts of the individual metabolites were formed. No differences in the metabolite profiles were observed between strains that could account for differences in susceptibility to skin tumor promotion. Interestingly, the major metabolite

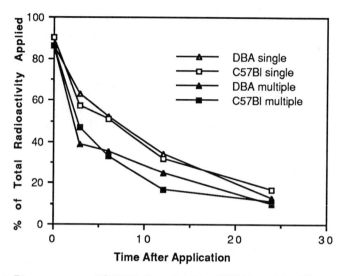

Figure 8. Disappearance of [³H]TPA from the skin of DBA/2 and C57BL/6 mice after a single treatment or the last of four treatments with the promoter. Groups of three mice each per time point were treated topically with 3.4 nmol [³H]TPA in acetone. Groups of mice were then killed at the time points indicated. Their skins were then removed and extracted with homogenization as described by Berry et al. (149). Values represent an average of two separate experiments. Open symbols are for the single application experiment, closed symbols for the multiple application experiment. For the latter experiment, mice were treated with unlabeled TPA until the last treatment, when they received [³H]TPA. Mice were treated twice weekly as in a typical tumor promotion protocol (151).

observed in skin from both strains of mice was phorbol-13-acetate (PA) (Fig. 9). Berry et al. (149) reported that phorbol-12-tetradecanoate (PT) (Fig. 9) was the major metabolite formed in skin in vivo and in epidermal homogenates in vitro from CD-1 mice. The reasons for this difference are still unknown.

There are many different chemical classes of skin tumor promoters (reviewed in refs. 159,160). For example, as compared with the potent phorbol esters, agents with strong tumor-promoting potency in mouse skin include croton oil, certain phorbol esters in croton oil, some synthetic phorbol esters, certain euphorbia lattices, 7-bromomethylbenz[a]anthracene, teleocidin B, aplysiatoxin, lyngbyatoxin A, and palytoxin. Those with moderate potency include anthralin, chrysarobin, extracts of unburned tobacco, tobacco smoke condensate, 1-fluoro-2,4-dinitrobenzene, benzo[e]pyrene, benzoyl peroxide, and lauroyl peroxide. Weak promoters include hydrogen peroxide, certain fatty acids and fatty acid methyl esters, certain long-chain alkanes, a number of phenolic compounds, surface active agents such as sodium lauryl sulfate and Tween 60,

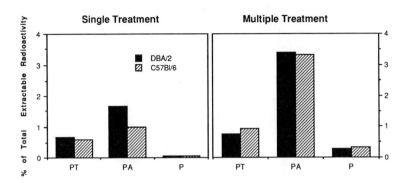

Figure 9. TPA metabolites produced in the skin of DBA/2 and C57Bl/6 mice 12 h after a single treatment or the last of four treatments with the promoter. Metabolites were analyzed by high-performance liquid chromatography (HPLC) of organic extracts from skins as described for Figure 8. HPLC procedures were similar to those described by Berry et al. (148). Abbreviations: PT, phorbol-12-O-tetradecanoate; PA, phorbol-13-acetate; P, phorbol.

citrus oils, and iodoacetic acid. These data are reviewed in refs. 159 and 160. Little information is available on potential metabolic pathways for these promoters. Hagiwara et al. (161) recently reported that the indole alkaloid promoter (–)-indolactam V is metabolized by the microsomal mixed-function oxidase system to several less biologically active derivatives. These data suggest that other indole alkaloids such as the teleocidins, which are believed to act by a mechanism similar to that of the phorbol esters (162), may follow similar metabolic pathways leading primarily to detoxification products. Because of marked species and strain differences in cytochrome P-450-mediated monooxygenase pathways, one might predict that indole alkaloids would not have the same species or strain distribution in terms of promoting activity as the phorbol esters. Further work on these questions seems warranted.

Another interesting class of skin tumor promoters are the naturally occurring anthrone derivatives (163-166), which seem to work by an initial mechanism different from that of the phorbol esters: anthrones do not compete for the phorbol ester receptor on mouse epidermal cells or in mouse epidermal particulate fractions (166,167) and do not activate partially purified preparations of mouse brain protein kinase C (PKC) in vitro nor do they induce the translocation of epidermal PKC from cytosol to membrane (DiGiovanni J, Hirabayashi N, Ashendel C, unpublished). And at optimal promoting doses, the time course and magnitude of induction of epidermal ornithine decarboxylase (ODC) by chrysarobin (1,8-dihydroxy-3-methyl-9-anthrone) is markedly different from that of TPA (169,170), the carcinoma:papilloma ratio in mice promoted with chrysarobin is higher than in mice treated with optimal papilloma promoting doses of TPA (171), chrysarobin does not function operationally as a stage I

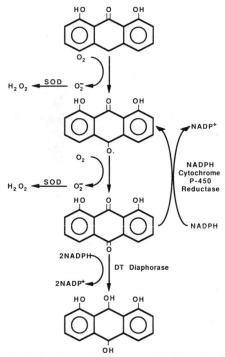

Figure 10. Hypothetical scheme for the autooxidation of anthrones (e.g., anthralin as shown) in biologic systems. Abbreviation: SOD, superoxide dismutase.

or stage II tumor promoter (169), and the ability of chrysarobin to increase epidermal polyamine levels and stimulate epidermal DNA synthesis may involve interconversion pathways possibly activated as a result of toxicity (172). In addition, the time courses for changes in epidermal DNA synthesis and induction of epidermal hyperplasia are markedly different following single topical applications of chrysarobin compared with TPA (172,173), and structure-activity studies for the induction of epidermal ODC and skin tumor promotion demonstrate an excellent correlation with the ability of several derivatives to undergo base-catalyzed oxidation in an in vitro system (174).

This latter evidence suggests that metabolic activation and detoxification pathways may play an important role in the mechanism of skin tumor promotion by anthrone derivatives. Figure 10 illustrates a hypothetical scheme for the oxidation and further metabolism of anthrone derivatives in skin tissues, making it readily apparent that many enzymatic pathways could influence the biologic activity of anthrones. Their metabolism, like that of the teleocidins and the other nonphorbol ester promoters, may be considerably different from that of the phorbol esters. A different spectrum of promoter activity may be expected, therefore, for the anthrone tumor promoters among species and strains.

These two examples of nonphorbol esters underline the need for further studies of the metabolism of tumor promoters in target tissues. Such studies will advance our understanding of potential mechanisms and provide information on trans-species and -strain differences in susceptibility to other environmentally relevant promoting agents.

SUMMARY

Mouse epidermal cells are a useful model system for studying chemical carcinogenesis in epithelial tissues. The available data suggest that some aspects of the metabolic activation and covalent binding of PAH carcinogens are similar in mouse and in human epidermis, whereas notable differences include conjugation pathways and wide interindividual differences, especially in adduct formation. Further work is necessary to determine the role of these differences in susceptibility to PAH carcinogenesis. Clearly, future in vitro assay systems for species extrapolation of epidermal carcinogenesis data must take into account the differentiation state of the cells, among other factors. We showed that the differentiation state of keratinocytes may profoundly influence the metabolic activation of PAHs. Also needed are in vivo assay systems in which quantitative data such as specific DNA adduct levels can be related to the biologic end point of cellular transformation. Several systems were discussed that may fulfill this need.

With regard to skin tumor promoters, much less is known about the role of metabolism in mediating species and strain differences in responsiveness. The data available for phorbol esters indicate that differences in the metabolic inactivation of TPA cannot explain the marked species differences in sensitivity to this class of promoters. Much less is known about other chemical classes of promoters, which also require further investigation.

ACKNOWLEDGMENTS

My thanks to Joyce Mayhugh for her excellent assistance in preparing this manuscript for publication. Original research was supported by grants CA 36979, CA 37111, and CA 38871 from the National Cancer Institute, U.S. Public Health Service.

REFERENCES

1. Heidelberger C. Chemical Carcinogenesis. Annu Rev Biochem 44:79-121, 1975.
2. Dipple A, Moschel RC, Bigger CAH. Polynuclear aromatic carcinogens. In Searle CE (ed): Chemical Carcinogens, Vol. 1. Washington, DC: American Chemical Society Monograph 182, 1984, pp 41-163.
3. Miller EC. Some current perspectives on chemical carcinogenesis in humans and experimental animals: Presidential address. Cancer Res 38:1479-1496, 1978.
4. Gelboin HV, Ts'o POP (eds): Polycyclic Hydrocarbons and Cancer. New York:

Academic Press, 1978.
5. Phillips DH, Sims P. Polycyclic aromatic hydrocarbon metabolites: Their reactions with nucleic acids. In Grover PL (ed): Chemical Carcinogens and DNA, Vol. 2. Boca Raton, FL: CRC Press, pp 29-57.
6. Sims P. The metabolic activation of chemical carcinogens. Br Med Bull 36:11-18, 1980.
7. Sims P, Grover PL. Epoxides in polycyclic aromatic hydrocarbon metabolism and carcinogenesis. Adv Cancer Res 20:165-274, 1974.
8. Jerina DM, Daly JW, Witkop B, Zaltzman-Nirenberg P, Underfriend S. 1,2-Napthalene oxide as an intermediate in the microsomal hydroxylation of napthalene. Biochemistry 9:147-156, 1970.
9. Jerina DM, Daly JW. Arene oxides: A new perspective of drug metabolism. Science 185:573-582, 1974.
10. Selkirk JK, Huberman E, Heidelberger C. An epoxide is an intermediate in the microsomal metabolism of the chemical carcinogen dibenz(a)anthracene. Biochem Biophys Res Commun 43:1010-1016, 1971.
11. Sims P. Polycyclic hydrocarbon epoxides as active metabolic intermediates. In Jollow DJ, Kocsis JJ, Snyder R, Vainio R (eds): Biologically Reactive Intermediates. New York: Plenum Press, 1977, pp 358-370.
12. Grover PL, Hewer A, Sims P. Formation of K-region epoxides as microsomal metabolites of pyrene and benzo[a]pyrene. Biochem Pharmacol 21:2713-2726, 1972.
13. Oesch F. Mammalian epoxide hydroses: Inducible enzymes catalyzing the inactivation of carcinogenic and cytotoxic metabolites derived from aromatic and objective compounds. Xenobiotica 3:305-340, 1973.
14. Boyland E, Chasseaud LF. The role of glutathione and glutathione S-transferases in mercapturic acid biosynthesis. Adv Enzymol 32:173-219, 1969.
15. Jerina DM, Bend JR. Glutathione S-transferases. In Jollow DJ, Kocsis JJ, Snyder R, Vainio H (eds): Biologically Reactive Intermediates. New York: Plenum Press, 1977, pp 207-236.
16. Bend JR, Ben-Zvi Z, Van Anda J, Dansette PM, Jerina DM. Hepatic and extrahepatic glutathione S-transferase activity toward several arene oxides and epoxides in the rat. In Freudenthal RI, Jones PW (eds): Carcinogenesis, Vol. 1. Polynuclear Aromatic Hydrocarbons: Chemistry, Metabolism, and Carcinogenesis. New York: Raven Press, 1976, pp 63-75.
17. Nemoto N, Gelboin HV. Enzymatic conjugation of benzo[a]pyrene oxide phenols and dihydrodiols with UDP-glucuronic acid. Biochem Pharmacol 25:1221-1226, 1976.
18. Baird WM, Chern CJ, Diamond L. Formation of benzo[a]pyrene-glucuronic acid conjugates in hamster embryo cell cultures. Cancer Res 37:3190-3197, 1977.
19. Nemoto N, Nirakawa T, Takayama S. Glucuronidation of benzo[a]pyrene in hamster embryo cells. Chem Biol Interact 22:1-14, 1978.
20. Boyland E, Sims P. The metabolism of phenanthrene in rabbits and rats: Dihydroxy compounds and related glucasiduronic acids. Biochem J 84:571-582, 1962.
21. Baird WM, Chemerys R, Chern CJ, Diamond L. Formation of glucuronic acid conjugates of 7,12-dimethylbenz[a]anthracene-treated hamster embryo cells. Cancer Res 38:3432-3437, 1978.
22. Sims P. Metabolism of polycyclic compounds, 19. The metabolism of phenanthrene in rabbits and rats: Phenols and sulphuric esters. Biochem J 84:558-563, 1962.

23.   Cohen GM, Haws SM, Moore BP, Bridges JW. Benzo[a]pyrene-3-yl hydrogen sulphate, a major ethyl acetate-extractable metabolite of benzo[a]pyrene in human, hamster, and rat lung cultures. Biochem Pharmacol 25:2561-2570, 1976.

24.   Nemoto N, Takayama S. Enzymatic formation and properties of a conjugate of sulfate with 3-hydroxybenzo[a]pyrene. Biochem Pharmacol 26:679-684, 1977.

25.   Moore BP, Cohen GM. Metabolism of benzo[a]pyrene and its major metabolites to ethyl acetate soluble and water-soluble metabolites by cultured rodent trachea. Cancer Res 38:3066-3075, 1978.

26.   Nemoto N, Takayama S. Modification of benzo[a]pyrene metabolism with microsomes by addition of uridine 5'-diphosphoglucuronic acid. Cancer Res 37:4125-4129, 1977.

27.   Cohen GM, Moore BP. Metabolism of benzo[a]pyrene, 7,8-dihydro-7,8-dihydroxybenzo[a]pyrene and 9,10-dihydro-9,10-dihydroxybenzo[a]pyrene by short-term organ cultures of hamster lung. Biochem Pharmacol 26:1481-1487, 1977.

28.   Nemoto N, Takayama S, Gelboin HV. Enzymic conversion of benzo[a]pyrene phenols, dihydrodiols, and quinones to sulfate conjugates. Biochem Pharmacol 26:1825-1829, 1977.

29.   Pelkonen O, Nebert DW. Metabolism of polycyclic aromatic hydrocarbons: Etiological role in carcinogenesis. Pharmacol Rev 34:189-222, 1982.

30.   Selkirk J. Analogous patterns of benzo[a]pyrene metabolism in human and rodent cells. In Huberman E, Barr SH (eds): Carcinogenesis, Vol. 10. The Role of Chemicals and Radiation in the Etiology of Cancer. New York: Raven Press, 1985, pp 123-133.

31.   Capdevila J, Jernsstrom B, Vadi H, Orreinus S. Cytochrome P-450-linked activation of 3-hydroxybenzo[a]pyrene. Biochem Biophys Res Commun 65:894-900, 1975.

32.   King HWS, Thompson MH, Brookes P. The role of 9-hydroxy-benzo[a]pyrene in the microsome mediated binding of benzo[a]pyrene to DNA. Int J Cancer 18:339-344, 1976.

33.   Sims P, Grover PL, Swaisland A, Pal K, Hewer A. Metabolic activation of benzo[a]pyrene proceeds by a diol-epoxide. Nature 252:326-328, 1974.

34.   Lubet RA, Capdevila J, Prough RA. The metabolic activation of benzo[a]pyrene and 9-hydroxybenzo[a]pyrene by liver microsomal fractions. Int J Cancer 23:353-357, 1979.

35.   Jerina DM, Daly JW. Oxidation of carbon. In Parke DV, Smith RL (eds): Drug Metabolism: From Microbe to Man. London: Taylor and Francis, Ltd., 1976, pp 13-32.

36.   Levin W, Wood AW, Wislocki PG, Chang RL, Kapitulnik J, Mah HD, Yagi H, Jerina DM, Conney AH. Mutagenicity and carcinogenicity of benzo[a]pyrene and benzo[a]pyrene derivatives. In Gelboin HV, Ts'o POP (eds): Polycyclic Hydrocarbons and Cancer. New York: Academic Press, 1978, pp 189-202.

37.   Conney AH. Induction of microsomal enzymes by foreign chemicals and carcinogenesis by polycyclic aromatic hydrocarbons: G.H.A. Clowes Memorial Lecture. Cancer Res 42:4875-4917, 1982.

38.   Wood AW, Levin W, Chang RL, Yagi H, Thakker DR, Lehr RE, Jerina DM, Conney AH. Bay-region activation of carcinogenic polycyclic hydrocarbons. In Jones PW, Leber P (eds): Polynuclear Aromatic Hydrocarbons. Ann Arbor, MI: Ann Arbor Science Publishers, 1979, pp 531-551.

39. Sims P, Grover PL. Involvement of dihydrodiols and diol-epoxides in the metabolic activation of polycyclic hydrocarbons other than benzo[a]pyrene. In Gelboin HV, Ts'o POP (eds): Polycyclic Hydrocarbons and Cancer, Vol. 3. New York: Academic Press, 1981, pp 117-174.

40. Weibel FJ, Leutz JC, Gelboin HV. Aryl hydrocarbon (benzo[a]pyrene) hydroxylase: A mixed-function oxygenase in mouse skin. J Invest Dermatol 64:184-189, 1975.

41. Akin FJ, Norred WP. Factors affecting measurement of aryl hydrocarbon hydroxylase activity in mouse skin. J Invest Dermatol 67:709-712, 1976.

42. Thompson S, Slaga TJ. Mouse epidermal aryl hydrocarbon hydroxylase. J Invest Dermatol 66:108-111, 1976.

43. Pohl RJ, Philpot RM, Fouts JR. Cytochrome P-450 content and mixed-function oxidase activity in microsomes isolated from mouse skin. Drug Metab Dispos 4:442-450, 1976.

44. Manil L, Van Cantfort J, Lapiere CM, Gielen JE. Significant variation in mouse-skin aryl hydrocarbon hydroxylase inducibility as a function of the hair growth cycle. Br J Cancer 43:210-221, 1981.

45. Eling TE, Krauss RS. Arachidonic acid-dependent metabolism of chemical carcinogens and toxicants. In Marnett LJ (ed): Arachidonic Acid Metabolism and Tumor Initiation. New York: Martinus Nijhoff, 1985, pp 83-124.

46. Marnett LJ, Reed GA, Dennison DJ. Prostaglandin synthetase dependent activation of 7,8-dihydro-7,8-dihydroxybenzo[a]pyrene to mutagenic derivatives. Biochem Biophys Res Commun 82:210-216, 1978.

47. Guthrie J, Robertson IGC, Zeiger E, Boyd JA, Eling TE. Selective activation of some dihydrodiols of several polycyclic aromatic hydrocarbons to mutagenic products by prostaglandin synthetase. Cancer Res 42:1620-1623, 1982.

48. Battista JR, Marnett LJ. Prostaglandin H synthase-dependent epoxidation of aflatoxin B_1. Carcinogenesis 6:1227-1229, 1985.

49. Robertson IGC, Sivarajah K, Eling TE, Zeiger E. Activation of some aromatic amines to mutagenic products by prostaglandin endoperoxide synthetase. Cancer Res 43:476-480, 1983.

50. Kondoh H, Sato Y, Kanoh H. Arachidonic acid metabolism in cultured mouse keratinocytes. J Invest Dermatol 85:64-69, 1985.

51. Wheeler EL, Berry DL. In vitro inhibition of mouse epidermal cell lipoxygenase by flavonoids: Structure-activity relationships. Carcinogenesis 7:33-36, 1986.

52. Nakadate T, Aizu E, Yamamoto S, Kato R. Some properties of lipoxygenase activities in cytosol and microsomal fractions of mouse epidermal homogenate. Prostaglandins Leukotrienes Med 21:305-309, 1986.

53. Fischer SM, Baldwin JK, Jasheway DW, Patrick KE, Cameron GS. Phorbol ester induction of 8-lipoxygenase in inbred Sencar (SSIN) but not C57BL/6J mice, correlated with hyperplasia, edema and oxidant generation but not ornithine decarboxylase induction. Cancer Res 48:658-664, 1988.

54. Nakadate T, Yamamoto S, Aizu E, Kato R. Inhibition of 12-O-tetradecanoylphorbol-13-acetate-induced increase in vascular permeability in mouse skin by lipoxygenase inhibitors. Jpn J Pharmacol 38:161-168, 1985.

55. Fischer SM, Mills GD, Slaga TJ. Inhibition of mouse skin tumor promotion by several inhibitors of arachidonic acid metabolism: A comparison between SENCAR and NMRI mice. Carcinogenesis 3:1243-1245, 1982.

56. Fischer SM, Furstenberger G, Marks F, Slaga TJ. Events associated with mouse skin tumor promotion with respect to arachidonic acid metabolism: A compari-

son between SENCAR and NMRI mice. Cancer Res 47:3174-3179, 1987.

57. Eling T, Curtis J, Battista J, Marnett LJ. Oxidation of (+)-7,8-dihydroxy-7,8-dihydrobenzo[a]pyrene by mouse keratinocytes: Evidence for peroxyl radical-and monooxygenase-dependent metabolism. Carcinogenesis 7:1957-1963, 1986.

58. Furstenberger G, Marks F. Early prostaglandin E synthesis is an obligatory event in the induction of cell proliferation in mouse epidermis in vivo by the phorbol ester TPA. Biochem Biophys Res Commun 42:749-756, 1980.

59. DiGiovanni J, Slaga TJ, Boutwell RK. Comparison of the tumor-initiating activity of 7,12-dimethylbenz[a]anthracene and benzo[a]pyrene in female SENCAR and CD-1 mice. Carcinogenesis 1:381-389, 1980.

60. Kahl GF, Kahl R, Kumaki K, Nebert DW. Association of the Ah locus with specific changes in metyrapone and ethylisocyanide binding to mouse liver microsomes. J Biol Chem 251:5397-5407, 1976.

61. Park SS, Fujino T, West D, Guengerich FP, Gelboin HV. Monoclonal antibodies that inhibit enzyme activity of 3-methylcholanthrene-induced cytochrome P-450. Cancer Res 42:1798-1808, 1982.

62. Marnett LJ. Hydroperoxide-dependent oxidations during prostaglandin biosynthesis. Free Radicals in Biology 6:63-93, 1984.

63. Slaga TJ, Bracken WM. The affects of antioxidants on skin tumor initiation and aryl hydrocarbon hydroxylase. Cancer Res 37:1631-1635, 1977.

64. DiGiovanni J, Slaga TJ, Berry DL, Juchau MR. Metabolism of 7,12-dimethylbenz[a]anthracene in mouse skin homogenates analyzed with high pressure liquid chromatography. Drug Metab Dispos 5:295-301, 1977.

65. Berry DL, Bracken WR, Slaga TJ, Wilson NM, Buty SG, Juchau MR. Benzo[a]pyrene metabolism in mouse epidermis: Analysis by high pressure liquid chromatography and DNA binding. Chem Biol Interact 18:129-142, 1977.

66. DiGiovanni J, Viaje A, Fischer S, Slaga TJ, Boutwell RK. Biotransformation of 7,12-dimethylbenz[a]anthracene by mouse epidermal cells in culture. Carcinogenesis 1:41-49, 1980.

67. DiGiovanni J, Miller DR, Singer J, Viaje A, Fischer SM, Slaga TJ. Benzo[a]pyrene metabolism in primary cultures of mouse epidermal cells and untransformed and transformed epidermal cell lines. Cancer Res 42:2579-2586, 1982.

68. Potten CS. Stem cells in epidermis from the back of the mouse. In Potten CS (ed): Stem Cells: Their Identification and Characterization. New York: Churchill-Livingston, 1983, pp 220-232.

69. Miller DR, Viaje A, Aldaz CM, Conti CJ, Slaga TJ. Terminal differentiation-resistant epidermal cells in mice undergoing two-stage carcinogenesis. Cancer Res 47:1935-1940, 1987.

70. Hennings H, Michael D, Cheng C, Steinert P, Holbrook K, Yuspa SH. Calcium regulation of growth and differentiation of mouse epidermal cells in culture. Cell 19:245-254, 1980.

71. Yuspa SH, Hawley-Nelson P, Stanley JR, Hennings H. Epidermal cell culture. Transplant Proc 12(Suppl 1):114-122, 1980.

72. Thakker DR, Yagi H, Akagi H, Kareeda M, Lu AYH, Levin W, Wood AW, Conney AH, Jerina DM. Metabolism of benzo[a]pyrene. VI. Stereoselective metabolism of benzo[a]pyrene and benzo[a]pyrene-7,8-dihydrodiol to diol epoxides. Chem Biol Interact 16:281-300, 1977.

73. Ashurst SW, Cohen GM. In vivo formation of benzo[a]pyrene diol epoxide-deoxyadenosine adducts in the skin of mice susceptible to benzo[a]pyrene-induced carcinogenesis. Int J Cancer 27:357-364, 1981.

74.   Ashurst SW, Cohen GM, Nesnow S, DiGiovanni J, Slaga TJ. Formation of benzo[a]pyrene/DNA adducts and their relationship to tumor initiation in mouse epidermis. Cancer Res 43:1024-1029, 1983.

75.   Koreeda M, Moore PD, Wislocki P, Levin W, Conney AH, Yagi H, Jerina DM. Binding of benzo[a]pyrene-7,8-diol-9,10-epoxides to DNA, RNA, and protein of mouse skin occurs with high stereoselectivity. Science 199:778-781, 1978.

76.   Nakayama J, Yuspa SH, Poire MC. Benzo[a]pyrene-DNA adduct formation and removal in mouse epidermis in vivo and in vitro: Relationship of DNA binding to initiation of skin carcinogenesis. Cancer Res 44:4087-4095, 1984.

77.   DiGiovanni J, Decina PC, Prichett WP, Fisher EP, Aalfs KK. Formation and disappearance of benzo[a]pyrene DNA-adducts in mouse epidermis. Carcinogenesis 6:741-747, 1985.

78.   Alexandrov K, Rojas M, Bourgeois Y, Chouroulinkov I. The persistence of benzo[a]pyrene diol-epoxide deoxyguanosine adduct in mouse skin and its disappearance in rat skin. Carcinogenesis 4:1655-1657, 1983.

79.   Huckle KR, Smith RJ, Watson WP, Wright AS. Comparison of hydrocarbon-DNA adducts formed in mouse skin in vivo and in organ culture in vitro following treatment with benzo[a]pyrene. Carcinogenesis 7:965-970, 1986.

80.   Fox CH, Selkirk JK, Price FM, Croy RG, Sanford KK, Cottler-Fox H. Metabolism of benzo[a]pyrene by human epithelial cells in vitro. Cancer Res 35:3551-3557, 1975.

81.   Kuroki T, Nemoto N, Kitano Y. Metabolism of benzo[a]pyrene in human epidermal keratinocytes in culture. Carcinogenesis 1:559-565, 1980

82.   Parkinson K, Newbold RF. Benzo[a]pyrene metabolism and DNA adduct formation in serially cultivated strains of human epidermal keratinocytes. Am J Cancer 26:289-299, 1980.

83.   Theall G, Eisinger M, Grunberger D. Metabolism of benzo[a]pyrene and DNA adduct formation in cultured human epidermal keratinocytes. Carcinogenesis 2:581-587, 1981.

84.   Hukkelhoven MWAC, Vromans LWM, Vermorken AJM, van Diepen CB, Bloemendal H. Determination of phenolic benzo[a]pyrene metabolites formed by human hair follicles. Anal Biochem 125:370-375, 1982.

85.   Hukkelhoven MWAC, Vermorken AJM, Vromans E, Bloemendal H. Human hair follicles: A convenient tissue for genetic studies on carcinogen metabolism. Clin Genet 21:53-58, 1982.

86.   Hukkelhoven MWAC, Vromans E, Vermorken AJM, Bloemendal H. A simple fluorometric microassay for DNA in hair follicles or fractions of hair follicles. Anticancer Res 2:89-94, 1982.

87.   Kuroki T, Hosomi J, Munakata K, Onizuka T, Terauchi M, Nemoto N. Metabolism of benzo[a]pyrene in epidermal keratinocytes and dermal fibroblasts of humans and mice with reference to variation among species, individuals and cell types. Cancer Res 42:1859-1865, 1982.

88.   Bickers DR, Kappas A. Human skin aryl hydrocarbon hydroxylase. J Clin Invest 62:1061-1068, 1978.

89.   Levin W, Conney AH, Alvares AP, Merkatz I, Kappas A. Induction of benzo[a]pyrene hydroxylase in human skin. Science 176:419-420, 1972.

90.   Alvares AP, Kappas A, Levin W, Conney AH. Inducibility of benzo[a]pyrene hydroxylase in human skin by polycyclic hydrocarbons. Clin Pharmacol Ther 14:30-40, 1973.

91.   Kouri RE. Relationship between levels of aryl hydrocarbon hydroxylase activity

and susceptibility to 3-methylcholanthrene and benzo[a]pyrene-induced cancers in inbred strains of mice. In Freudenthal R, Jones P (eds): Carcinogenesis: A Comprehensive Survey, Vol. 1. Chemistry, Metabolism and Carcinogenesis. New York: Raven Press, 1976, pp 139-141.

92. Nebert DW, Atlas SA, Guenther TH, Kouri RE. The Ah locus: Genetic regulation of the enzymes which metabolize polycyclic hydrocarbons and the risk for cancer. In Gelboin HV, Ts'o POP (eds): Polycyclic Hydrocarbons and Cancer, Vol. 2. New York: Academic Press, 1978, pp 346-390.

93. Nebert DW. Pharmacogenetics: An approach to understanding chemical and biologic aspects of cancer. JNCI 64:1279-1290, 1980.

94. Abbott P, Crew F. Repair of DNA adducts of the carcinogen 15,16-dihydro-11-methylcyclopenta[a]phenanthren-17-one in mouse tissues and its relation to tumor induction. Cancer Res 41:4115-4120, 1981.

95. Abbott P. Strain-specific tumorigenesis in mouse skin induced by the carcinogen, 15,16-dihydro-11-methyl-cyclopenta[a]phenanthren-17-one, and its relation to DNA adduct formation and persistence. Cancer Res 43:2261-2266, 1983.

96. Ashurst SW, Cohen GM. In vivo formation of benzo[a]pyrene diol epoxide deoxyadenosine adducts in the skin of mice susceptible to benzo[a]pyrene induced carcinogenesis. Int J Cancer 27:357-364, 1981.

97. Phillips DH, Grover PL, Sims P. The covalent binding of polycyclic hydrocarbons to DNA in the skin of mice of different strains. Int J Cancer 22:487-494, 1978.

98. DiGiovanni J, Slaga TJ, Juchau MR. Comparative epidermal metabolism in strains of mice with differing sensitivity to skin tumorigenesis by DMBA (abstract). Proceedings of the American Association of Cancer Research 20:134, 1979.

99. Dipple A, Pigott MA, Bigger AH, Blake DM. 7,12-Dimethylbenz[a]anthracene-DNA binding in mouse skin: Response of different mouse strains and effects of various modifiers of carcinogenesis. Carcinogenesis 5:1087-1090, 1984.

100. Nebert DW, Boobis AR, Yagi H, Jerina DM, Kouri RE. Genetic differences in mouse cytochrome P-450 mediated metabolism of benzo[a]pyrene in vitro and carcinogenic index in vivo. In Jollow DJ, Kocsis JJ, Snyder R, Vainio H (eds): Biologically Reactive Intermediates. New York: Plenum Press, 1977, pp 125-145.

101. Pelkonen O, Boobis AR, Levitt RC, Kouri RE, Nebert DW. Genetic differences in the metabolic activation of benzo[a]pyrene in mice: Attempts to correlate tumorigenesis with mutagenesis in vitro. Pharmacology 18:281-293, 1979.

102. Autrup H, Harris CC, Trump BF, Jeffrey AM. Metabolism of benzo[a]pyrene and identification of the major benzo[a]pyrene-DNA adducts in cultured human colon. Cancer Res 38:3689-3696, 1978.

103. Harris CC, Autrup H, Conner R, Barrett LA, McDowell EM, Trump BF. Interindividual variations in binding of benzo[a]pyrene to DNA in cultured human bronchi. Science 194:1067-1069, 1976.

104. Harris CC, Autrup H, Stoner GD, Trump BF, Hillman E, Schafer PW, Jeffrey AM. Metabolism of benzo[a]pyrene, N-nitrosodimethylamine, and N-nitrosopyrrolidine and identification of the major carcinogen-DNA adducts formed in cultured human esophagus. Cancer Res 39:4401-4406, 1979.

105 Dorman BH, Genta VM, Mass MJ, Kaufman DG. Benzo[a]pyrene binding to DNA in organ cultures of human endometrium. Cancer Res 41:2718-2722, 1981.

106. Mukhtar H, Del Tito BJ Jr, Marcelo CL, Das M, Bickers DR. Ellagic acid: A potent naturally occurring inhibitor of benzo[a]pyrene metabolism and its

subsequent glucuronidation, sulfation and covalent binding to DNA in cultured BALB/c mouse keratinocytes. Carcinogenesis 5:1565-1571, 1984.

107. Harris CC, Hsu IC, Stoner GD, Trump BF, Selkirk JK. Human pulmonary alveolar macrophages metabolize benzo[a]pyrene to proximate and ultimate mutagens. Nature 272:633-634, 1978.

108. Hsu IC, Stoner GD, Autrup H, Trump BF, Selkirk JK, Harris CC. Human bronchus-mediated mutagenesis of mammalian cells by carcinogenic polynuclear aromatic hydrocarbons. Proc Natl Acad Sci USA 75:2003-2007, 1978.

109. Reiners JJ, Nesnow S, Slaga TJ. Murine susceptibility to two-stage skin carcinogenesis is influenced by the agent used for promotion. Carcinogenesis 5:301-307, 1984.

110. Allen-Hoffman BL, Rheinwald JG. Polycyclic aromatic hydrocarbon mutagenesis of human epidermal keratinocytes in culture. Proc Natl Acad Sci USA 81:7802-7806, 1984.

111. Klein-Szanto AJP, Terzaghi M, Mirkin LD, Martin D, Shiba M. Propagation of normal human epithelial cell populations using an in vivo culture system. Am J Pathol 108:231-240, 1982.

112. Klein-Szanto AJP, Pal BC, Terzaghi M, Marchok AC. Heterotopic tracheal transplants: Techniques and applications. Environ Health Perspect 56:75-86, 1984.

113. Klein-Szanto AJP, Baba M, Trono D, Obara T, Resau J, Trump BF. Epidermoid metaplasias of xenotransplanted human tracheobronchial epithelium. Carcinogenesis 7:987-994, 1986.

114. Baba M, Klein-Szanto AJP, Trono D, Obara T, Yoakum GH, Masui T, Harris CC. Preneoplastic and neoplastic growth of xenotransplanted lung-derived human cell lines using deepithelialized rat tracheas. Cancer Res 47:573-578, 1987.

115. Yuspa SH, Morgan DL, Walker RJ, Bates RB. The growth of fetal mouse skin in cell cultures and transplantation of F1 mice. J Invest Dermatol 55:379-389, 1970.

116. Worst PKM, Valentine EA, Fusenig NE. Formation of epidermis after reimplantation of pure primary epidermal cell cultures from perinatal mouse skin. JNCI 53:1061-1064, 1974.

117. Fusenig NE, Valentine EA, Worst PKM. Growth behavior of normal and transformed mouse epidermal cells after reimplantation in vivo. In Richards RJ, Rajan KT (eds): Tissue Culture in Medical Research, No. II. Oxford: Pergamon Press, 1980, pp 87-95.

118. Worst PKM, Mackenzie IC, Fusenig NE. Reformation of organized epidermal structure by transplantation of suspensions and cultures of epidermal and dermal cells. Cell Tissue Res 225:65-77, 1982.

119. Conti CJ, Fries JW, Aldaz CM, Klein-Szanto AJP, Slaga TJ. Allogeneic transplantation of normal epidermal cells and squamous cell carcinomas in SENCAR mice. Environ Health Perspect 68:125-129, 1986.

120. Mackenzie IC, Hill MW. Maintenance of regionally specific patterns of cell proliferation and differentiation in transplanted skin and oral mucosa. Cell Tissue Res 219:597-607, 1981.

121. Gibson-D'Ambrosio RE, Leong Y, D'Ambrosio SM. DNA repair following ultraviolet and N-ethyl-N-nitrosourea treatment of cells cultured from human fetal brain, intestine, kidney, liver, and skin. Cancer Res 43:5846-5850, 1983.

122. Sutherland BM, Haber LC, Kochevar IE. Pyrimidine dimer formation and repair in human skin. Cancer Res 40:3181-3185, 1980.

123. Eggset G, Volden G, Krokan H. UV-induced DNA damage and its repair in human skin in vivo studied by immunohistochemical methods. Carcinogenesis 4:745-750, 1983.

124. Hosomi J, Kuroki T. UV-induced unscheduled DNA synthesis in cultured human epidermal and dermal cells. Gann 76:1072-1077, 1985.

125. Taichman LB, Setlow RB. Repair of ultraviolet light damage of the DNA of cultured human epidermal keratinocytes and fibroblasts. J Invest Dermatol 73:217-219, 1975.

126. Hanawalt PC, Liu S-C, Parsons S. DNA repair responses in human skin cells. J Invest Dermatol 77:86-90, 1981.

127. Epstein JH, Fukuyama K, Reed WB, Epstein WW. Defect in DNA synthesis in skin of patients with xeroderma pigmentosum demonstrated in vivo. Science 168:1477-1478, 1970.

128. Cleaver JE, Gruenert DC. Repair of psoralen adducts in human DNA: Differences among xeroderma pigmentosum complementation groups. J Invest Dermatol 82:311-315, 1984.

129. Lynch HT, Lynch PM, Guirgis HA. Host-environmental interaction and carcinogenesis in man. In Kouri RE (ed): Genetic Differences in Chemical Carcinogenesis. Boca Raton, FL: CRC Press, 1980, pp 185-209.

130. Bowden GT, Trosko JE, Shapas BG, Boutwell RK. Excision of pyrimidine dimers from epidermal DNA and nonsemiconservative epidermal DNA synthesis following ultraviolet irradiation of mouse skin. Cancer Res 35:3599-3607, 1975.

131. Bowden GT, Hohneck G, Fusenig NE. DNA excision repair in ultraviolet-irradiated normal and malignantly transformed epidermal cell cultures. Cancer Res 37:1611-1617, 1977.

132. Bowden GT, Giesselbach B, Fusenig NE. Postreplication DNA repair of DNA in ultraviolet light-irradiated normal and malignantly transformed mouse epidermal cell cultures. Cancer Res 38:2709-2718, 1978.

133. Kodama K, Ishakawa T, Takayama S. Dose response, wavelength dependence, and time course of ultraviolet radiation-induced unscheduled DNA synthesis in mouse skin in vivo. Cancer Res 44:2150-2154, 1984.

134. Ishikawa T, Sakarai J. In vivo studies on age dependency of DNA repair with age in mouse skin. Cancer Res 46:1344-1348, 1986.

135. Hennings H, Michael DM, Eaton S, Morgan DL. Purine-specific repair of 3-propiolactone-induced DNA damage in mouse skin. J Invest Dermatol 62:480-484, 1974.

136. Hennings H, Michael D. Guanine-specific DNA repair after treatment of mouse skin cells with N-methyl-N'-nitrosoguanidine. Cancer Res 36:2321-2325, 1976.

137. Ishikawa T, Kodama K, Ide F, Takayama S. Demonstration of in vivo DNA repair synthesis in mouse skin exposed to various chemical carcinogens. Cancer Res 42:5216-5221, 1982.

138. DiGiovanni J, Fisher EP, Sawyer TW. Kinetics of formation and disappearance of 7,12-dimethylbenz[a]anthracene: DNA adducts in mouse epidermis. Cancer Res 46:4400-4405, 1986.

139. Sawyer TW, Gill RD, Smith-Oliver T, Butterworth BE, DiGiovanni J. Measurement of unscheduled DNA synthesis in primary cultures of adult mouse epidermal keratinocytes. Carcinogenesis 9:1197-1202, 1988.

140. Potten CS. Stem cells in epidermis from the back of the mouse. In Potten CS (ed): Stem Cells: Their Identification and Characterization. New York: Churchill-Livingston, 1983, pp 220-232.

141. Bohr V, Mansbridge J, Hanawalt P. Comparative effects of growth inhibitors on DNA replication, DNA repair, and protein synthesis in human epidermal keratinocytes. Cancer Res 46:2929-2935, 1986.
142. Hewitt RR, Meyn RE. Applicability of bacterial models of DNA repair and recovery to UV-irradiated mammalian cells. Adv Radiat Biol 7:153-179, 1978.
143. Ootsuymama A, Tanooka H. Unscheduled DNA synthesis after β-irradiation of mouse skin in situ. Mutat Res 166:183-185, 1986.
144. Liu S-C, Parsons S, Hanawalt PC. DNA repair in cultured keratinocytes. J Invest Dermatol 81:179s-183s, 1983.
145. Slaga TJ, Bracken WJ, Gleason G, Levin W, Yagi H, Jerina DM, Conney AH. Marked differences in the skin tumor-initiating activities of the optical enantiomers of the diastereomeric benzo[a]pyrene-7,8-diol-9,10-epoxides. Cancer Res 39:67-71, 1979.
146. Slaga TJ, Bracken WM, Viaje A, Levin W, Yagi H, Jerina DM, Conney AH. Comparison of the tumor-initiating activities of benzo[a]pyrene arene oxides and diol-epoxides. Cancer Res 37:4130-4133, 1977.
147. Pelling C, Slaga TJ. Comparison of levels of benzo[a]pyrene diol epoxide diastereomeric covalently bound in vivo. Carcinogenesis 3:1135-1141, 1982.
148. Berry DL, Lieber MR, Fischer SM, Slaga TJ. Qualitative and quantitative separation of a series of phorbol-ester tumor promoters by high pressure liquid chromatography. Cancer Lett 3:125-132, 1977.
149. Berry DL, Bracken WM, Fischer SM, Viaje A, Slaga TJ. Metabolic conversion of 12-O-tetradecanoylphorbol-13-acetate in adult and newborn mouse skin and mouse liver microsomes. Cancer Res 38:2301-2306, 1978.
150. Kreibich G, Suss R, Kinzel V. On the biochemical mechanism of tumorigenesis in mouse skin. V. Studies of the metabolism of tumor promoting and non-promoting phorbol derivatives in vivo and in vitro. Zeitschrift für Krebsforschung 81:135-149, 1974.
151. DiGiovanni J. Genetic determinants of susceptibility to mouse skin tumor promotion in inbred mice. In Colburn NA (ed): Genes and Signal Transduction in Multistage Carcinogenesis. New York: Marcel Dekker, in press, 1989.
152. Reiners J, Davidson K, Nelson K, Mamrack M, Slaga TJ. Skin tumor promotion: A comparative study of several stocks and strains of mice. In Langenbach R, Nesnow S, Rice JM (eds): Organ and Species Specificity in Chemical Carcinogenesis. New York: Plenum Press, 1983, pp 173-188.
153. Barrett JC, Brown MT, Sisskin EE. Deacylation of 12-O-[³H]tetradecanoylphorbol-13-acetate and [³H]phorbol-12,13-didecanoate in hamster skin and hamster cells in culture. Cancer Res 42:3098-3101, 1982.
154. Sisskin EE, Gray T, Barrett JC. Correlation between sensitivity to tumor promotion and sustained epidermal hyperplasia of mice and rats treated with 12-O-tetradecanoylphorbol-13-acetate. Carcinogenesis 3:403-407, 1982.
155. Shoyab M, Warren RC, Todaro GJ. Phorbol-1,13-diester 12-ester hydrolase may prevent tumor promotion by phorbol diesters in skin. Nature 295:152-154, 1982.
156. Segal A, Van Duuren BL, Mate U. The identification of phorbolol myristate acetate as a new metabolite of phorbol myristate acetate in mouse skin. Cancer Res 35:2154-2159, 1975.
157. O'Brien TG, Saladik D, Sina JR, Mullin JM. Formation of a glucuronide conjugate of 12-O-tetradecanoylphorbol-13-acetate by LLC-PK1, renal epithelial cells in culture. Carcinogenesis 3:1165-1169, 1982.
158. DiGiovanni J, Prichett WP, Decina PC, Diamond L. DBA/2 mice are as sensitive

as SENCAR mice to skin tumor promotion by 12-O-tetradecanoylphorbol-13-acetate. Carcinogenesis 5:1493-1498, 1984.

159. Slaga TJ. Overview of tumor promotion in animals. Environ Health Perspect 50:3-14, 1983.

160. Fujiki H, Mori M, Nakayasu M, Terada M, Sugimura T, Moore RE. Indole alkaloids: Dihydroteleocidin B, teleocidin, and lyngbyatoxin A as members of a new class of tumor promoters. Proc Natl Acad Sci USA 78:3872-3876, 1981.

161. Hagiwara N, Irie K, Tokuda H, Koshimizu K. The metabolism of indole alkaloid tumor promoter, (–)-indolactam V, which has the fundamental structure of teleocidins, by rat liver microsomes. Carcinogenesis 8:963-965, 1987.

162. Umezawa K, Weinstein IB, Horowitz A, Fujiki H, Matsushima T, Sugimura T. Similarity of teleocidin B and phorbol ester tumor promoters in effects on membrane receptors. Nature 290:411-413, 1981.

163. Khan AA. The isolation of 1,8-dihydroxy-3-methyl-9-anthrone from the root of *Rumex crispus*. Can J Chem 41:1622-1623, 1963.

164. King FE, Grundon MF, Neill KG. The chemistry of extractives of hardwoods. IX. Constituents of heartwood of *Ferreirea spectabilis*. Journal of the Chemical Society 4580-4584, 1952.

165. Simatupang MH, Dietrichs HH, Gottwald H. Uber die hautreizenden Stoffe in Vataireaguianensis Aubl. Holzforschung 21:89-94, 1967.

166. Fairbairn JW. The anthracene derivatives of medicinal plants. Lloydia 22:79-87, 1964.

167. Blumberg PM, Dunn JA, Jaken S, Jeng AY, Leach KL, Sharkey NA, Yeh E. Specific receptors for phorbol ester tumor promoters and their involvement in biological responses. In Slaga TJ (ed): Mechanisms of Tumor Promotion, Vol. 3. Boca Raton, FL: CRC Press, 1984 , pp 143-184.

168. DiGiovanni J, Kruszewski FH, Chenicek KJ. Studies on the skin tumor promoting actions of chrysarobin (1,8-dihydroxy-3-methyl-9-anthrone). In Butterworth B, Slaga TJ (eds): Banbury Report 25: Nongenotoxic Mechanisms in Carcinogenesis. Cold Spring Harbor, NY: Cold Spring Harbor Laboratory, 1987, pp 25-39.

169. DiGiovanni J, Decina PC, Prichett WP, Cantor J, Aalfs KK, Coombs MM. Mechanism of mouse skin tumor promotion by chrysarobin. Cancer Res 45:2584-2589, 1985.

170. Kruszewski FH, Chenicek KJ, DiGiovanni J. Effect of application frequency on epidermal ornithine decarboxylase induction by chrysarobin in SENCAR mice. Cancer Lett 32:263-269, 1986.

171. Kruszewski FJ, Conti CJ, DiGiovanni J. Characterization of skin tumor promotion and progression by chrysarobin. Cancer Res 47:3783-3790, 1987.

172. Kruszewski F, Naito M, Naito Y, DiGiovanni J. Histological alterations produced by the tumor promoting anthrone, chrysarobin, in mouse skin. J Invest Dermatol (in press) 1989.

173. Kruszewski FH, DiGiovanni J. Changes in epidermal polyamine levels and DNA synthesis following topical treatment of mouse skin with chrysarobin. Cancer Res 48:6390-6395, 1988.

174. DiGiovanni J, Kruszewski FH, Coombs MM, Bhatt TS, Pesezkh A. Structure-activity relationship for skin tumor promotion by anthrones. Carcinogenesis 9:1437-1443, 1988.

Skin Carcinogenesis: Mechanisms and Human Relevance, pages 201–212

The Protein Kinase C Pathway in Tumor Promotion

*Peter M. Blumberg, George R. Pettit, Barbour S. Warren,
Arpad Szallasi, Loretta D. Schuman, Nancy A. Sharkey,
Hideki Nakakuma, Marie L. Dell'Aquila,
and David J. de Vries*

*Molecular Mechanisms of Tumor Promotion Section, Laboratory of Cellular
Carcinogenesis and Tumor Promotion, National Cancer Institute, Bethesda,
Maryland 20892 (P.M.B., B.S.W., A.S., L.D.S., N.A.S., H.N., M.L.D., and
D.J.D.) and Cancer Research Institute and Department of Chemistry,
Arizona State University, Tempe, Arizona 85287 (G.R.P.)*

Protein kinase C, which is the major receptor for the phorbol ester tumor promoters, also binds and is activated by phorbol esters that are only second-stage tumor promoters or are nonpromoting. Bryostatins, macrocyclic lactones isolated from marine bryozoans, afford an opportunity to study such heterogeneity of response within the protein kinase C pathway. Bryostatins, like phorbol esters, bind to protein kinase C and stimulate its activity. However, bryostatins induce only a subset of the responses phorbol esters typically do, and they block those phorbol ester responses that they themselves fail to induce. Particularly, bryostatins showed only weak activity when assayed as tumor promoters and partially blocked promotion by phorbol esters. A more transient duration of action for bryostatins, associated with accelerated breakdown of protein kinase C, may explain some of these differences. In other cases, the responses tested differed in their intrinsic abilities to be stimulated. In C3H/10T1/2 cells, for example, arachidonic acid release, measurable at 30 min, is stimulated by phorbol esters but not by bryostatin 1, whereas epidermal growth factor binding is blocked by both ligands. Two indirect arguments suggest that bryostatins may interact at sites other than the high-affinity binding site on protein kinase C. Bryostatins block the inhibitory effect of phorbol esters on Friend erythroleukemia cell differentiation in an apparently noncompetitive fashion. In HL-60 cells, bryostatins induce the phosphorylation of all the proteins that phorbol esters do, as well as that of two unique proteins. Structure-activity analysis of naturally occurring bryostatin derivatives indicates that they differ in their relative phorbol ester-like and phorbol ester antagonistic activities. Bryostatin 3, for example, induces arachidonic acid release in C3H/10T1/2 cells at up to 60% of the level induced by phorbol esters, whereas bryostatin 1 blocks this response

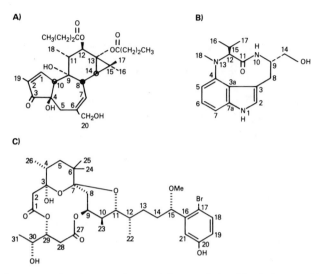

Figure 1. Structure of activators of protein kinase C. (A) Phorbol 12,13-dibutyrate, a semisynthetic phorbol derivative optimized for analysis of binding to protein kinase C. (B) (–)-Indolactam V, the basic ring structure for the indole alkaloid class of tumor promoters. (C) Aplysiatoxin, a representative of the polyacetate class of tumor promoters.

to bryostatin 3 as well as the response to phorbol esters. Computer modeling of bryostatins indicates structural homology with the phorbol ester pharmaco-phore model and is consistent with structure-activity analysis for binding and biological response.

Over the past 10 years, great progress has been made in advancing understanding of the initial events in the action of the phorbol ester tumor pro-moters (1-3) (Fig. 1). The major, and possibly exclusive, target of the phorbol esters is protein kinase C, an enzyme that mediates one arm of the phosphatidyl-inositol signal transduction pathway (4,5). For the many hormones and other cellular effectors that use this pathway, occupancy of their individual membrane receptors leads to activation of a cytosolic phospholipase C activity in what is thought to be a GTP-binding protein-mediated process. Phospholipase C cleaves a specific phospholipid, phosphatidylinositol 4,5-bisphosphate, to generate two products—sn-1,2-diacylglycerol and inositol 1,4,5-trisphosphate. Inositol 1,4,5-trisphosphate causes mobilization of intracellular calcium and the diacylglyc-erol binds to protein kinase C and activates it (4,5), apparently functioning as an endogenous phorbol ester analogue (6-8).

Unfortunately, this level of understanding is insufficient to allow accurate prediction of the consequences of treating an animal with a protein kinase C activator. Rather, considerable evidence suggests a heterogeneity in responses throughout the protein kinase C pathway (9). The analysis of phorbol ester binding to mouse skin particulate preparations indicates three binding sites with different affinity and structure-activity relations rather than a single binding site (10). In biological studies, different spectra of response have been observed for different phorbol esters. One of the best characterized examples is the comparison of mezerein and phorbol 12-myristate 13-acetate (PMA). Mezerein is similar in potency to PMA in terms of acute inflammatory and hyperplastic activity, but chronic treatment with mezerein fails to cause the sustained hyperplasia characteristic of PMA treatment (11).

Such heterogeneity could reflect either the existence of other phorbol ester targets than protein kinase C or heterogeneity within the protein kinase C system. The failure to identify other targets for the phorbol esters, together with much evidence that structurally distinct classes of activators of protein kinase C, in particular the indole alkaloids and polyacetates, share the same spectrum of biological responses as the phorbol esters (12), favor the latter possibility.

For protein kinase C, five mechanisms have been identified that could contribute to heterogeneity. First, protein kinase C is now known to be not a single enzyme but rather a family of related isozymes (13,14). As yet, the differences in the biochemical properties of these isozymes have not been characterized. Second, protein kinase C is not an enzymatically active moiety but rather is an apoenzyme that requires cofactors, namely anionic phospholipids and calcium, in order to be active. The nature of the phospholipids associated with protein kinase C largely determines the binding characteristics of the phospholipid-protein complex (15). Third, phospholipids determine not only the binding affinity of ligands for protein kinase C but also the consequences of that binding. Depending on the associated phospholipid, binding of a phorbol ester causes a greater or lesser degree of protein kinase C enzymatic activity (16). Fourth, different activators may induce different subcellular locations of activated protein kinase C. In the unstimulated cell, protein kinase C is largely found in the cytosol. Treatment of cells with a phorbol ester causes translocation of the enzyme to the membrane, where it can interact with the phorbol ester and, upon activation, phosphorylate substrates (17,18). Presumably, the substrates to which protein kinase C has access and, hence, the biological consequences of activation will depend on the cell membrane location at which the enzyme is activated. In turn, this will depend on the subcellular location of the activator. Finally, protein kinase C possesses two functional domains, a regulatory domain that binds calcium, phospholipid, and phorbol esters and an enzymatic domain responsible for kinase activity (4,5). Nishizuka and coworkers have shown that mild proteolytic treatment of the enzyme leads to cleavage of the two domains, liberating the enzymatic domain in an activated state. This proteolysis also occurs in intact cells, and the rate of breakdown of protein kinase C is enhanced in the presence of phorbol esters. As the phospholipid binding site responsible for membrane association of the intact kinase is on the regulatory domain, proteolytic cleavage of protein kinase C thus generates a catalytically active moiety that is present in the cytosol rather than on the membrane surface and that therefore has access to a different spectrum of substrates. Although each of the

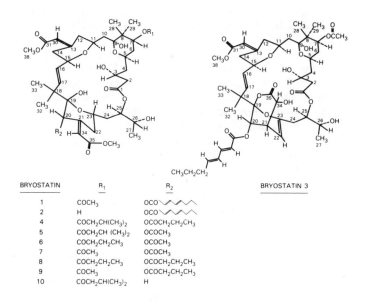

BRYOSTATIN	R₁	R₂
1	COCH₃	OCO ∿∿∿
2	H	OCO ∿∿
4	COCH₂CH(CH₃)₂	OCOCH₂CH₂CH₃
5	COCH₂CH (CH₃)₂	OCOCH₃
6	COCH₂CH₂CH₃	OCOCH₃
7	COCH₃	OCOCH₃
8	COCH₂CH₂CH₃	OCOCH₂CH₂CH₃
9	COCH₃	OCOCH₂CH₂CH₃
10	COCH₂CH(CH₃)₂	H

Figure 2. Structure of the bryostatins.

five mechanisms could contribute to the kinase's heterogeneity in response to the phorbol esters, as yet the relative contributions of these different mechanisms to the diversity in biological response have not been defined.

A class of compounds that promises to be of the utmost value in clarifying mechanisms of heterogeneity within the protein kinase C pathway is the bryostatins. In contrast to the phorbol esters, which are tetracyclic diterpenes, the bryostatins are macrocyclic lactones (19) (Fig. 2). They were isolated from marine bryozoans, in particular *Bugula neritina* and *Amathia convoluta*, on the basis of their antineoplastic activity in the P388 cell system. Initial studies demonstrated that the bryostatins blocked phorbol ester binding and activated protein kinase C (20,21). In addition, they induced similar biological responses to those of the phorbol esters. They activated neutrophils (22) and were mitogenic in Swiss 3T3 cells (20). Remarkably, however, in HL-60 promyelocytic leukemia cells, bryostatin 1 was reported not to induce differentiation, a typical phorbol ester response in these cells; bryostatin 1 also blocked the induction of differentiation in response to phorbol esters (21).

To explore the nature of this apparent antagonism between bryostatins and phorbol esters, we wished to distinguish between two possibilities: that the bryostatins were blocking differentiation responses themselves or, alternatively, that the bryostatins were blocking certain responses to the phorbol esters, including differentiation. To examine this question, we compared the activity of the phorbol esters and bryostatin 1 in Friend erythroleukemia cells (23). In this system, the phorbol esters cause the opposite response from that seen in the HL-60 cells; namely, the phorbol esters inhibit differentiation, whether spontaneous or induced by agents such as hexamethylene bisacetamide. Bryostatin 1 alone failed to inhibit differentiation in the Friend cell system; when present in combination with a phorbol ester, nanomolar concentrations of bryostatin 1 reversed the blockade of inhibition caused by phorbol ester treatment. These results strongly argued that the effect of bryostatins is to block specific phorbol ester responses rather than to block differentiation per se.

A second differentiating system that we examined was that of primary mouse epidermal cells. This system was chosen because different subpopulations of the cells respond to phorbol ester treatment by proliferation and by differentiation (24). We therefore thought we could use this cell type to distinguish within a single cell type between bryostatins' effects on phorbol ester-induced differentiation and on other responses. Ornithine decarboxylase is stimulated by phorbol esters and is a marker of the proliferative pathway. Bryostatin 1 at nanomolar concentrations induced ornithine decarboxylase activity, although not quite to the same level as did phorbol esters (25). Epidermal transglutaminase and cornified envelope formation are markers of the differentiation pathway in the primary epidermal cells. Bryostatin 1 induced neither transglutaminase activity nor cornified envelope formation and suppressed both the responses to phorbol ester treatment (25). These results suggest that bryostatins can distinguish between phorbol ester responses related to proliferation and those related to differentiation.

Further studies with mouse primary epidermal cells, however, suggested an alternative interpretation (26). Disruption of intercellular communication has been considered as a short-term assay for tumor-promoting activity. Intercellular communication can be measured by several techniques. We used microinjection of the fluorescent dye Lucifer yellow into a single cell and determined the number of cells into which the dye spread over a subsequent 10-min incubation period. In control epidermal cells, dye from a single injection spread into 30 to 40 adjacent cells. Phorbol ester treatment caused the rapid suppression of dye transfer, and this suppression was prolonged, lasting 12 to 24 h. Bryostatin 1, like the phorbol esters, caused rapid suppression of dye transfer. In marked contrast, however, suppression by bryostatin 1 only lasted 90 min, after which levels of dye transfer rapidly returned to control values. At the same time that bryostatin 1 lost its ability to inhibit dye transfer, the ability of phorbol esters to inhibit dye transfer in the presence of bryostatin 1 was also lost. These results suggest that one difference between the mechanisms of bryostatin and phorbol ester action may be that the duration of action for the bryostatins is shorter than that of the phorbol esters. The other results in the mouse primary epidermal cells can also be explained in terms of this model; ornithine decarboxylase induction was assayed at 3 h and was thus an early response, whereas the two differentiation responses—induction of epidermal transglutaminase and cornified envelope formation—were much later, at 9 and 24 h, respectively.

Although a shorter duration of action may explain some of the differences between bryostatins and phorbol esters, in other cases end points differ intrinsically in responsiveness (27). The C3H/10T1/2 fibroblast line is another cultured cell line that has been used for studying the in vitro action of tumor promoters. In this system, phorbol ester treatment causes the rapid release of labeled arachidonic acid from the cells, and this release can be measured for incubation times as short as 30 min. Bryostatin 1 causes only 15% of the release observed with phorbol ester treatment and upon coincubation suppresses the release induced by phorbol esters down to the level of release induced by bryostatin 1 alone. These results cannot be explained by an ultrashort duration of action for bryostatin 1 because for a different response—inhibition of epidermal growth factor binding—both the phorbol esters and bryostatin 1 caused inhibition that lasted many hours.

Not only do different end points within the same cell type differ intrinsically in their response to bryostatins but, reciprocally, the same end point responds differently in different cell types. This pattern has been best characterized for epidermal growth factor binding. As described above, in the C3H/10T1/2 cells, bryostatin 1 treatment caused the rapid inhibition of epidermal growth factor binding, and the level of binding recovered only to 25% of control values by 16 h of incubation. In contrast, in primary mouse epidermal cells, although the other biological responses reflected a transient duration of action, epidermal growth factor binding had largely recovered to control values by 4-6 h of incubation (25).

Most of the biological studies with bryostatins have been done with bryostatin 1. The characterization of related natural products has yielded a wealth of derivatives with modified functions. Using arachidonic acid release in the C3H/10T1/2 system, we have compared the activities of these different bryostatin derivatives with those of bryostatin 1 and of phorbol esters (27). We found that the different bryostatin derivatives varied in the degree to which they were bryostatin-like, that is, behaving like bryostatin 1, as compared with phorbol ester-like. Whereas bryostatin 1 caused only 15% of the level of arachidonic acid release induced by phorbol 12,13-dibutyrate, bryostatin 3 caused 60% of the phorbol ester-induced level of release. As we previously observed that bryostatins block those phorbol ester responses that bryostatins do not induce, we also examined the question of whether a bryostatin-like bryostatin such as bryostatin 1 would inhibit the release of arachidonic acid induced by a more phorbol ester-like bryostatin such as bryostatin 3. Consistent with the hypothesis that phorbol ester-like and bryostatin-like responses are mediated by different mechanisms, bryostatin 1 indeed blocked the enhanced response to bryostatin 3. An objective of future studies will be to clarify which structural features are responsible for the distinction between phorbol ester-like and bryostatin-like properties.

The differences in the behavior of different classes of protein kinase C agonists, as most forcefully illustrated in the case of the bryostatins, argue for the importance of extensive structure-activity analysis. Unfortunately, this approach has been limited by the lack of availability and by the chemical complexity of many of the naturally occurring agonists. An attractive complementary approach is the design of entirely synthetic agonists. As a guide to such synthesis, Dr. Paul Wender's laboratory in the Department of Chemistry at Stanford University has compared the x-ray crystallographic structures of phorbol esters, structurally related diterpenes, and indole alkaloids to identify the functional groups that are isospatial between these different classes of agonists (28). Results of this comparison suggest that the phorbol ester pharmacophore comprises a hydrophobic region, together with the hydroxyl groups of phorbol at the 4, 9, and 20 positions. Computer comparison of this model with the x-ray structure of bryostatins indicates excellent overlap and implicates a role for the hydroxyl groups at the 19 and 26 positions of bryostatin, together with the carbonyl at the 1 position (29). The modeling is consistent with our structure-activity analysis. Esterification of the 26 hydroxyl on the bryostatins causes loss of binding and biological activity. On the other hand, deletion of the ester groups at the 7 and 20 positions causes no loss of activity. Although the 19-oxygen atom occurs in a lactone in bryostatin 3, unlike the other bryostatins, this does not lead to a significant change in its three-dimensional position. The close fit of the bryostatins to the phorbol ester pharmacophore model and its agreement with the bryostatin structure-activity relations provide further support for the validity of this model.

Efforts to understand the biochemical basis for the heterogeneity of bryostatin action in different cell systems are still in early stages. Nonetheless, at least four mechanistic differences between bryostatins and phorbol esters have been identified that may contribute to this heterogeneity.

First, we have demonstrated by immunoblotting analysis that bryostatin treatment causes accelerated degradation of protein kinase C relative to the rate of degradation seen in phorbol ester-treated cells (Rivedal, Dell'Aquila, Leach, Yuspa, Herald, Pettit, and Blumberg, in preparation). This is true for Friend erythroleukemia cells, for primary mouse epidermal cells, and for C3H/10T1/2 cells. Accelerated degradation of protein kinase C would readily explain the transient duration of action of the bryostatins.

Second, the kinetics of ligand release from protein kinase C differ dramatically between bryostatins and phorbol esters (30). We have previously shown that the rate of release of phorbol esters from protein kinase C at 37°C is rapid. The kinetics of release of radioactively labeled bryostatin 4 from protein kinase C are heterogeneous, and the second phase of the release is very slow, with a half-life of several hours. The rapid rate of release of the phorbol ester should permit protein kinase C that has been translocated to one membrane compartment to reequilibrate and move to another membrane compartment. In contrast, a consequence of the slow rate of bryostatin release is that protein kinase C should be anchored at the membrane site where it first comes in contact with the bryostatin. We refer to this as the glue-trap model for bryostatin action.

Third, the bryostatins may have an additional class of targets that do not recognize the phorbol esters, at least at normal concentrations. Two lines of evidence support this possibility. First, in the Friend erythroleukemia cell system, in which bryostatins restore the differentiation response inhibited by phorbol esters, the amount of phorbol ester present in the assay was varied and its effect on the bryostatin dose-response curve for restoration was determined

(23). Because the assays were carried out over 5 days, equilibration should not have been a complicating factor. The result was clear cut: the antagonism of phorbol ester action by bryostatins was noncompetitive. The most straightforward interpretation is that the antagonistic action of the bryostatins is mediated by a high-affinity site that does not recognize phorbol esters with good efficiency. Further evidence for a bryostatin-specific site that does not recognize phorbol esters efficiently comes from studies of phosphorylation in the HL-60 cell system. In this system, we compared the ability of bryostatin 1 and phorbol 12,13-dibutyrate to induce phosphorylation of HL-60 proteins at 2-60 min after treatment (31). Our motivation was that the ability of bryostatins to induce only a subset of typical phorbol ester responses could reflect activation by bryostatin of only some of the protein kinase C isozymes. If this explanation were correct, then bryostatin treatment of the HL-60 cells would be predicted to induce phosphorylation of only some of the proteins phosphorylated in response to phorbol esters. In contrast, treatment with bryostatin 1 led to phosphorylation of all the proteins phosphorylated in response to phorbol 12,13-dibutyrate treatment. In addition, however, bryostatin 1 treatment caused the phosphorylation of two proteins that were not phosphorylated in response to the usual concentrations of phorbol esters. These results, like the evidence for noncompetitive antagonism of phorbol ester action in the Friend erythroleukemia cells, are consistent with bryostatins' having a site or sites of action in addition to using those of phorbol esters.

A fourth difference between bryostatins and phorbol esters is in their absolute affinities for protein kinase C. Both direct-binding measurements using radioactive bryostatin 4 and competition experiments using nonradioactive bryostatins suggest that the real potency of bryostatins for protein kinase C, at least under appropriate conditions of reconstitution into phosphatidylserine, may reflect a picomolar dissociation constant rather than the nanomolar dissociation constants typical for phorbol esters (32). If this is true for protein kinase C in biological membranes as well, then the structure-activity analysis in biological systems may be dominated by other factors that determine apparent potency. These factors might include dilution into the lipid phase of membranes, absorption onto the walls of the culture vessel, and titration of receptors, which are typically present at levels of 0.1-1 nM, depending on culture conditions. If such factors, rather than intrinsic binding affinity, determine the nanomolar concentrations of bryostatin required for many biological responses, then the biological systems potentially compress both the picomolar affinity responses to bryostatins and nanomolar affinity responses into a similar concentration range. Because the affinity of phorbol esters for protein kinase C is in the nanomolar range, responses to phorbol esters at micromolar concentrations might be equivalent to the situation observed with the bryostatins at nanomolar concentrations. The consequences of this model are still being explored, but initial studies suggest that micromolar concentrations of phorbol esters can indeed lead to some of the bryostatin-like effects described above. For example, the unique substrates phosphorylated by bryostatin in the HL-60 system are also phosphorylated in response to micromolar concentrations of phorbol 12,13-dibutyrate.

The relative contributions of these four mechanisms to the unique spectrum of responses induced by bryostatins are currently under evaluation. An important question is how the different isozymes of protein kinase C fit with the different rates of degradation or response.

The biological observation that in mouse primary epidermal cells, independent of the biochemical details of their mechanism, bryostatins failed to induce markers of differentiation and inhibited the induction of differentiation markers by phorbol esters is of the greatest interest. Yuspa and coworkers have postulated that induction of differentiation is a critical cellular feature of tumor promoters in mouse skin (24). Twin predictions of their model, therefore, are that bryostatins themselves should lack tumor-promoting activity and that bryostatins should antagonize tumor promotion by phorbol esters. Experiments using SENCAR mice confirm these predictions (33). Bryostatin 1 itself was not a complete tumor promoter and showed only weak activity relative to mezerein as a second-stage promoter. Application of bryostatin 1 and PMA at the same time led to a 50% suppression of tumor response relative to the PMA controls. The inhibition experiments were done with coapplication of bryostatin and PMA. From what we now know about the transient duration of bryostatin action in epidermal cell systems, we predict that application of bryostatin before PMA will lead to still more dramatic effects. Unfortunately, as in many of the bryostatin studies, the limited quantities of bryostatin currently restrict experimental design.

Great progress has been made in understanding how phorbol ester tumor promoters function. At the superficial level, therefore, one can predict that protein kinase C activators are candidate tumor promoters, as are those agents that act indirectly by elevating diglyceride or possibly calcium levels, leading to protein kinase C activation. Further analysis, however, demonstrates that our understanding is insufficient for reliable prediction. Phorbol ester-related analogues such as mezerein and other compounds such as bryostatins do not function as complete tumor promoters and may indeed antagonize a tumor promoter's action. Progress is being made toward understanding what is responsible for such differences in outcome. Nonetheless much remains to be done.

ACKNOWLEDGMENT

We thank Dr. Stuart H. Yuspa for critical reading of the manuscript.

OPEN FORUM

Dr. Stuart Yuspa: It is interesting to speculate that irradiation influences cell-cell communication in all cells, in addition to causing a mutation in a minor subpopulation. The change in cell-cell communication would then provide the permissive conditions to express the transformed phenotype at confluence.

Dr. Peter Blumberg: We don't know. You could visualize, for example, that you require both intact protein kinase C for part of the response and the proteolytically generated fragment of protein kinase C for another part of the response. The rate of breakdown of protein kinase C would determine whether the phorbol ester would be active. If you had too rapid or too slow breakdown of the enzyme, you might not get a hyperplastic response. If, in the C57 Bl6 mouse, protein kinase C broke down more slowly, for example, then bryostatin, which causes accelerated breakdown of protein kinase C, might give hyperplasia in that strain. We could presumably test the hypothesis by using immunoblotting to determine protein kinase C levels as a function of treatment and response.

Dr. Thomas J. Slaga: Although benzoyl peroxide does not seem to work through protein kinase C, you can give it at about any frequency to the C57 Black mice and get tumors.

Dr. Susan Fischer: Have you tried treating with bryostatin on a daily basis to see whether it would promote under those conditions?

Dr. Blumberg: No, we haven't because of the limited supply of bryostatin. The first step would be to examine hyperplasia because we could use fewer animals for a shorter period of time, which would require less bryostatin.

REFERENCES

1. Slaga TJ (ed): Mechanisms of Tumor Promotion. Boca Raton, FL: CRC Press, 1984.
2. Blumberg PM. Protein kinase C as the receptor for the phorbol ester tumor promoters: Sixth Rhoads Memorial Award Lecture. Cancer Res 48:1-8, 1988.
3. Aschendel CL. The phorbol ester receptor: A phospholipid-regulated protein kinase. Biochim Biophys Acta 822:219-242, 1985.
4. Nishizuka Y. The role of protein kinase C in cell surface signal transduction and tumor promotion. Nature 308:693-698, 1984.
5. Nishizuka Y. Studies and perspectives of protein kinase C. Science 233:305-312, 1986.
6. Sharkey NA, Leach KL, Blumberg PM. Competitive inhibition by diacylglycerol of specific phorbol ester binding. Proc Natl Acad Sci USA 81:607-610, 1984.
7. Sharkey NA, Blumberg PM. Kinetic evidence that 1,2-diolein inhibits phorbol ester binding to protein kinase C via a competitive mechanism. Biochem Biophys Res Commun 133:1051-1056, 1985.
8. Konig B, DiNitto PA, Blumberg PM. Stoichiometric binding of diacylglycerol to the phorbol ester receptor. J Cell Biochem 29:37-44, 1985.
9. Blumberg PM, Jaken S, Konig B, Sharkey NA, Leach KL, Jeng AY, Yeh E. Mechanism of action of the phorbol ester tumor promoters: Specific receptors for lipophilic ligands. Biochem Pharmacol 33:933-940, 1984.
10. Dunn JA, Blumberg PM. Specific binding of [20-^{3}H]12-deoxyphorbol 13-isobutyrate to phorbol ester receptor subclasses in mouse skin particulate preparations. Cancer Res 43:4632-4637, 1983.
11. Argyris TS. Nature of the epidermal hyperplasia produced by mezerein, a weak tumor promoter, in initiated skin of mice. Cancer Res 43:1768-1773, 1983.
12. Fujiki H, Sugimura T. New classes of tumor promoters: Teleocidin, aplysiatoxin, and palytoxin. Adv Cancer Res 49:223-264, 1987.
13. Coussens L, Parker PJ, Rhee L, Yang-Feng TL, Chen E, Waterfield MD, Franke U, Ullrich A. Multiple, distinct forms of bovine and human protein kinase C suggest

diversity in cellular signaling pathways. Science 233:859-866, 1986.

14. Knopf JL, Lee MH, Sultzman LA, Kriz RW, Loomis CR, Hewick RM, Bell RM. Cloning and expression of multiple protein kinase C cDNAs. Cell 46:491-502, 1986.

15. Konig B, DiNitto PA, Blumberg PM. Phospholipid and Ca^{++} dependency of phorbol ester receptors. J Cell Biochem 27:255-265, 1985.

16. Nakadate T, Blumberg PM. Modulation by palmitoylcarnitine of protein kinase C activation. Cancer Res 47:6537-6542, 1987.

17. Kraft AS, Anderson WB. Phorbol esters increase the amount of Ca^{++}, phospholipid-dependent protein kinase associated with plasma membrane. Nature 301:621-623, 1983.

18. Kraft AS, Anderson WB, Cooper HL, Sando JJ. Decrease in cytosolic calcium/phospholipid-dependent protein kinase activity following phorbol ester treatment of EL4 thymoma cells. J Biol Chem 257:13193-13196, 1982.

19. Pettit GR, Herald CL, Doubek DL, Herald DL, Arnold E, Clardy J. Isolation and structure of bryostatin 1. J Am Chem Soc 104:6846-6848, 1982.

20. Smith JA, Smith L, Pettit GR. Bryostatins: Potent, new mitogens that mimic phorbol ester tumor promoters. Biochem Biophys Res Commun 132:939-945, 1985.

21. Kraft AS, Smith JB, Berkow RL. Bryostatin, an activator of the calcium phospholipid-dependent protein kinase, blocks phorbol ester-induced differentiation of human promyelocytic leukemia cells HL-60. Proc Natl Acad Sci USA 83:1334-1338, 1986.

22. Berkow RL, Kraft AS. Bryostatin, a non-phorbol macrocyclic lactone, activates intact human polymorphonuclear leukocytes and binds to the phorbol ester receptor. Biochem Biophys Res Commun 131:1109-1116, 1985.

23. Dell'Aquila ML, Nguyen HT, Herald CL, Pettit GR, Blumberg PM. Inhibition by bryostatin 1 of the phorbol ester-induced blockage of differentiation in hexamethylene bisacetamide-treated Friend erythroleukemia cells. Cancer Res 47:6006-6009, 1987.

24. Yuspa SH, Hennings H, Lichti U. Initiator and promoter induced specific changes in epidermal function and biological potential. J Supramol Struct Cell Biochem 17:245-257, 1981.

25. Sako T, Yuspa SH, Herald CL, Pettit GR, Blumberg PM. Partial parallelism and partial blockade by bryostatin 1 of effects of phorbol ester tumor promoters on primary mouse epidermal cells. Cancer Res 47:5445-5450, 1987.

26. Pasti G, Rivedal E, Yuspa SH, Herald CL, Pettit GR, Blumberg PM. Transient inhibition of cell-cell communication in primary mouse epidermal cells by bryostatin 1. Cancer Res 48:447-451, 1988.

27. Dell'Aquila ML, Herald CL, Kamano Y, Pettit GR. Differential effects of bryostatins and phorbol esters on arachidonic acid metabolite release and epidermal growth factor binding in C3H10T1/2 cells. Cancer Res 48:3702-3708, 1988.

28. Wender PA, Koehler KF, Sharkey NA, Dell'Aquila ML, Blumberg PM. Analysis of the phorbol ester pharmacophore on protein kinase C as a guide to the rational design of new classes of analogs. Proc Natl Acad Sci USA 83:4214-4218, 1986.

29. Wender PA, Cribbs CM, Koehler KF, Sharkey NA, Herald CL, Kamano Y, Pettit GR, Blumberg PM. Modeling of the bryostatins to the phorbol ester pharmacophore on protein kinase C. Proc Natl Acad Sci USA 85:7197-7201, 1988.

30. Sharkey NA, de Vries DJ, Kamano Y, Pettit GR, Blumberg PM. Binding of [^{3}H]bryostatin 4 to protein kinase C (PKC) (abstract). Proceedings of the American Association for Cancer Research 29:160, 1988.

31. Warren BS, Herald CL, Pettit GR, Blumberg PM. Bryostatins 1 and 9 induce phos-

phorylation of a unique series of 70 kDa proteins in HL-60 cells. J Cell Biochem 11A:47, 1987.

32. de Vries DJ, Herald CL, Pettit GR, Blumberg PM. Demonstration of subnanomolar affinity of bryostatin 1 for the phorbol ester receptor in rat brain. Biochem Pharmacol (in press) 1988.

33. Hennings H, Blumberg PM, Pettit GR, Herald CL, Shores R, Yuspa SH. Bryostatin 1, an activator of protein kinase C, inhibits tumor promotion by phorbol esters in SENCAR mouse skin. Carcinogenesis 8:1343-1346, 1987.

Skin Carcinogenesis: Mechanisms and Human Relevance, pages 213–231

Regulation of Ornithine Decarboxylase in Normal and Neoplastic Mouse and Human Epidermis

Thomas G. O'Brien, Leonard Dzubow, Andrzej A. Dlugosz, Susan K. Gilmour, Kevin O'Donnell, and Oili Hietala

Wistar Institute, Philadelphia, Pennsylvania 19104 (T.G.O., S.K.G., K.O., O.H.), and Department of Dermatology, Hospital of the University of Pennsylvania, Philadelphia, Pennsylvania 19104 (L.D., A.A.D.)

Research into mouse skin carcinogenesis over the last 15 years has established an important, although still not completely defined, role for greatly elevated rates of polyamine biosynthesis in the tumor promotion stage of neoplastic development (1-3). Experimentally, this has been inferred from data showing that strong tumor promoters such as the phorbol esters cause induction of large amounts of the enzyme ornithine decarboxylase (ODC) within a few hours after treatment. ODC is the presumed rate-limiting enzyme for polyamine biosynthesis, and, in fact, large increases in epidermal polyamine levels have been measured in mouse epidermis after treatment with a strong inducer of ODC such as 12-O-tetradecanoylphorbol-13-acetate (TPA). Epidermal tumors produced by tumor initiation and promotion protocols have basal levels of ODC much higher than the basal level present in normal epidermis (1,4). Furthermore, limitation of polyamine biosynthesis during tumor promotion by a specific inhibitor of ODC, α-difluoromethylornithine (DFMO), substantially reduced skin tumor incidence and multiplicity (5,6).

Recent work from this laboratory has demonstrated the presence in epidermal tumors of a form of ODC that is structurally and functionally different from the ODC induced by phorbol esters in normal epidermis (4). This new form is characterized by a higher apparent molecular weight according to gel filtration chromatography and, most surprisingly, its activation by GTP (7). Mammalian ODC has never been reported to be affected by nucleotides such as GTP, and we have never detected a GTP-stimulable form of ODC in any normal mouse tissue, embryonic or postnatal, examined (O'Brien TG, O'Donnell K, unpublished data). Our working hypothesis is that as a result of tumor initiation and promotion in mouse skin, a new form of ODC is produced (via mutation, expression of a silent gene, posttranslational modifications, or other possible means), which is no longer subject to the tight control of ODC characteristic of normal tissues. This relatively unregulated ODC would then confer on cells containing it a selective growth advantage or a decreased propensity to enter into a differentiation pathway. Seen in this highly speculative light, ODC is a gene product that, if unregulated, can help to drive a cell from the initiation stage to a clone of cells observed visually and histopathologically as a papilloma. Of course, other gene products are undoubtedly differentially expressed during this stage of carcinogenesis and may be as important as, or more important than, ODC. We view the loss of control of genes critical to growth and differentiation as one of the key elements in tumor promotion. The study of how ODC regulation differs in normal and neoplastic epidermal cells may reveal more general mechanisms involved in the altered control of other genes important to the carcinogenic process.

It is virtually axiomatic among basic researchers that knowledge gained from experimental carcinogenesis models (largely in vitro systems and in vivo studies in rodents) will eventually be applied to the treatment and prevention of cancer in humans. But is this axiom necessarily true? If one considers the postinitiation stages of carcinogenesis as the most amenable to intervention/prevention strategies, what rational therapies for the treatment or prevention of epithelial cancers have been devised as a result of the extensive research with experimental models? A few examples come to mind, retinoids being perhaps the most prominent, but the overall results so far with respect to human cancer treatment have been disappointing. Does this mean that basic research is flawed or, perhaps more ominous, the rodent models are not relevant to human cancer development and progression? To distinguish these possibilities, it is the basic researchers' responsibility, albeit a difficult one, to attempt to validate their findings from experimental animal models in a relevant human model whenever possible. Therefore, to test the relevance of aberrant ODC expression to human cancer, we decided to analyze the properties of ODC in the closest human equivalent of the end result of two-stage carcinogenesis in mice, i.e., squamous cell carcinoma. The specific activities and the enzymatic properties of ODC from human cutaneous squamous cell carcinomas were compared with those of the enzyme present in normal skin. Because of evidence that aberrant regulation of ODC can drive tumor promotion in mouse skin, we sought to find evidence for disturbances in ODC regulation in human skin tumors. Our results strongly support the view that data from experimental carcinogenesis models in rodents can be extrapolated to human cancer.

MATERIALS AND METHODS

Animals and Treatment

Female CD-1 mice were used, beginning at 7 weeks of age. The dorsal hair was shaved at least 2 days prior to treatment, and all chemicals were applied percutaneously to the shaved area. For papilloma induction, mice received a single treatment with 7,12-dimethylbenz[a]anthracene (DMBA), followed 1 week later by twice-weekly applications of 17 nmol TPA. When at least some of the multiple tumors in an animal reached 5 mm, TPA treatment was stopped for at least 1 week before the animals were killed and tumors were harvested for ODC determinations. To obtain sufficient enzyme activity from epidermis, it was necessary to induce the enzyme with either a single or multiple (five) treatments with 17 nmol TPA. In either case, mice were killed 4.5 h later, and epidermal extracts were prepared.

Human Tissue

Histologically proven human squamous cell carcinomas from various skin sites were surgically excised, and portions were either quick frozen for ODC analysis or fixed and processed for immunocytochemistry as described (8). None of the tumors used in this study exhibited signs of infection, and the surgical areas were thoroughly swabbed with 70% isopropyl alcohol prior to excision. Normal human skin was obtained from the scalps of adult patients undergoing hair transplant surgery and from excised foreskins of newborns.

Biochemical Procedures

Crude extracts of normal and tumor tissue were prepared as described (4) from either fresh tissue or from samples that had been quick frozen in liquid N_2 and stored at $-80°C$. Procedures for gel filtration chromatography, kinetic analyses, and immunocytochemistry have been described in detail elsewhere (4,7,8).

RESULTS

Our experimental work with mouse skin model systems and carcinogen-induced epidermal tumors has been directed toward explaining tumor promotion in human skin in particular and human epithelial tissues in general. Although most of our results in the mouse skin system have been either the subjects of reviews or recently published (1,3,4,7), we will briefly summarize these findings before discussing results of our work on human tissues.

It has been known for more than 10 years that epidermal tumors produced by a two-stage protocol have much higher basal levels of ODC than does unstimulated mouse epidermis, even weeks after the last promoter treatment (1,4,9). In general, malignant squamous cell carcinomas have higher enzyme levels than do benign papillomas. Such results are not surprising, as similar data have been reported for other tumor and normal tissue comparisons (10). What is somewhat surprising is the finding that much of this elevated level of ODC within tumors is concentrated in a very few cells, as determined by in situ immunocytochemistry with an anti-ODC antibody (8). Such a high level of ODC at the cellular level has only been observed in normal tissue after it has been exposed to a strong inducing stimulus such as chronic TPA treatment of the skin (1) or androgen treatment of the mouse kidney (11). These immunocytochemical results strongly suggest that the control of enzyme synthesis and/or degradation is altered in at least some cells within these tumors.

In considering possible explanations for the relative loss of control of ODC expression in tumors, we investigated the possibility that tumor-specific structural alterations occur in the ODC protein itself. The rationale for these studies was that because ODC turns over very rapidly in epidermis (half-life of approximately 17 minutes) and apparently quite slowly in epidermal papillomas (1,9), a structural difference in tumor ODC might allow it to evade the specific degradative system responsible for ODC turnover. Thus the enzyme, once made by the cell, would be quite stable, in contrast to the rapidly turned over protein in normal mammalian cells. To test this idea, the enzymatic and structural properties of epidermal ODC and epidermal tumor ODC were compared. As explained in detail in our earlier publications (4,7), the epidermal tumor ODCs clearly differ in their enzymatic and structural properties from the enzyme present in normal epidermis. To obtain enough enzyme activity from normal epidermis for analysis, we compared the characteristics of TPA-induced ODC from normal epidermis and constitutively expressed epidermal tumor ODC. All of the tumors analyzed were induced by DMBA initiation and TPA promotion protocols. Most of the data have been obtained from papillomas, but results with squamous cell carcinomas were qualitatively similar. In all cases, promotion with TPA was stopped at least a week prior to harvesting epidermal tumors to eliminate any residual effects of the last promoter application on ODC activity. Table 1 summarizes the differences so far detected in the properties of ODC isolated from normal epidermis and epidermal tumors. One of the surprising differences observed was an apparent alteration in the active site of the papilloma enzyme, since the apparent K_m values for substrate L-ornithine and cofactor pyridoxal-5'-phosphate were substantially higher for tumor ODC than for epidermal ODC (Table 2). Based on these and other data, it was concluded that individual epidermal tumors produced by a tumor initiation-promotion protocol contain multiple active ODC isoforms, at least one of which has only been found in tumors. Another salient difference observed was the presence of a unique size of ODC in tumor extracts and the ability of the tumor enzyme, but not the epidermal ODC, to be activated by GTP.[1] This was most clearly seen when crude extracts of epidermal ODC and individual papillomas were chromatographed on an Ultrogel AcA34 column (LKB Products), which separates proteins according to molecular size. As shown in Figure 1, the epidermal enzyme chromatographed as a single peak with an approximate molecular weight of 100,000. When a crude extract of pooled papillomas was chromatographed, two peaks of enzyme activity were observed when the usual assay was conducted (Fig. 2). The major peak coincided with the position of the single peak of activity from the epidermal extract, while a smaller peak of higher molecular weight was consistently observed in this and several other experiments with epidermal tumor extracts. When a crude extract made from a single papilloma was analyzed, the same two peaks of ODC activity were detected (Hietala O, O'Brien TG, unpublished data), suggesting that both

---

[1] Activation refers to an increased activity of ODC in a cell-free extract upon addition of GTP without implying a specific mechanism.

Table 1. Properties of Mouse Ornithine Decarboxylase

Epidermis	Epidermal tumors
Heat labile	Heat resistant
Low K_m L-ornithine	High K_m L-ornithine
No effect of nucleotides	Activated by GTP
One form on native gels	Two forms on native gels
Super-inducible in perifollicular cells	Constitutively elevated in minor cell population
Subunit MW 54,500	Subunit MW 54,500
PIs 6.2–6.5	PIs 5.2–5.5

Table 2. Kinetic Properties of Mouse Epidermal and Papilloma ODC*

Tissue	Properties of ODC			
	L-Ornithine K_m (mM)	V_{max} (units/mg)	Heat sensitivity†	PLP K_m (μM)
Epidermis	0.07	10.4	++++	0.20
Papilloma				
A	1.10	10.2	+	
B	0.28	3.5	+	
C	1.00	7.7	+	1.7
D	0.31	3.7	++	
E	0.36	13.6	++	1.5
F	1.20	18.3	ND	
G	0.36	3.8	ND	
H	0.80	24.4	+	

* K_m and V_{max} values were obtained from Lineweaver-Burk reciprocal plots. The values for epidermis are the average of two different preparations.
† ++++, >95% inactivation after 4 min (at 55°C); ++, >50%<90% inactivation after 4 min; +, <50% inactivation after 4 min. (From O'Brien et al. Proc Natl Acad Sci USA 1986; 83:9448–9452.)
Abbreviations: ND, not determined; ODC, ornithine decarboxylase; PLP, pyridoxal 5′-phosphate.

peaks of enzyme activity can be obtained from a single tumor. When the column fractions were assayed in the presence of GTP, moreover, an interesting pattern emerged: the early-eluting higher-molecular-weight form of ODC was greatly stimulated by GTP, but the second peak was not. We have termed the GTP-activable form peak I ODC and the second form peak II.

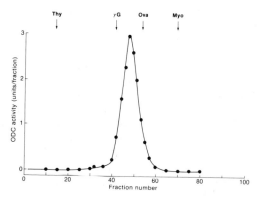

Figure 1. Gel filtration chromatography of epidermal ornithine decarboxylase (ODC). A crude extract of epidermis derived from mice treated five times with 17 nmol TPA was chromatographed on Ultrogel AcA34 as described in ref. 7. Fraction 1 is taken as the first fraction after the void volume of the column. Some of the peak fractions containing ODC activity were also assayed in the presence of 0.1 mM GTP. No effect was observed (data not shown). The elution positions of standard proteins (molecular weights in parentheses) are indicated: Thy, thyroglobulin (670,000); γG, immunoglobulin (158,000); Ova, ovalbumin (44,000); and Myo, myoglobin (17,000). (From O'Brien et al. Proc Natl Acad Sci USA 1987; 84:8927–8931.)

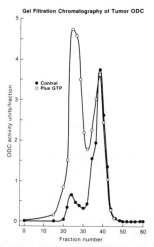

Figure 2. Gel filtration chromatography of papilloma ornithine decarboxylase (ODC). A crude extract derived from several pooled papillomas was chromatographed on the same column used in the experiment described in Figure 1. Fractions containing ODC activity were assayed in the presence (o) or absence (•) of 0.1 mM GTP at an L-ornithine concentration of 0.125 mM.

The activation of epidermal tumor ODC by GTP has heretofore not been described for mammalian ODC. We have studied the mechanism of this activation in some detail (7). As shown in Figure 3, enzyme kinetic analyses clearly indicate in unfractionated crude extracts that GTP causes a substantial reduction in the apparent K_m for L-ornithine from the aforementioned atypically high values of the tumor enzyme to apparent K_m values characteristic of mammalian ODC (0.076 ± 0.013 mM, $n=5$). If a crude tumor extract is chromatographed as in Figure 2, kinetic analyses indicate that peak I ODC has a very high K_m for L-ornithine (1.25 mM), which is reduced to 0.05 mM in the presence of GTP, whereas the K_m of peak II ODC is 0.05 mM and is unaffected by GTP. Peaks I and II ODC also differ in their sensitivity to heat inactivation and whether the presence of GTP can protect against heat inactivation (7).

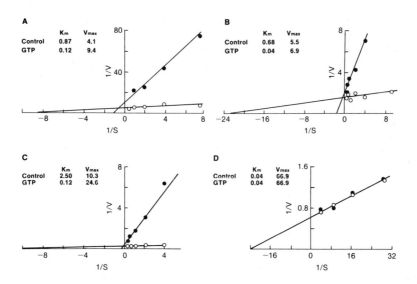

Figure 3. The kinetics of activation of epidermal tumor ornithine decarboxylase (ODC) by GTP. The enzyme activity of crude extracts of individual papillomas (A and B), a squamous cell carcinoma (C), and epidermis treated five times with 12-O-tetradecanoylphorbol-13-acetate (TPA) (D) was measured at various L-ornithine concentrations in the presence (o) or absence (•) of 0.1 mM GTP. The data are expressed as Lineweaver-Burk plots, and the lines have been derived from linear regression analysis. The units for the kinetic parameters are mM K_m and units/mg protein for V_{max}. (From O'Brien et al. Proc Natl Acad Sci USA 1987; 84:8927–8931.)

Properties of ODC in Normal Human Skin and Human Squamous Cell Carcinomas of the Skin

If our results with experimental mouse skin carcinogenesis suggest an important role for constitutively elevated ODC levels in tumor promotion, what predictions would follow if human squamous cell carcinoma development were analogous to the mouse model, that is, exhibited a tumor promotion-like stage? With respect to ODC, several predictions can be made. First, the basal levels of ODC activity would be much higher in tumor tissue than in normal skin. Second, some or all tumors may contain new, tumor-specific forms of ODC. Third, some or all tumor extracts will contain a GTP-activable ODC. Fourth, loss of the ability to regulate ODC levels might be detected in tumors at the cellular level by immunocytochemical methods using an anti-ODC antibody. We have designed our experiments (with the sometimes-limited amount of tumor tissue available) to test the above predictions.

Initial assays of crude extracts of both normal-appearing skin and histologically proved squamous cell carcinomas were done in the presence and absence of GTP because this is an easy and sensitive assay for the presence of a functionally altered ODC. Our preliminary results are summarized in Table 3. Compared with either adult or neonatal skin, all the tumor extracts contained elevated levels of ODC, as reported by others (12); in addition, four of the seven tumors examined contained ODC activity that could be stimulated by GTP. Enzyme kinetic analyses were done on most of these extracts, and the results are presented in Figure 4 and Table 4. As shown in Figure 4, panels A and B, GTP lowered the apparent K_m for L-ornithine in some tumor extracts, whereas in other tumors (Table 3; Fig. 4, panels C and D) GTP did not affect apparent K_m but did increase the V_{max} of the enzyme. These results differ somewhat from mouse epidermal tumors, in which GTP always lowered the apparent K_m of the tumor enzyme for L-ornithine and only sometimes increased the V_{max}. In subsequent work, the number of tumors examined has been increased to 18, with little change in the proportion of tumor ODCs that can be stimulated by GTP [10 of 18 (56%) versus 4 of 7 (57%) in Table 3; Hietala O, O'Brien TG, unpublished results].

Gel filtration analysis of crude tumor extracts has been difficult because of the limited amount of enzyme activity available and the lack of sufficient normal tissue ODC for comparison. Nevertheless, results with some of the tumor extracts listed in Table 3 have been informative. For example, chromatography of the crude extract of tumor D revealed multiple peaks of activity (Fig. 5), only one of which could be stimulated by GTP (see inset, Fig. 5). It is important to point out that although the crude extract of this tumor was only stimulated 50% by GTP, once the active forms were separated by chromatography, the activation of one of the peaks (peak I) was approximately 300%. The human tumor extracts appear to exhibit more complexity upon chromatographic analysis than the mouse epidermal tumor extracts previously examined, but two important similarities remain: multiple species of active ODC are present in tumors, and apparently only one of the forms present is activated by GTP.

Table 3. ODC Activity in Normal Human Skin and Squamous Cell Carcinomas*

Tissue	ODC activity (units/mg protein)		
	−GTP	+GTP (0.1 mM)	Ratio +GTP/−GTP
Normal scalp	0.042	0.044	1.0
Foreskin	0.093	0.077	0.8
Squamous cell carcinoma			
A	13.40	80.20	6.0
B	0.92	7.34	8.0
C	0.29	0.45	1.6
D	1.13	1.69	1.5
E	10.70	10.70	1.0
F	3.98	3.66	0.9
G	0.22	0.22	1.0

* Crude extracts of normal tissue or cutaneous squamous cell carcinomas were assayed for enzyme activity in the presence or absence of 0.1 mM GTP at a L-ornithine concentration of 0.125 mM.
Abbreviation: ODC, ornithine decarboxylase.

Table 4. Kinetic Properties of Human Epidermal and Squamous Cell Carcinoma ODC

Tissue	ODC kinetic parameters*			
	L-Ornithine K_m (mM)		V_{max} (units/mg)	
	−GTP	+GTP	−GTP	+GTP
Normal scalp	0.036	ND	0.104	ND
Squamous cell carcinoma				
A	1.430	0.048	72.70	87.60
B	0.200	0.023	0.18	6.90
C	0.034	0.033	0.35	0.40
D	0.066	0.068	1.72	2.04
E	0.064	ND	14.54	ND
F	0.013	ND	4.69	ND
G	ND	ND	ND	ND

* Kinetic parameters were determined graphically from Lineweaver-Burk reciprocal plots of data from at least 4 L-ornithine concentrations. If GTP did not stimulate ornithine decarboxylase (ODC) activity in the initial assay (see Table 3), kinetic analyses were not determined in the presence of GTP.
Abbreviation: ND, not determined.

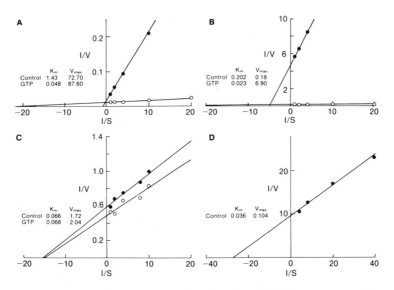

Figure 4. Kinetic analyses of ornithine decarboxylase (ODC) from tumors and normal skin. Crude extracts of tumors A, B, and D (Table 3) were assayed for ODC activity at varying L-ornithine concentrations in the presence (o) or absence (•) of 0.1 mM GTP (panels A, B, and C). Results are expressed as double reciprocal plots and the calculated kinetic parameters are shown in the inset to each panel. The enzyme from normal scalp skin (panel D) was analyzed in the absence of GTP because preliminary assays with this extract as well as ODC from other normal skin extracts showed no effect of GTP addition (data not shown). (From Hietala et al. Cancer Res 48:1252-1257, 1988, with permission.)

At the cellular level, immunolocalization studies using anti-ODC antibodies have detected a minor population of cells within some human squamous cell carcinomas (especially those with high ODC content measured enzymatically) that exhibit intense specific staining for ODC (13; S. Gilmour, unpublished data). Attempts to detect specific ODC staining in normal skin by this technique were uniformly negative. Thus we have evidence in human squamous cell carcinomas for a constitutively high expression of ODC at the cellular level, a situation also observed in mouse epidermal tumors (8). We attribute this high level of expression in both mouse and human tumors to so-far-unexplained disturbances in control mechanisms that normally tightly regulate the level of ODC. By contrast, high levels of ODC expression at the cellular level can be observed in tumor-promoter-treated normal mouse epidermis, but this induced enzyme is quite transient in nature compared with the apparently long-lived enzyme found in tumors. It is our impression from examining a limited number of tumors that high levels of ODC expression at the cellular level are most readily observed in human tumors containing a GTP-activable ODC, suggesting that a

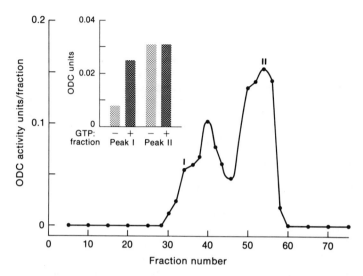

Figure 5. Gel filtration analysis of ornithine decarboxylase (ODC) from a squamous cell carcinoma. An Ultrogel AcA34 column (1.6 x 55 cm) was equilibrated with buffer, and a crude extract of tumor was chromatographed as described in the legend to Figure 1. The peak fractions containing ODC activity were pooled, concentrated, and assayed for enzyme activity in the presence or absence of 0.1 mM GTP (inset). (From Hietala et al. Cancer Res 48:1252-1257, 1988, with permission.)

functionally different form of ODC may be the actual enzyme species that is overexpressed in these tumors.

It was of interest to correlate the biologic behavior of the cutaneous squamous cell carcinomas we have obtained with the properties of ODC contained therein. Several factors are known to influence the clinical features of these tumors, including tumor size and depth, etiology (actinic versus nonactinic), and anatomic site (14). In the limited series of tumors listed in Table 3, it appears that the presence of a GTP-activable ODC correlates with an aggressive biologic behavior. For example, tumor A was a large tumor that arose at the site of a prior burn scar. Tumor C was a very large tumor arising in a non-sun-exposed area (the groin). Tumor D also was a very large tumor, of the penis. In contrast, tumors E, F, and G were small tumors found on sun-exposed areas and were clinically nonaggressive. A more extensive tumor series is needed to draw firm conclusions, but these preliminary data indicate a possible correlation between the presence of a GTP-activable ODC within a tumor and its biological behavior.

DISCUSSION

Over the last 30 years, much of the experimental work on skin carcinogenesis has focused on the mechanism of tumor promotion because if an analogous stage exists in human carcinogenesis, as is most likely, understanding the principles of the process may be easily translated into cancer intervention or prevention strategies in humans, at least for certain high-risk populations. Given what is known about the early (tumor initiation) and late (metastasis) stages of neoplastic development, it seems less likely that strategies designed to intervene in these processes will be successful. Clearly, the vast middle period of tumor development (encompassing tumor promotion and the early stage of tumor progression) is more susceptible to modulation by exogenous agents in rodents and, it is hoped, in humans as well.

Our attempts to understand tumor promotion in mouse skin have been guided by two basic questions. First, the activation or enhanced/inhibited expression of which genes drives the continued proliferation of initiated cells? Second, what accounts for the selective proliferation of initiated cells, and perhaps other cell populations, relative to other cells within the epidermis? With regard to the first question, it has been widely assumed since it was first articulated by Boutwell in 1974 (15) that gene activation is an important attribute of tumor promotion. The question is, which genes? While much attention in mouse skin and other carcinogenesis models has focused on the class of genes termed proto-oncogenes, and deservedly so, our laboratory has considered the possibility that another class of genes, which might be termed cellular growth-regulatory genes (with no homology to known viral genes), might also be involved in tumor promotion. Our hypothesis has been that tumor initiation might introduce a heritable alteration into a few cells, with the result being the inability to properly regulate one of these important growth-related genes. Tumor promoters, by virtue of their ability to increase the expression of this key gene or genes, would stress the initiated cell by elevating the level of a gene product that the cell was now unable to regulate normally. Because the gene is involved in growth control, one would expect disturbances in growth and/or differentiation to ensue as a consequence of tumor initiation plus promotion protocols. Promoter treatment alone should not result in abnormal growth behavior, as none of the cells would have the tumor initiation-induced regulatory defect. ODC is a good candidate for this class of cellular growth-regulatory genes because polyamines are essential for growth (16), ODC is one of the key enzymes regulating polyamine biosynthesis (17), the levels of ODC and its mRNA are very tightly controlled in most normal tissues including epidermis (18, 19), and effective tumor promoters are very potent inducers of ODC in mouse epidermis (20, 21).

What has been lacking until recently is evidence that the control of ODC synthesis and/or its degradation is specifically altered in tumors as compared with normal skin. There has been suggestive but not definitive evidence for 12 years or more that the characteristically short half-life of ODC (17 min in normal epidermis) is abnormally long in epidermal papillomas (9). With the recent availability of molecular reagents specific for the ODC protein (22) and its mRNA

(23, 24), it has become clear that some aspects of the regulation of ODC have become deranged in mouse epidermal tumors, at least in certain cell populations within these tumors (8).

Our data concerning ODC regulation in mouse epidermis also bear on the second question—that concerning the mechanism of promoter-driven clonal expansion of cells treated with tumor-initiating agents relative to other cells in the tissue. The literature gives the impression that cells that have undergone initiation are the only cells in the chronically promoter-treated epidermis that expand relative to the total epidermal cell population. This is a natural conclusion, as the neoplastic phenotype is usually the end point being scored (papillomas). However, the results of ODC immunolocalization studies of previously uniniti-ated skin treated five times with TPA emphasize that promoters can cause the clonal expansion of other cells as well. In this case, chronic (but not single) treat-ment with TPA leads to the appearance of a cell population that is hyperinducible for ODC and perhaps other genes as well. Thus, the ability of promoters to clonally expand certain cell populations within the epidermis is an intrinsic property of this class of agents and is not dependent on whether the tissue has been exposed to tumor-initiating agents or not. The original, rather simplistic view of effective promoters as agents capable of stimulating cell division within the epidermis, then, can be modified to incorporate three distinct proliferation-related properties: after acute exposure, a global epidermal hyperplasia occurs that most likely is regenerative in nature; with chronic exposure, effective pro-moters produce sustained hyperplasia, whereas weak promoters or nonpromot-ers do not; and within the overall hyperplastic epidermis, certain cell popula-tions increase in number relative to others, i.e., clonal expansion occurs. This process is obvious in skin treated with a tumor initiation and promotion protocol but nevertheless occurs in skin treated only with tumor promoters as well.

Given the highly specialized nature of the multistage mouse skin carcino-genesis model, extrapolations of research results to skin cancer in humans can be risky. For example, phorbol esters and related TPA-type promoters probably play a vanishingly small role in human skin cancer. How much of what we know about how these agents work is applicable to the action of promoters on human skin, whatever they may be? A better question might be whether any of the phenotypic changes produced in mouse skin by promoters and thought to be important to tumor promotion can be observed in humans. This is a difficult question to pursue experimentally for obvious reasons, but the recent advances in serial culture of keratinocytes (25), as well as human skin grafting techniques (see the chapter in this book by JG Rheinwald), present promising experimental systems for future study. We have taken a different approach in attempting to extrapolate our findings on ODC regulation in normal and neoplastic mouse skin to humans. Our rationale was that if disturbances in ODC regulation confer a selective growth advantage on human epidermal cells that have undergone tumor initiation, then human cutaneous squamous cell carcinomas should exhibit some of the same changes in ODC activity/structure/function/expression seen in mouse tumors, even though the former have not received tumor-promoting treatment with a strong inducer of ODC such as TPA. In other words, if loss of control of ODC is important in the process of neoplastic development, it should be possible to detect such alterations in at least some human premalignant or malignant lesions. We chose to study human squamous cell carcinomas rather than the more common basal cell carcinomas because they are the closest human equivalent in histopathologic terms of the end point of neoplastic development to multistage mouse carcinogenesis.

The results of our analyses of human squamous cell carcinomas have been encouraging. Confirming the results of others (12), we found that the tumors have a much higher ODC activity level than normal skin does. And, of greater interest in approximately 60% of the tumors examined, a GTP-activable ODC could be detected. This is a minimal estimate of the percentage of tumors containing this isoform of ODC because in human tumors, as opposed to the mouse tumors we have analyzed previously, there is the possibility of sampling error—only a fraction of the tumor is made available for biochemical analysis. So the unanalyzed portion of negative tumors (generally the margins) may have contained a GTP-activable form of ODC. The chromatographic profiles of human tumor ODC reveal multiple peaks of active enzyme, as in the mouse tumors analyzed, including separate peaks that are or are not stimulated by GTP. Finally immunocytochemical staining of tumor sections demonstrates the presence of cells with high levels of constitutive ODC expression, a situation never detected in normal skin. Although our sample size is small, our results so far indicate that the only tumors in which ODC-positive cells could be detected were those in which GTP stimulated enzyme activity, suggesting that a functionally and structurally different ODC may be the actual isoform of the enzyme that is overexpressed at the cellular level in these tumors (Gilmour S, O'Brien T, unpublished observations). It is also intriguing that the presence of a GTP-activable ODC is correlated with more aggressive biologic behavior of the squamous cell carcinomas that we have studied so far, although a more extensive series of tumors will have to be studied to rigorously document this observation. In summary, the results of our comparison of ODC regulation in normal and neoplastic human epidermis are remarkably similar to what we have previously found in the mouse skin system.

Our conclusion that similar changes in ODC regulation can be found in both mouse and human skin undergoing neoplastic development has several important implications for both basic research and clinical medicine. First, at least some research findings from experimental carcinogenesis in rodents are relevant to human carcinogenesis. This should be reassuring to basic researchers, clinical practitioners, policymakers, and the general public—that eventually understanding of cancer at the cellular and molecular level in experimental models will lead to improvements in cancer diagnosis, treatment, and prevention. Second, there are important cellular regulatory genes, exemplified by ODC, with no known homology to viral oncogenes that if aberrantly regulated by a cell may predispose or contribute to that cell's progression toward a malignant phenotype. The heavy research emphasis on the structure and function of proto-oncogenes in neoplasia, although warranted in most cases, should not limit our search for other important genes, especially those that may act only in certain stages of the neoplastic process. Third, the identification of a functionally and/ or structurally altered ODC present only in tumors raises the possibility of designing drugs to specifically interfere with the function of a tumor-specific protein. For instance, once the structure of the GTP-activable ODC is known in greater detail, it may be possible to design specific inhibitors of only this form of the enzyme for use in cancer chemotherapy. A potent irreversible inhibitor of ODC, DFMO, has been used in clinical trials with disappointing results so far (26). The relative lack of success with this inhibitor may be attributable to its inability to inhibit a novel tumor-specific form of ODC.

In conclusion, we have identified a gene product, ODC, whose regulation in neoplastic mouse epidermis differs from the usual tight controls on the level of this protein in normal mouse epidermis. We have used the multistage mouse skin carcinogenesis model to investigate how this gene is regulated in normal and neoplastic cells and to devise ways to modulate tumor promotion by interfering with polyamine biosynthesis. Our preliminary analysis of human squamous cell carcinomas has revealed great similarities to the results in mouse epidermal tumors despite the presumably different etiological agents involved. Our studies so far reinforce our bias that the broad features of tumor promotion and some of the specific molecular changes, as defined in mouse skin, will be relevant to the process of neoplastic development in human skin and perhaps other epithelia as well.

OPEN FORUM

Dr. Claudio M. Aldaz: Do you have any information on the hyperplastic skin surrounding the tumors?

Dr. Thomas O'Brien: With respect to ODC expression, we have never seen increased levels of ODC using immunocytochemical methods unless that tissue was treated 4.5 h earlier with TPA. We have not taken the hyperplastic skin surrounding papillomas and made crude extracts to see whether there is a GTP-activated form of the enzyme. We have looked at lots of different hyperplastic and fetal tissues, and we have never been able to detect any altered properties of ODC in any of those rapidly growing fetal or adult tissues. So we have no evidence that it is expressed, other than in the tumors that we have looked at.

We have also done combined [³H]thymidine labeling and ODC immunocytochemistry. The percentage of labeled cells in the tumor versus the corresponding hyperplastic epidermis is not much different in many cases, whereas the uninduced level of expression of ODC is quite different in these two tissues. It is very low in hyperplastic epidermis, so you do not expect to see immunostaining, but the labeling index can be quite high. In tumors, the labeling index and the constitutive level of ODC are high as well.

In summary, we have not seen any consistent relationship between cells that express high levels of ODC versus cells that are cycling, in either normal or tumor tissue. We see no obvious relationship between the cells that are staining for ODC versus cells that are in S phase. However, in these experiments we are taking snapshots of tumors, so we do not know whether cells with a lot of enzyme might have entered S phase some time after the animal had been killed.

Dr. G. Tim Bowden: You are probably aware of work from Gene Gerner's lab, and probably Tony Pegg, indicating a possible translational level of regulation. There is an indication that in the 5' untranslated regions, polyamines may interact and actually block translation.

Dr. O'Brien: That work is still somewhat controversial. The mRNA for ODC is somewhat unusual in that there are multiple alternative initiation codons—multiple AUG codons. Some people have suggested, based on analogy to a yeast message, that is, the GCN-4 message, which is quite similar in its 5' untranslated region, that there may be translation control of ODC mRNA. However, when much of that leader sequence has been deleted, no difference has been seen in the translatability of that message in in vitro systems. The experiments you mentioned and the deletion studies have not yet been conducted in vivo. Multiple mechanisms probably account for high levels of ODC in tumors. As I showed for human squamous cell carcinomas, there are some tumors with very high levels of ODC activity that apparently have a functionally normal enzyme, suggesting high steady-state levels of ODC mRNA that is translationally active. Whether these tumors have lost a form of translational control is an interesting question for future work.

Dr. Claudio J. Conti: Do you think that those strongest-stained cells in the papillomas may represent different stages of the cell cycle, different stages of differentiation, or different cell populations?

Dr. O'Brien: That is the basic question. It is possible that the positive-staining cells overexpress ODC at a specific point in their cell cycle, and if one looked 2 or 4 h later, that level of expression would be down, and perhaps other cells' expression would be up.

Dr. Conti: That can probably be shown by combining autoradiography and immunohistochemistry.

Dr. O'Brien: At a specific time point, certainly. We have not seen any consistent association of ODC overexpression with S-phase cells, for instance. In fact we have not seen any cell with high levels of expression of ODC that was clearly in S phase. We have done this experiment with tritiated thymidine and autoradiography, followed by immunocytochemistry. This does not mean that if we looked at that same tumor 30 min later, the ODC-positive cell might not have entered S phase. But at the time we do the tumor "snapshot," we have not seen any cells that are in S phase that also have high levels of expression of ODC.

Dr. Helen Gensler: Have you looked at the effect of retinoids on this particular protein? Is the abnormal ODC influenced by retinoids?

Dr. O'Brien: That would be interesting, but it is hard to do those kinds of experiments. We are dealing with tumors, and the proportion of the two peaks that I showed, as well as the absolute level of enzyme, varies from tumor to tumor. So one cannot, for instance, treat one group of mice with papillomas with vehicle and one with retinoids and ask whether there is any inhibition of ODC expression. We would love to have an in vitro model that expressed this particular form of the enzyme, so that we could do experiments like that, but right now I think that they are very difficult to do in the in vivo model.

Dr. Stuart Yuspa: I presume that the small number of cells that are highly stained by the antibody do not explain the high activity in tumors. I presume that most of the tumor cells have high activity and these have super-high activity. I wonder if that small number of highly positive cells might have reduced GTPase activity, so that they have high intracellular GTP levels making the GTP-dependent enzyme particularly active in those cells. Certainly, changes in GTPase activity have been associated with transformation.

Dr. O'Brien: Our antibody recognizes both forms of the enzyme that are present in tumors, so when we see cells expressing high levels, we do not know which form or forms are present. It is difficult to say whether GTP might be increasing the immunoreactivity of the antibody if it is bound to the enzyme. That is one possibility. All of our western blots are done with denatured enzyme. There may be a confirmation change that persists in fixed tissue that allows that particular form to be more immunoreactive under certain conditions, but we have no evidence for that. Certainly, we would like to know more about other differences in those cells—both in normal epidermis that is chronically treated with TPA and in tumors. For instance, we would like to do anti-P21 immunocytochemistry in combination with ODC.

Dr. Yuspa: There is a considerable variation in activity from tumor to tumor, so maybe crude lysates could be used to measure GTPase activity in general to see if there is a correlation.

Dr. O'Brien: I believe there is a lot of GTPase around, so I am not sure how I would interpret that result.

Dr. Kenneth Kraemer: Are there any clinical differences between the half of the tumors that showed the abnormality and the half that did not?

Dr. O'Brien: Yes, the two human squamous cell tumors with high levels of GTP-activated ODC were most unusual. One arose from a burn scar and was very aggressive. The other was also aggressive clinically and was from a non-sun-exposed area. So there may be something to the association between the form of ODC and either etiology or biologic behavior of the tumor. We have not gotten extensive clinical and family histories yet, but we will when we have enough tumors to look at.

REFERENCES

1. O'Brien TG. The induction of ornithine decarboxylase as an early, possibly obligatory, event in mouse skin carcinogenesis. Cancer Res 36:2644-2653, 1976.
2. Boutwell RK. Evidence that an elevated level of ornithine decarboxylase is an essential component of tumor promotion. Advances in Polyamine Research 4:127-134, 1983.
3. Takigawa M, Boutwell RK, Verma AK. Evidence that an elevated level of ornithine decarboxylase may be essential to tumor promotion by phorbol esters. In Imahori K, Suzuki F, Suzuki O, Bachrach U (eds): Polyamines: Basic and Clinical Aspects. Utrecht: VNU Science Press, 1985, pp 1-8.
4. O'Brien TG, Madara T, Pyle JA, Holmes M. Ornithine decarboxylase from mouse

epidermis and epidermal papillomas: Differences in enzymatic properties and structure. Proc Natl Acad Sci USA 84:9448-9452, 1986.

5. Takigawa M, Verma AK, Simsiman RC, Boutwell RK. Polyamine biosynthesis and skin tumor promotion: Inhibition of 12-O-tetradecanoylphorbol-13-acetate-promoted mouse skin tumor formation by the irreversible inhibitor of ornithine decarboxylase α-difluoromethylornithine. Biochem Biophys Res Commun 105:969-976, 1982.

6. Weeks CE, Herrmann AL, Nelson FR, Slaga TJ. α-Difluoromethylornithine, an irreversible inhibitor of ornithine decarboxylase, inhibits tumor promoter-induced polyamine accumulation and carcinogenesis in mouse skin. Proc Natl Acad Sci USA 79:6028-6032, 1982.

7. O'Brien TG, Hietala O, O'Donnell K, Holmes M. Activation of mouse epidermal tumor ornithine decarboxylase by GTP: Evidence for different catalytic forms of the enzyme. Proc Natl Acad Sci USA 84:8927-8931, 1987.

8. Gilmour SK, Aglow E, O'Brien TG. Heterogeneity of ornithine decarboxylase expression in 12-O-tetradecanoylphorbol-13-acetate-treated mouse skin and in epidermal tumors. Carcinogenesis 7:943-947, 1986.

9. Astrup EG, Boutwell RK. Ornithine decarboxylase activity in chemically induced mouse skin papillomas. Carcinogenesis 3:303-308, 1982.

10. Scalabrino G, Ferioli ME. Polyamines in mammalian tumors. Part I. Adv Cancer Res 35:151-268.

11. Henningsson S, Persson L, Rosengren E. Polyamines and nucleic acids in the mouse kidney induced to growth by testosterone propionate. Acta Physiol Scand 102:385-393, 1978.

12. Scalabrino G, Pigatto P, Ferioli ME, Modena D, Paerari M, Caru A. Levels of activity of the polyamine biosynthetic decarboxylases as indicators of the degree of malignancy of human cutaneous epitheliomas. J Invest Dermatol 73:122-124, 1980.

13. Hietala O, Dzubow L, Dlugosz AA, Pyle JA, Jenney F, Gilmour SK, O'Brien JA. Activation of human squamous cell carcinoma ornithine decarboxylase activity by GTP. Cancer Res 48:1252-1257, 1988.

14. Friedman HI, Cooper PH, Wanebo HJ. Prognostic and therapeutic use of microstaging of cutaneous squamous cell carcinoma of the trunk and extremities. Cancer 56:1099-1105, 1985.

15. Boutwell RK. The function and mechanism of promoters of carcinogenesis. CRC Crit Rev Toxicol 2:419-443, 1974.

16. Tabor CW, Tabor H. Polyamines. Ann Rev Biochem 53:749-790, 1984.

17. Pegg AE. Recent advances in the biochemistry of polyamines in eukaryotes. Biochem J 234:249-262, 1986.

18. Verma AK, Erickson D, Dolnick BJ. Increased mouse epidermal ornithine decarboxylase activity by the tumor promoter 12-O-tetradecanoylphorbol-13-acetate involves increased amounts of both enzyme protein and messenger RNA. Biochem J 237:297-300, 1986.

19. Gilmour SK, Verma AK, Madara T, O'Brien TG. Regulation of ornithine decarboxylase gene expression in mouse epidermis and epidermal tumors during two-stage carcinogenesis. Cancer Res 47:1221-1225, 1987.

20. O'Brien TG, Simsiman RC, Boutwell RK. Induction of the polyamine-biosynthetic enzymes in mouse epidermis by tumor-producing agents. Cancer Res 35:1662-1670, 1975.

21. O'Brien TG, Simsiman TC, Boutwell RK. Induction of the polyamine biosynthetic enzymes in mouse epidermis and their specificity for tumor promotion. Cancer Res 35:2426-2433, 1975.
22. Persson L, Rosengren E, Sandler F. Localization of ornithine decarboxylase by immunocytochemistry. Biochem Biophys Res Commun 104:1196-1201, 1982.
23. McConlogue L, Gupta M, Wu L, Coffino P. Molecular cloning and expression of the mouse ornithine decarboxylase gene. Proc Natl Acad Sci USA 81:540-544, 1984.
24. Kahana C, Nathans D. Isolation of cloned cDNA encoding mammalian ornithine decarboxylase. Proc Natl Acad Sci USA 81:3645-3649, 1984.
25. Rheinwald JG, Green H. Serial cultivation of strains of human epidermal keratinocytes: The formation of keratinizing colonies from single cells. Cell 6:331-344, 1975.
26. Abeloff M, Rosen ST, Luk GD, Baylin SB, Zetzman M, Sjoerdsma A. Phase II trials of α-difluoromethylornithine, an inhibitor of polyamine synthesis, in advanced small cell lung cancer and colon cancer. Cancer Treat Rep 70:843-845, 1986.

Skin Carcinogenesis: Mechanisms and Human Relevance, pages 233–248
© 1989 Alan R. Liss, Inc.

Role of Free Radicals in Tumor Promotion and Progression

Thomas W. Kensler, Patricia A. Egner, Bonita G. Taffe, and Michael A. Trush

Division of Toxicological Sciences, Department of Environmental Health Sciences, Johns Hopkins School of Hygiene and Public Health, Baltimore, Maryland 21205

Substantial evidence implicates free radicals, particularly those derived from molecular oxygen, in chemical carcinogenesis; this has been the subject of several recent reviews (1-4). This chapter focuses on the role of free radical species in tumor promotion, principally in murine skin. Five major lines of experimental evidence implicate free radicals in tumor promotion: (1) tumor promoters stimulate the production of reactive oxygen species from endogenous sources in a variety of cell types, (2) reactive oxygen-generating systems can mimic the biochemical actions of tumor promoters, (3) free radical-generating compounds such as organic peroxides are tumor promoters, (4) tumor promoters modulate cellular antioxidant defense systems, and (5) free radical scavengers and detoxifiers inhibit tumor promotion. These observations collectively serve to implicate free radicals strongly in the process of tumor promotion, but the molecular mechanisms of their participation in tumor promotion are unknown. In many instances, tumor promoters override the homeostatic regulatory mechanisms used by growth factors, and there is some evidence that free radicals can modify phenotypic expression and differentiation of cells by affecting signal-transduction cascades. However, as a tissue response, tumor promotion mediated through free radical mechanisms probably results from an altered homeostatic equilibrium produced by increased cytotoxicity, increased terminal differentiation, and phenotypic reprogramming, which in summation result in the clonal expansion of initiated cells.

ACTIVATION OF CELLULAR SOURCES OF REACTIVE OXYGEN BY TUMOR PROMOTERS

Oxygen-centered free radicals, which may be produced by all respiring cells, have been studied extensively because of their apparent central role in a number of pathological states, including cancer. The sequential one-electron reduction of molecular oxygen that yields reactive oxygen is depicted in Figure

EXCITATION AND REDUCTION OF OXYGEN

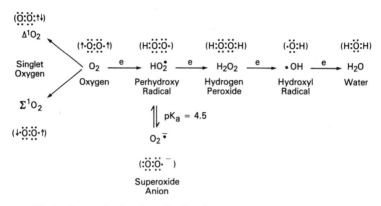

Figure 1. Excitation and reduction of molecular oxygen.

1. The one-electron reduction of molecular oxygen produces superoxide anion (O_2^{-}), which is not very reactive toward cellular molecules, although its protonated form ($HO_2\cdot$) is more so. Superoxide anion can also reduce species such as transition metals and disulfides, thereby regenerating molecular oxygen. If O_2^{-} is further reduced, hydrogen peroxide (H_2O_2) is formed, which, although it is not a radical, can be involved in the redox cycling of electrons via transition metals such as iron. The one-electron reduction product of H_2O_2 is the hydroxyl radical ($\cdot OH$), which is extremely reactive toward biomolecules. Finally, one-electron reduction of $\cdot OH$ yields water. Molecular oxygen can also undergo energy transfer to form the excited-state singlet oxygen species ($^1O_2$); however, the actual formation of $^1O_2$ in biological systems remains ambiguous at this time.

Free radicals can be generated in vivo as by-products of normal metabolism during the catalytic cycling of numerous enzymes (5). In several instances, it appears that tumor promoters accentuate the elaboration of reactive oxygen species by these endogenous sources to create a cellular pro-oxidant state. The best-characterized example of this action is the stimulation of the oxidative burst in inflammatory cells. In response to tumor promoters, neutrophils and macrophages increase their oxygen consumption, oxidize glucose via the hexose monophosphate shunt, and generate O_2^{-}, H_2O_2, and chemiluminescence (6-8). In the case of 12-*O*-tetradecanoylphorbol-13-acetate (TPA), these processes appear to be mediated through the interaction of the phorbol diester and its receptor, protein kinase C (9,10) and the subsequent activation of a pyridine nucleotide-dependent oxidase system localized to the plasma membrane. Structure-activity studies comparing phorbol diester analogues of varying tumor promoter activity with their ability to act as stimulators of reactive oxygen metabolism, as monitored by O_2^- production and chemiluminescence, have shown a strong concordance between the two processes. Other classes of epidermal tumor promoters such as the indole alkaloids (teleocidin, lyngbyatoxin A, and dihydroteleocidin) and polyacetates (aplysiatoxin and debromoaplysiatoxin) (11,12), which are chemically distinct from the phorbol diesters, also activate protein kinase C and stimulate O_2^- production in inflammatory cells. Additionally, some promoters such as palytoxin and thapsigargin, which do not appear to activate the protein kinase C signal-transduction cascade, also evoke an oxidative burst in neutrophils (13), while others such as anthralin, iodoacetic acid, and benzoyl peroxide do not. Other promoters that stimulate O_2^- production are mezerein (11), bryostatin (14), and retinoids (15).

Oxygen radicals derived from inflammatory cells may be a critical component of the tumor promotion process (16,17). This conclusion is derived from the observations that these cells produce copious quantities of reactive oxygen, that inflammation appears to be an obligatory component of promotion in the epidermis (18), and that most inhibitors of tumor promotion in vivo block the oxidative burst seen in phorbol diester-stimulated neutrophils. Notable examples of these antipromoters include protease inhibitors, inhibitors of the arachidonate cascade, retinoids, steroids, and antioxidants (4,16,19-25). However, Fischer and her colleagues have demonstrated that the putative target cells, the basal keratinocytes, can also produce oxygen radicals in response to tumor promoters (26). Addition of phorbol diesters to primary keratinocytes results in the rapid generation of a chemiluminescent response that appears to be mediated through the protein kinase C cascade (27). As is the case with activated neutrophils, chemiluminescence generated by keratinocytes can be blocked by most antipromoters; however, studies of these inhibitors suggest primary involvement of the cyclooxygenase and lipoxygenase pathways in the generation of oxidants. Tumor promotion in a complex organ such as the skin undoubtedly involves interactions between multiple cell types, with epithelial, mesenchymal, and immune cells all participating in the response.

Another source of reactive oxygen in phorbol diester-treated skin may be xanthine oxidase, which generates O_2^- during the reduction of oxygen to H_2O_2. Reiners et al. (28) have observed a threefold increase in xanthine oxidase activity that appears to be due to de novo synthesis of xanthine dehydrogenase and conversion of both newly synthesized and preexisting dehydrogenases to the oxidase form. This increase in xanthine oxidase activity requires several days to reach its maximum and is probably related to cell hyperplasia and terminal differentiation of the keratinocytes (29). Consistent with this view, Hartley et al. (30) have noted an association of DNA strand breaks with accelerated terminal dif-ferentiation in mouse epidermal cells exposed to tumor promoters. DNA strand breaks can also be induced by addition of xanthine/xanthine oxidase to cells in culture (16).

FREE RADICAL-GENERATING SYSTEMS THAT MIMIC THE ACTION OF TUMOR PROMOTERS

A number of systems have been proposed as models of in vitro promotion; mouse embryo fibroblast C3H/10T1/2 cells and JB6 mouse epidermal cells are the two most thoroughly studied. Exposure of C3H/10T1/2 cells to carcinogenic agents such as polycyclic aromatic hydrocarbons or ultraviolet or x-ray irradiation followed by sustained exposure to phorbol diesters results in augmented formation of transformed foci. Zimmerman and Cerutti (31) have reported that reactive oxygen acts directly as a promoter of transformation in C3H/10T1/2 cells. Cells initiated with either x-rays or benzo[a]pyrene-diol-epoxide I at doses that produce minimal transformation show a strong enhancement of formation of malignant foci following daily treatment for 3 weeks with xanthine oxidase and xanthine. Addition of this extracellular O_2^- generating system produces an effect comparable to that engendered by TPA addition, and like the TPA response, is inhibited by simultaneous addition of superoxide dismutase (SOD). Additionally, neutrophils themselves can mediate the transformation of these cells (32).

The murine JB6 epidermal cell line can undergo irreversible transformation to an anchorage-independent growth phenotype in the presence of different classes of promoters (33,34). Only those cells expressing the transformed phenotype grow in soft agar and are tumorigenic when injected into syngeneic newborn mice. As shown in Table 1, anchorage-independent growth can also be induced in these cells by xanthine/xanthine oxidase. Transfection studies between promotion-sensitive and -resistant variants suggest that specific genes may determine sensitivity to promotion of neoplastic transformation in these preneoplastic cells (35). However, studies on the effects of reactive oxygen-generating systems on selective gene activation and expression await more intense attention.

One gene product that might be useful in this type of study is the enzyme ornithine decarboxylase (ODC), the rate-limiting step in polyamine biosynthesis. There is an excellent correlation between the tumor-promoting ability of various compounds and their activity as inducers of ODC in mouse epidermis. Similarly, many antipromoters block the induction of this enzyme. The induction of ODC activity is a prominent, early, and transient event following exposure to epidermal tumor promoters. Xanthine/xanthine oxidase will induce the activity of ODC in primary murine keratinocytes in a manner analogous to that observed with TPA (36). Induction of this enzyme can also be accomplished by addition of either diacylglycerol or phospholipase C to these cells, implicating protein kinase C in the signaling mechanism (37,38).

TUMOR PROMOTION BY FREE RADICAL-GENERATING COMPOUNDS

A number of free radical-generating dialkylperoxides and hydroperoxides used in the chemical and pharmaceutical industries are skin irritants and tumor promoters. Benzoyl peroxide, lauroyl peroxide, decanoyl peroxide, and dicumyl peroxide are active in the initiation-promotion model of the mouse epidermis,

Table 1. Induction of Anchorage-Independent Growth in JB6 Murine Epidermal Cells by a Superoxide Anion-Generating System

Treatment	Colonies/dish*
None	322 ± 12[†]
Xanthine (15 μM)	360 ± 14
Xanthine oxidase (XO)	374 ± 19
Xanthine (5 μM) + XO	579 ± 40[‡]
Xanthine (10 μM) + XO	628 ± 40[‡]
Xanthine (15 μM) + XO	696 ± 62[‡]
TPA (3 ng/ml)	3854 ± 326[‡]

* Suspensions (1.5 ml) of 1×10^4 JB6 cells (Cl22) in 0.33% agar containing TPA or xanthine as indicated were plated over a layer of 0.5% agar containing the same agents. Xanthine oxidase (0.2 mU/ml) was added to the upper layer on days 0, 1, and 2. Soft agar colonies of 8 or more cells were scored after 14 days.
† Mean ± SE (n=3).
‡ Differs from control; $P<0.01$.

whereas *tert*-butyl hydroperoxide, cumene hydroperoxide, butylated hydroxytoluene (BHT) hydroperoxide, and methyl ethyl ketone peroxide can be described as weak promoters (39,40). Although they are active as tumor promoters and progressors, these peroxides are largely inactive as either initiators or complete carcinogens (41).

Promoter activity of these peroxides is ascribed to their ability to generate free radical derivatives, although they are generally quite stable to unimolecular homolysis at body temperature (42). Several hydroperoxides undergo accelerated decomposition in the presence of hematin to form radical species that can be detected by spin trapping and electron-spin resonance (43). Free radical products of the organic hydroperoxides *tert*-butyl hydroperoxide and cumene hydroperoxide have recently been characterized during incubation with isolated murine keratinocytes (44). Methyl radicals were the primary species observed. The generation of radicals from the diacylperoxide promoters has also been demonstrated in human and murine keratinocytes; however, full characterization of the radical products is incomplete. A proposed scheme for the activation of benzoyl peroxide to alkoxyl and alkyl radical species is shown in Figure 2. The peroxide and hydroperoxide tumor promoters require cell-mediated activation to free radical products that may be catalyzed by a variety of hemoproteins, including peroxidases, as well as by nonenzymatic metal-mediated reactions between endogenous reductants and peroxides.

Once formed, primary radicals can undergo fragmentation, addition, abstraction, or substitution reactions. Fragmentation occurs because the radicals' instability is similar to that of tertiary alkoxyl radicals, which undergo β-scission to produce an alkyl radical and a ketone or aldehyde. Formation of methyl radicals from keratinocyte-activated *tert*-butyl and cumene hydroperoxides occurs in

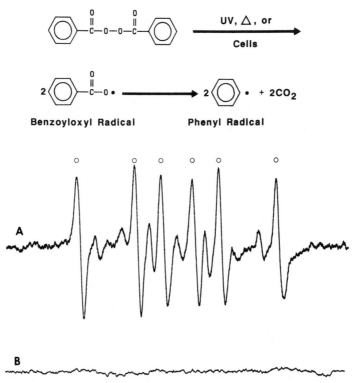

Figure 2. Proposed scheme for the activation of benzoyl peroxide to free radicals by keratinocytes. (A) Electron spin resonance spectrum of DMPO–benzoyl peroxide adducts in neonatal mouse epidermal cells. The predominant six-line signal is characteristic of alkyl radical adducts (O). (B) No signals are obtained when benzoyl peroxide is omitted or when cells are heat inactivated.
Abbreviations: DMPO, 5,5'-dimethyl-1-pyrroline-N-oxide; UV, ultraviolet.

this manner and raises the question of a possible role of alkylation of cellular macromolecules in modulating the cell phenotype during promotion or progression. Methylation reactions, for example, are implicated in eukaryotic gene expression, posttranslational modification of proteins, and alteration of membrane fluidity. Addition reactions with alkyl radicals occur at sites of high electron density, such as the double bonds that are found in a variety of biological molecules. These molecules include unsaturated lipids, aromatic amino acid residues, and nucleotides. Addition reactions can also occur either at nitrogen centers such as those found in the basic amino acids or with molecular oxygen. The result of addition of a free radical to a biomolecule is the formation of a cellular radical, whereas addition to molecular oxygen results in the formation of a new peroxyl radical. Hydrogen abstraction by alkoxyl or alkyl radicals results in the generation of a reduced nonradical product and a cellular radical. Cellular species that are susceptible to hydrogen abstraction include reduced cofactors such as glutathione, nicotinamide adenine dinucleotide phosphate, nicotinamide adenine dinucleotide, ascorbate, α-tocopherol, and possibly flavins, as well as polyunsaturated lipids containing allylic hydrogens. The resulting product is a cellular radical such as a glutathione or a lipid radical that may be significantly longer lived than the primary radical. Finally, aromatic substitution is a possible reaction of alkyl radicals and would result in formation of a hydrogen radical, but whether this reaction occurs in biological systems has not been determined.

MODULATION OF OXIDANT DEFENSE MECHANISMS BY TUMOR PROMOTERS

Cells have multiple defense mechanisms for coping with oxidants. Protection of cellular constituents from damage from oxygen and its metabolites can be accomplished through enzymatic and nonenzymatic means. SOD, catalase, and peroxidases (particularly glutathione peroxidase) catalyze reactions to remove O_2^- or H_2O_2. Enzymes that catalyze the removal of $\cdot OH$ or $^1O_2$ are unknown; these species must be removed by quenching molecules such as glutathione and vitamins A, C, and E. Maintenance of cellular pro-/antioxidant homeostasis involves a complex interaction between cellular enzyme activity, availability of reducing equivalents, and levels of scavengers in the cells. Alteration of any of these components of the oxidant defense system, as can occur following promoter exposure, modulates the fate of reactive oxygen species in the cell. An early response of the epidermis to tumor promoters is a rapid decrease in the specific activity of SOD (45). The decline in SOD activity occurs within 3 h after application of a single dose of TPA and is maximal at 16 h. As shown in Figure 3, multiple TPA treatments, as are required to produce papillomas, sustain the SOD depression, even after cessation of promoter exposure. SOD activities are diminished in papillomas as well (45). The role of lowered SOD activity in neoplasia has been reviewed by Oberley et al. (46).

Catalase activity has also been reported to decrease following treatment with TPA (45). By contrast, glutathione peroxidase activity increases transiently in mouse skin following TPA treatment, followed by a depression to below control levels by 1 h. This suppression of activity is sustained over 12 h (47), but activity becomes elevated over the control level several days after a single exposure (48). Multiple treatments lead to maintenance of elevated glutathione peroxidase activity (48). Glutathione reductase activity is depressed throughout a multidose exposure (48). Perchellet et al. (49) also have observed that addition of TPA to isolated epidermal cells leads rapidly to a fourfold increase in the levels of oxidized glutathione. Preincubation with either reduced glutathione or its constituent amino acids blocks this response. The increased levels of oxidized glutathione presumably reflect oxidant stress resulting from both an altered balance in the production and detoxification of oxygen radicals and retarded

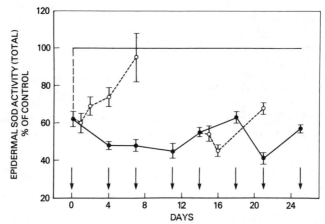

Figure 3. Effect of repetitive tumor promoter treatment on the diminution of epidermal SOD activity. Epidermis was isolated and assayed for total SOD activity 3 h after application of 4 nmol TPA. Arrows indicate days of TPA exposure. Closed circles represent mice receiving repeated doses of TPA, and open circles represent mice receiving no further treatment with TPA.
Abbreviations: SOD, superoxide dismutase; TPA, 12-O-tetradecanoylphorbol-13-acetate.

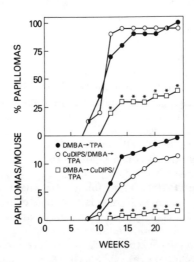

Figure 4. Effects of the biomimetic superoxide dismutase CuDIPS on tumorigenesis in the skin of CD-1 mice induced by an initiation-promotion regimen. Mice were treated with 2 µmol CuDIPS either 15 min before initiation with a single 0.2 µmol dose of DMBA or 15 min before twice-weekly promotion with 4 nmol TPA.
Abbreviations: CuDIPS, copper(II)(3,5-diisopropylsalicylate)$_2$; DMBA, 7,12-dimethylbenz-[a]anthracene.

reduction of oxidized glutathione. Such development of a pro-oxidant state in a subpopulation of basal cells could lead to either enhanced cytotoxicity upon sustained promoter exposure or increased entry of these cells into the terminally differentiating population. Either possibility allows for the clonal expansion of initiated cells that are resistant to terminal differentiation. In this regard, Hartley et al. (50) have recently observed that murine keratinocytes derived from initiated skin or from papillomas are resistant to DNA strand breakage induced by and cytotoxic effects of benzoyl peroxide, as compared with normal keratinocytes.

INHIBITION OF TUMOR PROMOTION BY FREE RADICAL SCAVENGERS AND DETOXIFIERS

Substantial, albeit indirect, evidence for the involvement of free radicals in tumor promotion derives from the use of inhibitors. Free radical scavengers, in particular natural and synthetic phenolic antioxidants, as well as oxidant detoxification enzymes such as SOD and catalase can inhibit numerous actions of tumor promoters both in vivo and in vitro (51). As shown in Figure 4, involvement of reactive oxygen in tumor promotion can be inferred from the observation that a biomimetic SOD, copper(II)(3,5-diisopropylsalicylate)$_2$(CuDIPS), was an effective inhibitor of promotion in mouse skin (52,53). This agent is a low-molecular-weight, lipophilic copper coordination complex that catalytically dispro-portionates O_2^- at rates comparable to CuZn SOD. Analogues lacking SOD-mimetic activity, namely, the ligand diisopropylsalicylate (DIPS), the corresponding zinc complex ZnDIPS, and copper-EDTA, were without antipromoter activity, underscoring the probable role of O_2^- in promotion. That this copper complex can participate in the reduction of other reactive oxygen species has not been ruled out. However, other studies using in vitro models for promotion have consistently demonstrated an inhibitory effect of CuDIPS, SOD, or SOD and catalase additions on cell transformation (32,54,55).

In a comprehensive survey of structural analogues of butylated hydrox-yanisole (BHA), Kozumbo et al. (24,56) found a strong correlation between the ability of BHA congeners to inhibit phorbol diester-mediated induction of ODC in mouse epidermis and both the lipophilic and antioxidant properties of these compounds. Experiments in which the time of addition of antioxidant was varied suggested that the antioxidant needed to be present at the time of exposure to the promoter and served to rule out the possibility of secondary effects of BHA, such as elevation of intracellular thiol levels, in the protective mechanism. However, agents that elevate glutathione levels, such as the constituent amino acids glutamate, cysteine, and glycine, can protect against phorbol diester-mediated induction of ODC and tumor promotion (57). In contrast to the endogenous antioxidants glutathione and α-tocopherol, which can scavenge O_2^- as well as other radicals (58,59), phenolic antioxidants, such as BHA, show no reactivity toward O_2^- (24,60). This suggests that other reactive oxygen species such as peroxyl, alkoxyl, and hydroxyl radicals also may be involved in promotion. Studies demonstrating that organic peroxide and hydroperoxide tumor promoters generate a different spectrum of radicals, namely, alkoxyl and alkyl radicals, also substantiate this view.

A POSSIBLE ROLE FOR INFLAMMATION IN TUMOR PROGRESSION

Papillomas induced by standard initiation-promotion protocols progress to carcinomas at a low frequency. The conversion to malignancy can be greatly accelerated by the exposure of papillomas to a variety of compounds, including initiating agents and peroxides. Given the spectrum of agents that facilitate this conversion, a supposition is that DNA damage, particularly clastogenesis, may be important to the process. DNA base modifications, strand breaks, and chromosomal rearrangements have been observed in eukaryotic cells exposed to oxidants (3,4). Additionally, reactive oxygen species are mutagenic and enhance the transformation of cells in vitro. Thus, oxidants, whether produced by activated inflammatory cells or from free radical derivatives of the agents themselves, can provoke macromolecular damage consonant with this stage of carcinogenesis. The possibility that chronic inflammation could contribute to this process is inferred from the sizable clinical experience indicating that human malignancies often occur at sites of ongoing inflammation. Table 2 presents several chronic inflammatory disorders that are associated with a high risk for cancer in man. The role of inflammation in the pathogenesis of cancer has recently been reviewed (4,61,62).

Table 2. Chronic Inflammatory Disorders Associated with High Cancer Risk*

Malignancy	Inflammatory disorder
Alimentary tract	
Gastric carcinoma	Atrophic gastritis
Adenocarcinoma of colon/rectum	Chronic ulcerative colitis
Hepatocellular carcinoma	Hepatic cirrhosis
Gallbladder carcinoma	Cholelithiasis
Biliary tract carcinoma	*Clonorchis sinensis* infestation
Adenocarcinoma of pancreas	Chronic pancreatitis
Squamous cell carcinoma of mouth	Oral inflammation/ulceration secondary to denture problems
Respiratory tract	
Bronchioalveolar carcinoma or mesothelioma	Asbestosis
Urinary tract	
Carcinoma of skin	Urethral fistula
Carcinoma of urinary bladder	*Schistosoma haematobium* infestation

*Adapted from ref. 62.

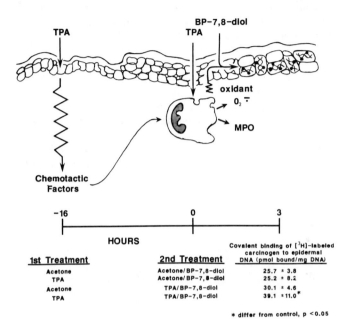

Figure 5. Role of neutrophil recruitment in the metabolic activation of polycyclic aromatic hydrocarbons in mouse skin. Mice were treated with TPA (17 nmol in acetone) and 400 nmol [³H]*trans*-7,8-dihydroxy-7,8-dihydrobenzo[a]pyrene (BP-7,8-diol) at the indicated times. Mice were killed 3 h after the last treatment, and DNA was isolated from epidermal cells. Adapted from ref. 64.
Abbreviations: MPO, myeloperoxidase.

Oxidants produced during an inflammatory state could also participate in genetic alteration through an indirect mechanism. Activated neutrophils can participate in the metabolic activation of proximate carcinogens to genotoxic species. For example, human neutrophils stimulated with TPA mediate the activation of *trans*-7,8-dihydroxy-7,8-dihydrobenzo[a]pyrene (BP-7,8-diol) to species that elicit mutagenesis in *Salmonella typhimurium*, induce sister chromatid exchanges in cocultured V-79 fibroblasts, and bind to the DNA of cocultured murine keratinocytes (63,64). This pathway for the metabolic activation of BP-7,8-diol is dependent upon both oxidant production and myeloperoxidase release by the neutrophils. Figure 5 depicts a model system that has been used to investigate the influence of an inflammatory state on the metabolic activation of carcinogens in vivo. Application of TPA to mouse skin leads to an enormous increase in the influx of neutrophils into the dermis between 12 and 20 h after exposure. This influx is presumably mediated by the release of chemotactic factors from the epidermis. Activation of the treated neutrophils by a second application of TPA followed immediately by treatment with the penultimate carcinogen BP-7,8-diol results in a 50% increase in the amount of carcinogen irreversibly associated with epidermal DNA as compared with the amount in mice treated with either a single application of TPA or only the acetone vehicle. The requirement for two doses of TPA would militate against the involvement of epithelial systems in the enhancement process because a single dose of TPA should maximally, if at all, influence these pathways. In this regard, it is worth noting that endogenous peroxyl radical-dependent pathways appear paramount in the metabolic activation of BP-7,8-diol in naive murine keratinocytes (65). These observations provide a possible molecular basis for the observed association between the development of malignancies and sites of ongoing inflammation, but the biological significance of enhanced carcinogen binding to malignant conversion remains to be established.

ACKNOWLEDGMENTS

The authors gratefully acknowledge financial support from the National Institutes of Health (CA44530, ES00454, and ES03760) and the American Cancer Society (SIG-3). T.W.K. is the recipient of a Research Career Development Award (CA01230).

OPEN FORUM

Dr. John DiGiovanni: Can you rule out the possibility that you simply stimulated arachidonic acid metabolism in the keratinocytes in your experiments and hence increased cooxidation of the diol directly in the cells, rather than its being the inflammatory infiltrate?

Dr. Thomas Kensler: No. I cannot completely rule out this possibility in the in vivo setting, as we have not used any inhibitors to arachidonic acid processing. However, arachidonic metabolism is also an integral part of the oxidative burst in neutrophils. If you shut that down, you blunt that response. My conclusion is based in part on the analogy to the in vitro situation, in which neutrophils cocultured with keratinocytes modify keratinocyte DNA and on the observation that one dose of TPA alone coadministered with the BP diol has no effects on covalent binding. Thus, mere activation of the arachidonate cascade in keratinocytes by TPA is insufficient to enhance covalent binding of BP-diol. You need the two-dose exposure to TPA. I interpret this to require the initial infiltration of neutrophils and then their subsequent activation, as opposed to a direct effect of TPA on keratinocytes.

Dr. DiGiovanni: Is there no infiltration of neutrophils with a single dose of TPA?

Dr. Kensler: There are plenty of neutrophils in the dermis several hours after a single dose of TPA, but I don't know anything about their metabolic capacity 16 h after they have been recruited. I would expect them to be reasonably inactive, so our second dose of TPA presumably activates these newly recruited cells.

REFERENCES

1.   Cerutti PA. Prooxidant states and tumor promotion. Science 227:375-381, 1985.
2.   Kensler TW, Trush MA. In Oberley LW (ed): Superoxide Dismutase, Vol. III. Pathological States. Boca Raton, FL: CRC Press, 1985, pp 191-236.
3.   Kensler TW, Taffe BG. Free radicals in tumor promotion. Advances in Free Radical Biology and Medicine 2:347-387, 1986.
4.   Troll W, Wiesner R. The role of oxygen radicals as a possible mechanism of tumor promotion. Annu Rev Pharmacol Toxicol 25:509-528, 1985.
5.   Freeman BA, Crapo JD. Biology of disease, free radicals and tissue injury. Lab Invest 47:412-426, 1982.
6.   Kensler TW, Trush MA. Inhibition of phorbol ester-stimulated chemiluminescence in human polymorphonuclear leukocytes by retinoic acid and 5,6-epoxyretinoic acid. Cancer Res 41:216-222, 1981.
7.   Repine JE, White JG, Clawson CC, Holmes BM. The influence of phorbol myristate acetate on oxygen consumption by polymorphonuclear leukocytes. J Clin Lab Med 83:911-920, 1974.
8.   DeChatelet LR, Shirley PS, Johnson RB Jr. Effect of phorbol myristate acetate on the oxidative metabolism of human polymorphonuclear leucocytes. Blood 47:545-554, 1976.
9.   Patriarca P, Zatti M, Cramer R, Rossi F. Stimulation of the respiration of polymorphonuclear leukocytes by phospholipase C. Life Sci 9:841-849, 1970.
10. Fujita I, Irita K, Takeshige K, Minakami S. Diacylglycerol, 1-oleoyl-2-acetylglycerol, stimulates superoxide-generation from human neutrophils. Biochem Biophys Res Commun 120:318-324, 1984.
11. Goldstein BD, Witz G, Amoruso M, Stone DS, Troll W. Stimulation of human polymorphonuclear leukocyte superoxide anion radical production by tumor promoters. Cancer Lett 11:257-262, 1981.
12. Nishimura S, Ames BN. U.S.-Japan meeting on "Oxygen Radicals in Cancer." Jpn J Cancer Res 77:843-848, 1986.
13. Berkow RL, Kraft AS. Bryostatin, a non-phorbol macrocyclic lactone, activates intact human polymorphonuclear leukocytes and binds to the phorbol ester receptor. Biochem Biophys Res Commun 131:1109-1116, 1985.
14. Kano S, Iizuka T, Ishimura Y, Fujiki H, Sugimura T. Stimulation of superoxide anion formation by the non-TPA type tumor promoters palytoxin and thapsigargin in porcine and human neutrophils. Biochem Biophys Res Commun 143:672-677, 1987.
15. Lochner JE, Badwey JA, Horn W, Karnovsky ML. All-trans-retinol stimulates superoxide release and phospholipase C activity in neutrophils without significantly blocking protein kinase C. Proc Natl Acad Sci USA 83:7673-7677, 1986.
16. Birnboim HC. Importance of DNA strand-break damage in tumor promotion. In Nygaard OF and Simic MG (eds): Radioprotectors and Anticarcinogens. New York: Academic Press, 1983, pp 539-556.

17. Troll W, Frenkel K, Teebor G. Free oxygen radicals: Necessary contributors to tumor promotion and cocarcinogenesis. In Fujiki H, Hecker E, Moore RE, Sugimura K, Weinstein IB (eds): Cellular Interactions by Environmental Tumor Promoters. Utrecht:VNU Science Press, 1984, pp 207-218.

18. Slaga TJ, Fischer SM, Viaje A, Berry DL, Bracken WM, LeClerc S, Miller DR. Inhibition of tumor promotion by anti-inflammatory agents: An approach to the biochemical mechanism of promotion. In Slaga TJ, Sivak A, Boutwell RK (eds): Carcinogenesis: A Comprehensive Survey, Vol. 2. Mechanisms of Tumor Promotion and Cocarcinogenesis. New York: Raven Press, 1978, pp 173-195.

19. Goldstein BD, Witz G, Amoruso M, Troll W. Protease inhibitors antagonize the activation of polymorphonuclear leukocyte oxygen consumption. Biochem Biophys Res Commun 88:854-860, 1979.

20. Hoffman M, Autor AP. Effect of cyclooxygenase inhibitors and protease inhibitors on phorbol-induced stimulation of oxygen consumption and superoxide production by rat pulmonary macrophages. Biochem Pharmacol 31:775-780, 1982.

21. Blackburn WD Jr, Heck LW, Wallace RW. The bioflavonoid quercetin inhibits neutrophil degranulation, superoxide production, and the phosphorylation of specific neutrophil proteins. Biochem Biophys Res Commun 144:1229-1236, 1987.

22. Witz G, Goldstein BD, Amoruso M, Stone DS, Troll W. Retinoid inhibition of superoxide anion radical production by human polymorphonuclear leukocytes stimulated with tumor promoters. Biochem Biophys Res Commun 97:883-888, 1980.

23. Whitcomb JM, Schwartz AG. Dehydroepiandrosterone and 16 α-Br-epiandrosterone inhibit 12-O-tetradecanoylphorbol-13-acetate stimulation of superoxide radical production by human polymorphonuclear leukocytes. Carcinogenesis 6:333-335, 1985.

24. Kozumbo WJ, Trush MA, Kensler TW. Are free radicals involved in tumor promotion? Chem Biol Interact 54:199-207, 1985.

25. Kensler TW, Trush MA. Inhibition of oxygen radical metabolism in phorbol ester-activated polymorphonuclear leukocytes by an antitumor promoting copper complex with superoxide dismutase-mimetic activity. Biochem Pharmacol 32:3485-3487, 1983.

26. Fischer SM, Adams LM. Suppression of tumor promoter-induced chemiluminescence in mouse epidermal cells by several inhibitors of arachidonic acid metabolism. Cancer Res 45:3130-3136, 1985.

27. Fischer SM, Baldwin JK, Adams LM. Phospholipase C mimics tumor promoter-induced chemiluminescence in murine epidermal cells. Biochem Biophys Res Commun 131:1103-1108, 1985.

28. Reiners JJ Jr, Pence BC, Barcus MCS, Cantu AR. 12-O-Tetradecanoylphorbol-13-acetate-dependent induction of xanthine dehydrogenase and conversion to xanthine oxidase in murine epidermis. Cancer Res 47:1775-1779, 1987.

29. Pence BC, Reiners JJ Jr. Murine epidermal xanthine oxidase activity: Correlation with degree of hyperplasia induced by tumor promoters. Cancer Res 47:6388-6392, 1987.

30. Hartley JA, Gibson NW, Zwelling LA, Yuspa SH. Association of DNA strand breaks with accelerated terminal differentiation in mouse epidermal cells exposed to tumor promoters. Cancer Res 45:4864-4870, 1985.

31. Zimmerman R, Cerutti P. Active oxygen acts as a promoter of transformation in mouse embryo C3H/10T1/2/Cl8 fibroblasts. Proc Natl Acad Sci USA 81:2085-2087, 1984.

32. Weitzman SA, Weitberg AB, Clark EP, Stossel TP. Phagocytes as carcinogens: Malignant transformation produced by human neutrophils. Science 227:1231-1233, 1985.

33. Gindhart TD, Srinivas L, Colburn NH. Benzoyl peroxide promotion of transformation of JB6 mouse epidermal cells: Inhibition by ganglioside GT but not retinoic acid. Carcinogenesis 6:309-311, 1985.

34. Gindhart TD, Nakamura Y, Stevens LA, Hegameyer GA, West MW, Smith BM, Colburn NH. Genes and signal transduction in tumor promotion: Conclusions from studies with promoter resistant variants of JB-6 mouse epidermal cells. In Mass MJ, Nesnow S, Siegfried JM, Steele VE (eds): Carcinogenesis: A Comprehensive Survey, Vol. 8. Cancer of the Respiratory Tract: Predisposing Factors. New York: Raven Press, 1985, pp 341-367.

35. Colburn NH, Talmadge CB, Gindhart TD. Transfer of sensitivity to tumor promoters by transfection of DNA from sensitive into insensitive mouse JB6 epidermal cells. Mol Cell Biol 3:1182-1186, 1983.

36. Fischer SM, Cameron GS, Baldwin JK, Jasheway DW, Patrick K. Reactive oxygen in the tumor promotion stage of skin carcinogenesis. Lipids 23:592-597, 1988.

37. Sasakawa N, Ishii K, Yamamoto S, Kato R. Induction of ornithine decarboxylase activity by 1-oleoyl-2-acetyl-glycerol in isolated mouse epidermal cells. Biochem Biophys Res Commun 28:913-920, 1985.

38. Jeng AY, Lichti U, Strickland JE, Blumberg PM. Similar effects of phospholipase C and phorbol ester tumor promoters on primary mouse epidermal cells. Cancer Res 45:5714-5721, 1985.

39. Slaga TJ, Klein-Szanto AJP, Triplett LL, Yotti LP, Trosko JE. Skin tumor promoting activity of benzoyl peroxide, a widely used free radical generating compound. Science 213:1023-1025, 1981.

40. Slaga TJ, Solanki V, Logani M. Studies on the mechanism of action of antitumor promoting agents: Suggestive evidence for the involvement of free radicals in promotion. In Nygaard OF, Simic MG (eds): Radioprotectors and Anticarcinogens. New York: Academic Press, 1983, pp 471-485.

41. Watts P. Peroxides, genes and cancer. Food Chem Toxicol 23:957-960, 1985.

42. Pryor WA. The role of free radical reactions in biological systems. In Pryor WA (ed): Free Radicals in Biology, Vol. 1. New York: Academic Press, 1975, pp 1-49.

43. Kalyanaraman B, Mottley C, Mason RP. A direct electron spin resonance and spin-trapping investigation of peroxyl free radical formation by hematin/hydroperoxide systems. J Biol Chem 258:3855-3858, 1983.

44. Taffe BG, Takahashi N, Kensler TW, Mason RP. Generation of free radicals from organic hydroperoxide tumor promoters in isolated mouse keratinocytes: Formation of alkyl and alkoxyl radicals from tert-butyl hydroperoxide and cumene hydroperoxide. J Biol Chem 62:12143-12149, 1987.

45. Solanki V, Rana RS, Slaga TJ. Diminution of mouse epidermal superoxide dismutase and catalase activities by tumor promoters. Carcinogenesis 2:1141-1146, 1981.

46. Oberley LW, Oberley TD, Buettner GR. Cell division in normal and transformed cells: The possible role of superoxide and hydrogen peroxide. Med Hypotheses 7:21-42, 1981.

47. Perchellet JP, Perchellet EM, Orten DK, Schneider BA. Inhibition of the effects of 12-O-tetradecanoylphorbol-13-acetate on mouse epidermal glutathione peroxidase and ornithine decarboxylase activities by glutathione level-raising agents and selenium-containing compounds. Cancer Lett 26:283-293, 1985.

48. Taffe BG, Kensler TW. Modification of cellular oxidant defense mechanisms in mouse skin by multiple applications of TPA (abstract). Proceedings of the American Association for Cancer Research 27:148, 1986.

49. Perchellet JP, Perchellet EM, Orten DK, Schneider BA. Decreased ratio of reduced/oxidized glutathione in mouse epidermal cells treated with tumor promoters. Carcinogenesis 7:503-506, 1986.

50. Hartley JA, Gibson NW, Kilkenny A, Yuspa SH. Mouse keratinocytes derived from initiated skin or papillomas are resistant to DNA strand breakage by benzoyl peroxide: A possible mechanism for tumor promotion mediated by benzoyl peroxide. Carcinogenesis 8:1827-1830, 1987.

51. Kozumbo WJ, Cerutti PA. Antioxidants as antitumor promoters. In Shankel DM, Hartman PE, Kada T, Hollaender A (eds): Antimutagenesis and Anticarcinogenesis Mechanisms. New York: Plenum Press, 1986, pp 491-506.

52. Kensler TW, Bush DM, Kozumbo WJ. Inhibition of tumor promotion by a biomimetic superoxide dismutase. Science 221:75-77, 1983.

53. Egner PA, Kensler TW. Effects of a biomimetic superoxide dismutase on complete and multistage carcinogenesis in mouse skin. Carcinogenesis 6:1167-1172, 1985.

54. Nakamura Y, Colburn NH, Gindhart TD. Role of reactive oxygen in tumor promotion: Implication of superoxide anion in promotion of neoplastic transformation in JB-6 cells by TPA. Carcinogenesis 6:229-235, 1985.

55. Borek C, Troll W. Modifiers of free radicals inhibit in vitro the oncogenic actions of x-rays, bleomycin, and the tumor promoter 12-O-tetradecanoylphorbol-13-acetate. Proc Natl Acad Sci USA 80:1304-1307, 1983.

56. Kozumbo WJ, Seed JL, Kensler TW. Inhibition by 2(3)-tert-butyl-4-hydroxyanisole and other antioxidants of epidermal ornithine decarboxylase activity induced by 12-O-tetradecanoylphorbol-13-acetate. Cancer Res 43:2555-2559, 1983.

57. Perchellet JP, Owen MD, Posey TD, Orten DK, Schneider BA. Inhibitory effects of glutathione level-raising agents and D-α-tocopherol on ornithine decarboxylase induction and mouse skin tumor promotion by 12-O-tetradecanoylphorbol-13-acetate. Carcinogenesis 6:567-573, 1985.

58. Forman HJ, Fisher AB. Antioxidant defenses. In Gilbert DL (ed): Oxygen and Living Processes. New York: Springer-Verlag, 1981, pp 235-249.

59. Burton GW, Ingold KU. Mechanisms of antioxidant action: Studies on vitamin E and related antioxidants in biological systems. In Slater TF (ed): Protective Agents in Cancer. New York: Academic Press, 1983, pp 81-99.

60. Simic MG, Hunter EPL. Interaction of free radicals and antioxidants. In Nygaard OF, Simic MG (eds): Radioprotectors and Anticarcinogens. New York: Academic Press, 1983, pp 449-460.

61. Roman-Franco AA. Non-enzymatic extramicrosomal bioactivation of chemical carcinogens by phagocytes: A proposed new pathway. J Theor Biol 97:543-555, 1982.

62. Demopoulos HB, Pietronigro DD, Seligman ML. The development of secondary pathology with free radical reactions as a threshold mechanism. Journal of the American College of Toxicology 2:173-185, 1983.

63. Trush MA, Seed JL, Kensler TW. Oxidant-dependent metabolic activation of polycyclic aromatic hydrocarbons by phorbol ester-stimulated human polymorphonuclear leukocytes: Possible link between inflammation and cancer. Proc Natl Acad Sci USA 82:5194-5198, 1985.

64. Kensler TW, Egner PA, Moore KG, Taffe BG, Twerdok LE, Trush MA. Role of inflammatory cells in the metabolic activation of polycyclic aromatic hydrocarbons in mouse skin. Toxicol Appl Pharmacol 90:337-346, 1987.

65. Eling T, Curtis J, Battista J, Marnett LJ. Oxidation of (+)-7,8-dihydroxy-7,8-dihydrobenzo[a]pyrene by mouse keratinocytes: Evidence for peroxyl radical- and monooxygenase-dependent metabolism. Carcinogenesis 7:1957-1963, 1986.

Skin Carcinogenesis: Mechanisms and Human Relevance, pages 249–264

The Arachidonic Acid Cascade and Multistage Carcinogenesis in Mouse Skin

Susan M. Fischer, Gregory S. Cameron, James K. Baldwin, Daniel W. Jasheway, Kelly E. Patrick, and Martha A. Belury

Department of Carcinogenesis, Science Park, The University of Texas M. D. Anderson Cancer Center, Smithville, Texas 78957

Experimental chemical carcinogenesis studies in animals are valuable in identifying those biological events or agents that have either an essential or modulatory role in the development of neoplasias. Mouse skin has proved to be one of the best model systems in which to study the multistage nature of carcinogenesis, particularly 12-O-tetradecanoylphorbol-13-acetate (TPA) tumor promotion (1-5).

Investigation of the mechanism of action of TPA has been under way for many years and has been hampered in part by the fact that TPA causes a plethora of morphological and biochemical responses in the skin. Of all the observed effects, the induction of three events—epidermal cell proliferation and inflammation, ornithine decarboxylase (ODC) activity, and dark cell appearance—appear to best correlate with promoting activity (3,5). These correlations do not necessarily hold for promoters that are not of the phorbol diester series or for irritating but nonpromoting agents such as ethyl phenylpropiolate (6).

Investigations in this laboratory as well as others into the role of prostaglandins and the other arachidonic acid metabolites in tumorigenesis were prompted in part by the observation that TPA induces inflammation and vascular permeability changes (7,8). The essential nature of inflammation to phorbol ester promotion was suggested by several early studies using the anti-inflammatory steroids dexamethasone and fluocinolone acetonide. Fluocinolone acetonide in particular is extremely potent: repeated application of as little as 0.01 µg almost completely counteracts TPA tumor promotion (9,10). This drug also effectively counteracts TPA-induced cell proliferation and inflammation (10). Recently, anti-inflammatory steroids also have been shown to block the production of arachidonic acid metabolites by inhibiting phospholipase A_2 (11,12). This may be the underlying mechanism by which these agents act as strong inhibitors of TPA-induced inflammation and epidermal DNA synthesis (13,14).

ARACHIDONIC ACID METABOLISM

Free arachidonic acid (5,8,11,14-eicosatetraenoic acid) or the products of its metabolism, commonly referred to as eicosanoids, are not normally found intra- or extracellularly in the absence of chemical, physical, or hormonal stimulation. Arachidonate is usually stored as the fatty acid covalently bound to the second carbon of the glycerol backbone of phospholipids. As such, it is not a substrate for the metabolizing enzymes. It is, however, readily released as the free fatty acid by phospholipase A_2 or diacylglycerol lipase following phospholipase C action. In its free form, it is the substrate for the several enzymes constituting the arachidonate cascade, as shown in Figure 1. Generally, this pathway is divided into two major branches, the prostaglandin synthetase and lipoxygenase branches. The branches have in common the insertion of molecular oxygen into a polyunsaturated fatty acid with acyl chain rearrangement to form the various eicosanoid structures. Prostaglandin synthetase (cyclooxygenase, prostaglandin endoperoxidase) produces an intermediate prostaglandin, PGH_2, that is a substrate for the enzymes involved in the synthesis of the three major prostaglandins, PGE, PGF, and PGD, as well as thromboxane and prostacyclin. Lipoxygenases result in the formation of hydroperoxy fatty acids (commonly referred to as HPETEs), which lack the pentane ring of the prostaglandin synthetase pathway. The position of the hydroperoxy function is determined by the particular lipoxygenase; i.e., 5-lipoxygenase converts arachidonate to 5-hydroperoxyeicosatetraenoate (5-HPETE). The 5-HPETE is of particular interest because it can be further metabolized to the leukotrienes, which are commonly known as the slow-reacting substances involved in anaphylaxis.

ARACHIDONATE CASCADE AND TUMOR INITIATION

The initiation phase of carcinogenesis is generally believed to involve the covalent binding to or damage to DNA such that heritable genetic changes occur. There are two ways in which arachidonic acid metabolism may participate in the initiation process. The first, and least studied, is the binding of arachidonate metabolites to DNA (15,16). Although some metabolites, such as malondialdehyde, have been shown to be mutagenic (16), their relevancy to tumorigenesis in animal model systems has not been completely explored. Of perhaps more importance, and the second means by which arachidonate can participate in initiation, is the cooxidation of some carcinogens as a result of arachidonic acid oxygenation (17). One of the more studied examples is the cooxidation of 7,8-dihydroxy-7,8-dihydrobenzo[a]pyrene by prostaglandin synthetases to the diol epoxide form, which is mutagenic and carcinogenic. Other cooxidation products of benzo[a]pyrene and several other carcinogens and xenobiotics have been recently reviewed by Marnett (17).

That arachidonic acid metabolism may be important in the initiation phase of the mouse skin model has been suggested by work from this laboratory (18 and unpublished data). When arachidonic acid is applied prior (4 to 8 h) to

Arachidonic Acid Release and Metabolism

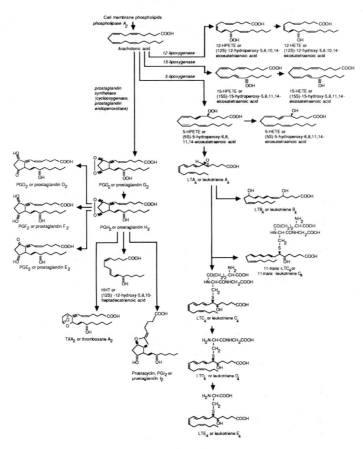

Figure 1. Arachidonic acid release and metabolism. This diagram illustrates the major enzymatic pathways involved in the production of the prostaglandins and lipoxygenase products.

dimethylbenz[a]anthracene initiation treatment, the tumor yield increases approximately 50%. If the anti-inflammatory indomethacin or flurbiprofen is also applied, the tumor yield is the same as with dimethylbenz[a]anthracene alone. This indicates that arachidonate metabolism increases the initiating efficacy of this carcinogen, although it remains to be shown whether this occurs via cooxidative metabolism or via altered cell physiology.

ARACHIDONATE CASCADE AND TUMOR PROMOTION

There is now substantial evidence to demonstrate that TPA elicits prostaglandin (and other eicosanoids) synthesis in mouse epidermal cells (reviewed in refs. 19 and 20). Studies by Bresnick et al. (21) and Verma et al. (22) suggest that PGE_2 is the principal prostaglandin affected by TPA. In addition, Verma et al. (23) demonstrated that the cyclooxygenase inhibitor indomethacin markedly inhibited TPA induction of ODC, an effect that could be reversed by application of PGE_2. More recently, Nakadate et al. (24,25) have used phospholipase A_2 and lipoxygenase inhibitors and found that lipoxygenase products also seem to be involved in the induction of ODC.

Results of these studies suggest that tumor promotion can be modified through the application of either exogenous prostaglandins or inhibitors of various parts of the arachidonate cascade. Our first approach to this possibility (26) was to determine the effect of individual prostaglandins when applied topically either alone or with TPA on initiated mouse skin. This series of experiments demonstrated that the effect of various prostaglandins on tumor production depends on both the particular agent used and the timing of its application relative to TPA. Specifically, $PGF_{2\alpha}$ enhances TPA tumor promotion in the SENCAR mouse by up to 60% with 10 µg applications, and PGE_1 reproducibly inhibits promotion at doses as low as 1 µg (26). None of the prostaglandins tested had promoting activity when applied repetitively to initiated SENCAR mice (22). Verma et al. (22) confirmed this with PGE_2 in CD-1 mice, as did Furstenberger and Marks (27) with PGE_2 and $PGF_{2\alpha}$ in NMRI mice.

The second approach that our laboratory and several others have taken in studying the role of increased arachidonate metabolism is to use inhibitors of various parts of the arachidonate cascade. Because of the role of prostaglandins in inflammation, it was originally thought that nonsteroidal anti-inflammatory agents, i.e., the cyclooxygenase inhibitors indomethacin and flurbiprofen, would inhibit promotion. In the SENCAR mouse, however, it was found that topical application of indomethacin enhanced TPA tumor promotion at doses of 25 to 100 µg but inhibited it at higher, probably toxic doses (28). This enhancing effect is even more pronounced using the multistage promotion protocol established by Slaga et al. (2), in which four applications of TPA (first stage) are followed by repetitive applications of the weak promoter mezerein (second stage). When indomethacin was applied 2 h before TPA in the first stage, the number of tumors was double that with TPA alone (29). This enhancement occurred in spite of the fact that indomethacin inhibited ODC induction by TPA (data not shown). Indomethacin has only a mildly enhancing effect on the second stage of promotion. Histological studies have shown that in SENCAR mice, indomethacin does not inhibit TPA-induced hyperplasia, inflammation, or dark cells (28).

Using other strains of mice, notably CD-1 and NMRI, Verma et al. (30) and Furstenberger and Marks (27) found only an inhibitory effect for indomethacin. To investigate the basis for this difference among stocks of mice, we determined the effects of both cyclooxygenase and lipoxygenase inhibitors on several promoter-elicited events in epidermis from NMRI and SENCAR mice. The parameters compared were TPA stimulation of PGE$_2$ synthesis, DNA synthesis, ODC activity, and tumor promotion (31).

The effect of arachidonate inhibitors on TPA-induced DNA synthesis was compared in the different mice both in vitro and in vivo. As shown in Figures 2 and 3, the cyclooxygenase inhibitors indomethacin and flurbiprofen enhanced TPA-induced DNA synthesis in cultures of SENCAR epidermis, but the same agents inhibited TPA-stimulated DNA synthesis in NMRI cultures. Similar results were found with in vivo treatments. The cyclooxygenase-lipoxygenase inhibitors eicosatetraynoic acid (ETYA) and phenidone and the phospholipase A$_2$ inhibitor dibromoacetophenone inhibited TPA-stimulated DNA synthesis in both stocks of mice (31). These findings establish a good correlation between the inhibitor's effects on promotion and on DNA synthesis.

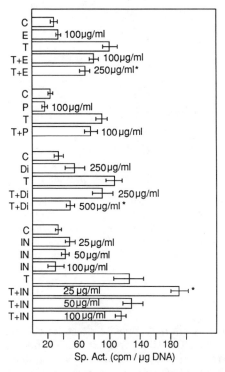

Figure 2. Effect of inhibitors of arachidonic acid metabolism on TPA-induced DNA synthesis in vivo in the SENCAR mouse. The specific activity was determined 24 h after topical application of acetone, 1 µg TPA, and/or the given doses of arachidonate inhibitors. Values, average of six mice; bars, SD; *, significant difference (P>.005, Student's t-test) from the TPA-only treated mice. Abbreviations: C, acetone control; T, 12-O-tetradecanoylphorbol-13-acetate; IN, indomethacin; P, phenidone; Di, dibromoacetophenone; and E, eicosatetraynoic acid. Reproduced with permission from Fischer SM, et al. Cancer Res 47:3174-3179, 1987.

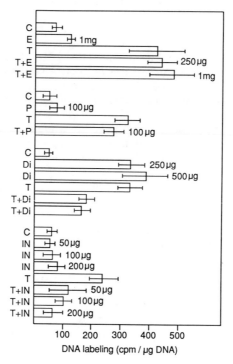

Figure 3. Effect of inhibitors of arachidonic acid metabolism on TPA-induced DNA synthesis in vivo in the NMRI mouse. The specific activity was determined 18 h after topical application of acetone, 6.16 µg TPA, and/or the given doses of arachidonate inhibitors that were applied 30 min prior to TPA. Values, average of 6 to 10 mice; bars, SD. Abbreviations: C, acetone control; T, 12-O-tetradecanoylphorbol-13-acetate; IN, indomethacin; P, phenidone; Di, dibromoacetophenone; and E, eicosatetraynoic acid. Reproduced with permission from Fischer SM, et al. Cancer Res 47:3174-3179, 1987.

Because indomethacin had opposite effects in the two stocks of mice, its effect on TPA-induced ODC activity was examined. Indomethacin was equally effective in both strains of mice in inhibiting TPA-induced ODC activity. In addition, the stimulation of PGE$_2$ synthesis by TPA was also nearly the same in the two strains of mice. PGE$_2$ synthesis, one of the earliest responses to TPA, has been thought to be involved in triggering epidermal hyperplasia of the type that is accompanied by inflammation (32). This, in turn, suggests that arachidonate metabolites are part of the endogenous growth-control mechanisms in these tissues. In the NMRI mouse, increased PGE$_2$ synthesis appears to be essential to subsequent events such as ODC induction, DNA synthesis, and tumor promotion, inasmuch as indomethacin suppresses all of these events. In the

SENCAR mouse, PGE_2 apparently does not have the same regulatory activity; one or more lipoxygenase products may serve this function. This is suggested by previous findings in SENCAR mice (25) that indomethacin elevated the levels of lipoxygenase products. In summary, this comparative study indicated that NMRI and SENCAR mice respond to TPA in a similar manner with respect to promotion, PGE_2 synthesis, and ODC induction. The function of the arachidonate metabolites in these processes in the two strains of mice may account for their different tumor responses to the cyclooxygenase inhibitor indomethacin. The apparent increased lipoxygenase activity in SENCAR mice may be responsible for the greater sensitivity of these mice to the phorbol ester tumor promoters.

Other cyclooxygenase and lipoxygenase inhibitors used in tumor promotion experiments in this laboratory and others are summarized in Table 1. Specifically, we have reported (33) that dual inhibitors such as phenidone and ETYA inhibit tumor promotion by up to 45%. The predominantly lipoxygenase inhibitors nordihydroguaiaretic acid (NDGA) and quercetin were shown by Nakadate et al. (34) and Kato et al. (35) to significantly inhibit TPA-induced tumor promotion. Additionally, inhibitors of phospholipase A_2, i.e., dibromoacetophenone and the anti-inflammatory steroids have been shown by several laboratories to have strong inhibitory activity (9,10,13,33-36).

These inhibitor studies strongly suggest not only that arachidonic acid

Table 1. Summary of Effects of Inhibitors of Arachidonate Metabolism on TPA Tumor Promotion

Inhibitor	Effect	Reference
Cyclooxygenase		
Indomethacin	Enhances	Fischer et al. (28)
	Inhibits	Furstenberger and Marks (27)
		Verma et al. (30)
Flurbiprofen	Enhances	Fischer et al. (28)
Dual cyclooxygenase/lipoxygenase		
Phenidone	Inhibits	Fischer et al. (33)
ETYA	Inhibits	Fischer et al. (33)
		Furstenberger and Marks (20)
NDGA	Inhibits	Nakadate et al. (34)
		Kato et al. (35)
Quercetin	Inhibits	Kato et al. (35,36)
Phospholipase A_2		
Anti-inflammatory steroids	Inhibits	Belman and Troll (13)
		Schwartz et al. (10)
		Slaga et al. (9)
Dibromoacetophenone	Inhibits	Fischer et al. (33)
		Nakadate et al. (34)
		Kato et al. (35,36)

Abbreviations: NDGA, nordihydroguaiaretic acid; ETYA, eicosatetraynoic acid.

256 / Fischer et al.

release and metabolism are important and perhaps essential to tumor promotion
but also that the most important metabolites may be not the prostaglandins
themselves but the lipoxygenase products.

STUDIES ON ARACHIDONATE METABOLISM IN SKIN

The precise roles of the prostaglandins and lipoxygenase products in either
the normal physiology of the skin or in pathological conditions, such as those
induced by TPA, have yet to be clearly elucidated. Given the volume of information on the involvement of eicosanoids in inflammation and proliferation/
differentiation, their greatly increased level of synthesis induced by TPA may
contribute to the biochemical and morphological manifestations of TPA application. Some of the suggested interactions between these products and cellular
components of the skin are shown diagrammatically in Figure 4.

We have initiated several studies that are designed to more clearly identify
the eicosanoids produced in mouse skin and their biological effects. The most
recent, and ongoing, such study is concerned with identifying the subpopulation
of keratinocytes that are responsible for prostaglandin and/or lipoxygenase

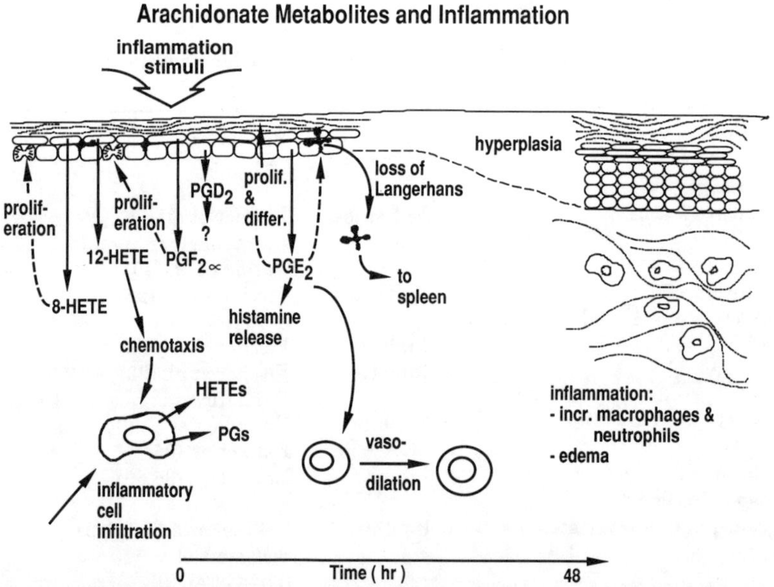

Figure 4. Arachidonic acid metabolism and inflammation. This diagram illustrates the
possible functions of the known major eicosanoids that can be produced by mouse
epidermal cells in response to inflammatory stimuli such as the tumor promoter 12-O-
tetradecanoylphorbol-13-acetate. Abbreviations: differ., differentiation; prolif., proliferation; HETE, hydroxyeicosatetranoic acid; PG, prostaglandin; incr., increase in.

product formation. In this study, epidermal cells from the SENCAR mouse were separated by Percoll gradient centrifugation into three fractions such that fraction I contained the most differentiated, squamous cells and fraction III almost exclusively contained the proliferative basal cells (details of these criteria are provided in ref. 37). Each of the three fractions was evaluated for its capacity to metabolize exogenous arachidonate to prostaglandins and hydroxyeicosate-traenoic acids (HETEs). This was done using both intact cells, in which competition between incorporation into phospholipids and metabolism occurs, and nonviable disrupted cells, where no or minimal incorporation occurs. Using either approach, we found (38) that the three major prostaglandins, PGE_2, $PGF_{2\alpha}$, and PGD_2, are produced principally by cells committed to differentiation (fraction II) and by differentiated cells (fraction I). The same distribution was found for the HETEs. This distribution of eicosanoid production is most likely a reflection of the presence of the metabolizing enzymes and suggests that eicosanoid production is a feature of differentiated or mature keratinocytes. This pattern also resembles that observed by John Reiners (personal communication) for the induction of xanthine oxidase by TPA. A pilot experiment indicated that TPA application to the skin 24 h before cell isolation caused the basal cells to express a greater eicosanoid synthesis capacity. Confirmation of this finding should contribute to our understanding of how TPA and perhaps other irritants cause extensive inflammation.

We have also been interested in why a single application of TPA to the backs of C57BL/6J mice elicits little inflammation or hyperplasia. The skins of these mice are only marginally responsive to TPA as a promoter, although they respond to benzoyl peroxide as a promoter to nearly the same extent as do SENCAR mice (39); this suggests that they are promotable but have an altered response specifically to phorbol esters. Since the necessity of arachidonate metabolism to inflammation and tumor promotion has been fairly well established, we hypothesized that C57BL/6J mice might be either quantitatively or qualitatively different from SENCAR mice in their production of arachidonate metabolites. For this reason, a comparative study was undertaken between inbred SENCAR (SSIN) mice and C57BL/6J mice with respect to arachidonic acid metabolism, the induction of hyperplasia, edema, and oxidant generation (40). As shown in Figure 5, TPA induced arachidonate release to nearly the same extent in epidermal cells from SSIN and C57BL/6J mice. The arachidonate was metabolized principally to PGE_2 and to the same extent in cells from both mice. Some minor differences were observed for PGD_2, the next most abundant prostaglandin, and for $PGF_{2\alpha}$, although the biological implications of this are not known. Because HETE production is most readily measured using cytosol preparations, the effects of TPA were monitored by using animals topically pretreated with TPA. Due to cochromatographic problems with the HETEs, it was necessary to use both reverse-phase and normal-phase high-performance liquid chromatography to identify and quantitate these lipoxygenase products. With this approach, we determined that both SSIN and C57BL/6J epidermis can produce the 12-, 15-, 8- and 5-HETEs to the same extent, as shown in Table 2. By approximately 24 h after a single application of TPA, however, an apparent

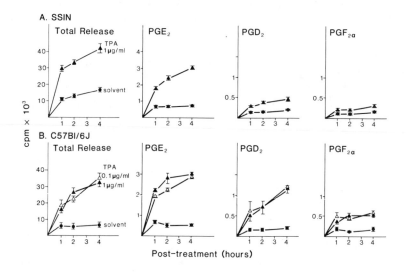

Figure 5. Effect of TPA on arachidonate release and on prostaglandin synthesis in cultured SSIN and C57BL/6J epidermal cells. Cultures were prelabeled with [^{14}C]arachidonic acid 12 h prior to replacement with fresh medium and treatment with either acetone or TPA. At the given times, medium was removed and metabolites separated by thin layer chromatography. Points, mean of duplicate cultures; bars, range; the experiment was repeated at least twice. Reproduced from Fischer SM, et al. Cancer Res 48:658-664, 1988.

induction of the 8-lipoxygenase was observed in the SSIN but not in the C57BL/6J mice. The correlation between TPA-induced hyperplasia (and inflammation) and 8-lipoxygenase induction in the SSIN mice and the lack of both effects in the C57BL/6J mouse suggests a role for the 8-HETE in proliferation. This is further strengthened by recent work in which we found that daily TPA applications for 3 to 5 days to the C57BL/6J mouse resulted in both an induction of 8-lipoxygenase and hyperplasia (as well as inflammation as identified histologically). In addition, we have recently found that when daily or thrice-weekly, but not biweekly (the standard protocol for TPA-promotion experiments) applications of TPA are made to C57BL/6J mice previously given initiating doses of carcinogens, a significant number of papillomas appear.

Another difference we have observed between the SSIN and C57BL/6J mouse is the oxidant response, as measured by chemiluminescence, to TPA or phospholipase C (40). The response of the C57BL/6J mice is considerably less than that of the SSIN mice. All lipoxygenase inhibitors tested so far (41) inhibit this oxidant response, although no evidence shows that lipoxygenase metabolism of arachidonate in epidermal cells is responsible for the measured oxidant

Table 2. Lipoxygenase Products from SSIN or C57BL/6J Epidermal Cells*

Strain by promoter and process		Metabolites (%)		
		15-HETE	12/8-HETE	5-HETE
Reverse-phase HPLC				
SSIN	-Acetone	1.2 ± 0.3	56.3 ± 10.7	0.8 ± 0.2
	-TPA	1.9 ± 0.6	58.0 ± 04.9	1.0 ± 0.3
C57BL/6J	-Acetone	1.4 ± 0.8	53.3 ± 08.2	0.9 ± 0.3
	-TPA	2.4 ± 0.5	49.7 ± 14.4	1.2 ± 0.6
Normal-phase HPLC		12/15-HETE	8-HETE	5-HETE
SSIN	-Acetone	80.8 ± 3.9	04.4 ± 1.6	<0.5
	-TPA	69.0 ± 8.7	16.6 ± 3.9	<0.5
C57BL/6J	-Acetone	74.3 ± 5.2	05.5 ± 1.2	<0.5
	-TPA	71.7 ± 2.5	00.5 ± 2.3	<0.5

*Cytosolic preparations of epidermis, treated 24 h earlier with acetone or 2 mg TPA, were incubated with [^{14}C]arachidonic acid, and the metabolites were extracted and separated by HPLC. Values represent the mean ± SD of three to five experiments using two mice each and are the percentage of the total metabolized arachidonic acid. The TPA-induced increase in the 8-HETE, as evaluated by normal-phase separation, is significantly different ($P < .001$, Student's t-test) from the acetone control value for the SSIN mice. Abbreviations: HPLC, high-performance liquid chromatography; HETE, hydroxyeicosatetraenoic acid. Reproduced from Fischer SM, et al. Cancer Res 48:658-664, 1988.

response. Recent work (41) indicates that this oxidant response may be mediated by protein kinase C, as protein kinase C inhibitors can suppress the responses induced by either TPA or phospholipase C. The difference in oxidant generation between SSIN and C57BL/6J mice and the correlation of this response to inflammation/hyperplasia in the respective mice suggest that the principal mediators of the inflammation seen in SSIN mice may be reactive oxygens rather than the metabolites of arachidonic acid. Reactive oxygens are mediators of other types of tissue damage and inflammation, including arthritis, ulcers, and ischemia. However, it remains to be determined whether the poor inflammatory response to TPA seen in the C57BL/6J mouse is caused by a defective response either to particular arachidonate metabolites or to other aspects of the TPA-elicited signaling mechanisms.

The final approach that we are taking toward elucidating the role of the eicosanoids is the modulation of the types of fatty acids comprising the membrane phospholipids that are potential substrates for prostaglandin synthetase and lipoxygenases. Specifically the n-6 (arachidonate) and n-3 (eicosapentaenoate) fatty acids are being compared, both in vitro and in vivo. The basis for this study is that the n-3 eicosanoids (e.g., PGE$_3$) are much less biologically active than are the n-6 (e.g., PGE$_2$). If the n-6 products mediate the excessive inflammation and hyperplasia induced by TPA, then substitution of n-3 for n-6 could have an ameliorating effect both on these parameters and on the final tumor

Table 3. Effect of Arachidonate (AA) vs. Eicosapentaenoate (EPA) on TPA-Induced ODC
In Vitro

Treatment	ODC activity*
Control	0.070 ± 0.032
+ TPA (1 µg/ml)	0.827 ± 0.195
AA†	0.054 ± 0.023
+TPA	1.118 ± 0.243
EPA	0.059 ± 0.022
+ TPA	0.688 ± 0.125

* nmol CO_2/mg protein/h.
†Fatty acids were used at a 1 µg/ml media concentration; they were complexed to fatty
acid free BSA prior to addition of serum free media. Values represent the mean$\pm$ SD ($n=5$
or 6). The difference in ODC activity between AA+TPA and EPA+TPA is statistically
significant ($P<0.01$; Student's t-test).
Abbreviations: ODC, ornithine decarboxylase; BSA, bovine serum albumin.

burden. In in vitro studies done to date, we have observed that epidermal cells
from SSIN mice incorporate into their phospholipids approximately equal
amounts of arachidonate and eicosapentaenoate (Larson, Patrick, Locniskar,
and Fischer, in preparation). After subsequent treatment with TPA, however,
more arachidonate than eicosapentaenoate is released. More striking is the
difference in prostaglandin production under these conditions: considerably
more PGE_2 is produced from arachidonate-fed cultures than is PGE_3 from
eicosapentaenoate-fed cultures. Similar findings were observed for PGD and
PGF. The biological significance of these findings is suggested by the effect of
these two fatty acids on TPA-induced ODC, as shown in Table 3. Arachidonic acid
addition enhanced TPA-induced ODC activity, but eicosapentaenoic acid had
little effect. This is in keeping with the findings of Verma et al. (23), who showed
that PGE_2 is needed for the induction of ODC. Whether dietary n-3 fatty acid
substitution results in comparable findings in vivo soon may be determined.

CONCLUSIONS

Taken together, the results of studies from this laboratory and others
clearly demonstrate that inhibition of arachidonic acid metabolism, and particularly inhibition of lipoxygenases, results in an inhibition of tumor promotion and
further suggest that at least some of the metabolites have an essential role in the
tumor promotion process. This, in turn, implies that any agent that induces
arachidonic acid release and metabolism may contribute to tumorigenesis. This
probably holds true for human neoplasias as well; thus, anti-inflammatory
agents or dietary regulation of fatty acids may be of chemopreventive value.

ACKNOWLEDGMENTS

This work was supported principally by NIH grants CA-43334, CA-42211, and CA-46886. The secretarial assistance of Carol Hildman is gratefully acknowledged.

OPEN FORUM

Dr. Thomas Argyris: When you took density gradients and isolated the squames from the basal layers, was that with normal epidermis?

Dr. Susan Fischer: Yes. We have not yet done the experiments looking at TPA-treated epidermis. That is our next project.

Dr. Andrew T. Huang: When you applied arachidonic acid alone to mouse skin, did that initiate tumors?

Dr. Fischer: No. Arachidonic acid alone will induce edema and a certain amount of inflammation, but it is not a promoter by itself. One of the reasons I mentioned histamine and some of these other mediators of inflammation is that inflammation is a complex process, and arachidonic acid is only part of it. Perhaps one reason that we do not see promotion with just arachidonic acid is that we are only looking at part of the process.

Dr. Huang: After repetitive application of arachidonic acid, did the skin appear to be damaged?

Dr. Fischer: It depends on the dose level. If you apply a high enough dose, you eventually get ulceration of the skin. You do get inflammation with arachidonic acid, and particularly edema.

Dr. Allan Balmain: We published some experiments a couple of years ago showing that TPA treatment of skin induces the granulocyte-macrophage colony stimulating factor (GM-CSF). You get a massive induction at the protein level in the epidermis of this hematopoietic growth factor. Ian Pragnell has also looked at the effects of indomethacin on this induction. It is interesting that you find that indomethacin increases promotion, because he has found that whereas dexamethasone completely eliminates the GM-CSF induction, indomethacin superinduces GM-CSF. That fits in very nicely with what you were saying. Is it possible to fit GM-CSF into your scheme of things? Is it known whether that induces any of the enzymes involved in arachidonic acid metabolism?

Dr. Fischer: I do not know.

Dr. Stuart Yuspa: I do not understand the experiments using C57/BL mice. Based on what we know about phorbol ester responses, why would painting TPA on mice for 3 days make the animal TPA-responsive? Do you have any ideas to explain this finding?

Dr. Fischer: At this point we do not know why this happens. We do know that when you treat with a single application of TPA, you get good ODC induction at low levels of TPA; the response is comparable to what we see in SENCAR mice. We do not get hyperplasia in the C57 black mouse, however. This suggests that for some reason there is a dissociation between ODC induction and proliferation.

We have done experiments in both the SENCAR and the C57 black where, if we treat with TPA, wait 24 h, and then treat with TPA again, we do not see ODC induction. Presumably this is because protein kinase C is downregulated. However, under those circumstances, if we continue to give TPA daily, we get hyperplasia in the black mouse. The suggestion is that it is due to something other than a protein kinase C-mediated mechanism. It may be due to these arachidonic acid metabolites, but I am only guessing at this point. But protein kinase C does not appear to be involved.

REFERENCES

1. Berenblum I, Shubik P. A new, quantitative approach to the study of the stages of chemical carcinogenesis in the mouse skin. Br J Cancer 1:373-391, 1947.
2. Slaga TJ, Fischer SM, Nelson K, Gleason GL. Studies on the mechanism of skin tumor promotion: Evidence for several stages in promotion. Proc Natl Acad Sci USA 77:3659-3663, 1980.
3. Slaga TJ, Fischer SM, Weeks CE, Klein-Szanto AJP. Cellular and biochemical mechanisms of mouse skin tumor promoters. In Hodgson JR, Bend RM, Philpot RM (eds): Reviews in Biochemical Toxicology, Vol 3. New York: Elsevier/North Holland, 1981, pp 231-282.
4. Slaga TJ, Klein-Szanto AJP, Fischer SM, Weeks CE, Nelson K, Major S. Studies on the mechanism of action of anti-tumor promoting agents: Their specificity in two-stage promotion. Proc Natl Acad Sci USA 77:2251-2254, 1980.
5. Slaga TJ, Fischer SM, Weeks CE, Klein-Szanto AJP. Multistage chemical carcinogenesis in mouse skin. Curr Probl Dermatol 10:193-218, 1980.
6. Slaga TJ. Mechanisms involved in two-stage carcinogenesis in mouse skin. In Slaga TJ (ed): Mechanisms of Tumor Promotion. Boca Raton, FL: CRC Press, 1984, pp 1-16.
7. Janoff A, Klassen A, Troll W. Local vascular changes induced by the cocarcinogen phorbol myristate acetate. Cancer Res 30:2568-2571, 1970.
8. Marks F, Berry DL, Bertsch S, Furstenberger G, Richter H. On the relationship between epidermal hyperproliferation and skin tumor promotion. In Hecker E, Marks F, Fusenig N, Slaga TJ (eds): Cocarcinogenesis and Biological Effects of Tumor Promoters. New York: Raven Press, 1982, pp 331-346.
9. Slaga TJ, Fischer SM, Viaje A, Berry DL, Bracken WM, LeClerc S, Miller DR. Inhibition of tumor promotion by anti-inflammatory agents: An approach to the biochemical mechanism of promotion. In Slaga TJ, Sivak A, Boutwell RK (eds): Mechanisms of Tumor Promotion and Cocarcinogenesis. Carcinogenesis: A Comprehensive Survey, Vol 2. New York: Raven Press, 1978, pp 173-195.
10. Schwartz JA, Viaje A, Slaga TJ, Yuspa SH, Hennings H, Lichti U. Fluocinolone acetonide: A potent inhibitor of mouse skin tumor promotion and epidermal DNA synthesis. Chem Biol Interact 17:331-347, 1977.
11. Hong SL, Levine L. Inhibition of arachidonic acid release from cells as the biochemical action of anti-inflammatory corticosteroids. Proc Natl Acad Sci USA 73:1730-1734, 1977.
12. Gryglewski RJ. Effects of anti-inflammatory steroids on arachidonate cascade. In Weissmann G, Samuelsson B, Paoletti R (eds): Advances in Inflammation Research, Vol. 1. New York: Raven Press, 1979, pp 505-514.

13. Belman S, Troll W. The inhibition of croton oil-promoted mouse skin tumorigenesis by steroid hormones. Cancer Res 32:450-454, 1972.

14. Scribner JD, Slaga TJ. Multiple effects of dexamethasone on protein synthesis and hyperplasia caused by a tumor promoter. Cancer Res 33:542-546, 1973.

15. Anderson MW, Crutchley DJ, Chaudhari A, Wilson AGE, Eling TE. Studies on the covalent binding of an intermediate(s) in prostaglandin biosynthesis to tissue macromolecules. Biochim Biophys Acta 573:40-50, 1979.

16. Basu A, Marnett LJ. Unequivocal demonstration that malondialdehyde is a mutagen. Carcinogenesis 4:331-333, 1983.

17. Marnett LJ. Arachidonic acid metabolism and tumor initiation. In Marnett LJ (ed): Arachidonic Acid Metabolism and Tumor Initiation. Boston: Martinus Nijhoff, 1985, pp 39-82.

18. Fischer SM, Gleason GL, Bohrman JS, Slaga TJ. Prostaglandin enhancement of skin tumor initiation and promotion. In Samuelsson B, Ramwell PW, Paoletti R (eds): Advances in Prostaglandin and Thromboxane Research, Vol 6. New York: Raven Press, 1980, pp 517-22.

19. Fischer SM. Arachidonic acid metabolism and tumor promotion. In Fischer SM, Slaga TJ (eds): Arachidonic Acid Metabolism and Tumor Promotion. Boston: Martinus Nijhoff, 1985, pp 49-72.

20. Furstenberger G, Marks F. Prostaglandins, epidermal hyperplasia and skin tumor promotion. In Fischer SM, Slaga TJ (eds): Arachidonic Acid Metabolism and Tumor Promotion. Boston: Martinus Nijhoff, 1985, pp 73-100.

21. Bresnick E, Meunier P, Lamden M. Epidermal prostaglandins after topical application of a tumor promoter. Cancer Lett 7:121-125, 1979.

22. Verma AK, Ashendel CL, Boutwell RK. Inhibition by prostaglandin synthesis inhibitors of the induction of epidermal ornithine decarboxylase activity, the accumulation of prostaglandins and tumor promotion caused by 12-O-tetrade-canoylphorbol-13-acetate. Cancer Res 40:308-315, 1980.

23. Verma AK, Rice HM, Boutwell RK. Prostaglandins and skin tumor promotion: Inhibition of tumor promoter-induced ornithine decarboxylase activity in epidermis by inhibitors of prostaglandin synthesis. Biochem Biophys Res Commun 79:1160-1166, 1977.

24. Nakadate T, Yamamoto S, Ishii M, Kato R. Inhibition of 12-O-tetradecanoylphorbol-13-acetate-induced epidermal ornithine decarboxylase activity by lipoxygenase inhibitors: Possible role of product(s) of lipoxygenase pathway. Carcinogenesis 3:1411-1414, 1982.

25. Nakadate T, Yamamoto S, Ishii M, Kato R. Inhibition of 12-O-tetradecanoylphorbol-13-acetate-induced epidermal ornithine decarboxylase activity by phospholipase A_2 inhibitors and lipoxygenase inhibitor. Cancer Res 42:2841-2845, 1982.

26. Fischer SM, Gleason GL, Bohrman JS, Slaga TJ. Prostaglandin modulation of phorbol ester skin tumor promotion. Carcinogenesis 1:245-248, 1980.

27. Furstenberger G, Marks F. Studies on the role of prostaglandins in the induction of cell proliferation and hyperplasia and in tumor promotion in mouse skin. In Hecker E et al. (eds): Symposium on Cocarcinogenesis and Biological Effects of Tumor Promoters. New York: Raven Press, 1982, pp 325-330.

28. Fischer SM, Gleason GL, Mills GD, Slaga TJ. Indomethacin enhancement of TPA tumor promotion in mice. Cancer Lett 10:343-350, 1980.

29. Fischer SM. The role of prostaglandins in tumor promotion. In Slaga TJ (ed): Mechanisms of Tumor Promotion. Tumor Promotion and Skin Carcinogenesis, Vol II. Boca Raton, FL: CRC Press, 1983, pp 113-126.

30. Verma AK, Ashendel CL, Boutwell RK. Inhibition by prostaglandin synthesis inhibitors of the induction of epidermal ornithine decarboxylase activity, the accumulation of prostaglandins and tumor promotion caused by 12-O-tetradecanoylphorbol-13-acetate. Cancer Res 40:308-315, 1980.

31. Fischer SM, Furstenberger G, Marks F, Slaga TJ. Events associated with mouse skin tumor promotion with respect to arachidonic acid metabolism: A comparison between SENCAR and NMRI mice. Cancer Res 47:3174-3179, 1987.

32. Marks F, Furstenberger G, Kownatzki E. Prostaglandin E-mediated mitogenic stimulation of mouse epidermis in vivo by divalent cation ionophore A 23187 and by tumor promoter 12-O-tetradecanoylphorbol-13-acetate. Cancer Res 41:696-702, 1981.

33. Fischer SM, Mills GD, Slaga TJ. Inhibition of mouse skin tumor promotion by several inhibitors of arachidonic acid metabolism. Carcinogenesis 3:1243-1245, 1982.

34. Nakadate T, Yamamoto S, Iseki H, Sonoda S, Takemura S, Ura A, Hosoda Y, Kato R. Inhibition of 12-O-tetradecanoylphorbol-13-acetate-induced tumor promotion by nordihydroguaiaretic acid, a lipoxygenase inhibitor and p-bromophenacyl bromide, a phospholipase A_2 inhibitor. Gann 73:841-843, 1982.

35. Kato R, Nakadate T, Yamamoto S. Involvement of lipoxygenase products of arachidonic acid in tumor-promoting activity of TPA. In Thaler-Dao H, dePaulet AC, Paoletti R (eds): Eicosanoids and Cancer. New York: Raven Press, 1984, pp 101-114.

36. Kato R, Nakadate T, Yamamoto S, Sugimura T. Inhibition of 12-O-tetradecanoylphorbol-13-acetate-induced tumor promotion and ornithine decarboxylase activity by quercetin: Possible involvement of lipoxygenase inhibition. Carcinogenesis 4:1301-1305, 1983.

37. Fischer SM, Nelson KDG, Reiners JJ, Viaje A, Pelling JC, Slaga TJ. Separation of epidermal cells by density centrifugation: A new technique for studies on normal and pathological differentiation. J Cutan Pathol 9:43-49, 1982.

38. Cameron GS, Baldwin JK, Jasheway DW, Patrick KE, Fischer SM. Distribution of arachidonic acid metabolism according to the state of differentiation in mouse epidermal cells (abstract). Proceedings of the American Association for Cancer Research 29:75, 1988.

39. Reiners JJ, Nesnow S, Slaga TJ. Murine susceptibility to two-stage carcinogenesis is influenced by the agent used for promotion. Carcinogenesis 5:301-307, 1984.

40. Fischer SM, Baldwin JK, Jasheway DW, Patrick KE, Cameron GS. Phorbol ester induction of 8-lipoxygenase in inbred SENCAR (SSIN) but not C57BL/6J mice correlated with hyperplasia, edema, and oxidant generation but not ornithine decarboxylase induction. Cancer Res 48:658-664, 1988.

41. Fischer SM, Cameron GS, Baldwin JK, Jasheway DW, Patrick KE. Reactive oxygen in the tumor promotion stage of skin carcinogenesis. Lipids 23:592-597, 1988.

Skin Carcinogenesis: Mechanisms and Human Relevance, pages 265–279
© 1989 Alan R. Liss, Inc.

Short-Term Assays to Detect Tumor-Promoting Activity of Environmental Chemicals

Hiroshi Yamasaki

International Agency for Research on Cancer, Lyon, France

Development of short-term assays to detect carcinogenic chemicals has been an important endeavor in view of the large number of chemicals humans are exposed to and the fact that rodent assays are too slow and too expensive to perform for each chemical. More than 100 different short-term tests have been developed (1-3). However, almost all of these test systems were designed to detect the so-called genotoxic activity of chemicals. As molecular and cellular mechanisms of multistage carcinogenesis became known through much intensive research, it became apparent that different stages could involve different mechanisms (4-6), and thus mechanisms of action of chemicals could also represent a wide spectrum, including nongenotoxic as well as genotoxic activity.

Identification of a family of cellular genes that is critically involved in carcinogenesis has helped in evaluating the validity of existing short-term tests. For example, carcinogen-specific induction of mutation in certain cellular oncogenes is implicated as a molecular determinant of carcinogenesis (7,8). A single exposure of rats to N-methyl-N-nitrosourea (MNU) induces mammary tumors that contain an activated oncogene shown to be the Harvey-*ras*-protooncogene mutated at the 12th codon (9); this oncogene is activated by a specific G to A transition. MNU is known to be a potent mutagen that preferentially induces G to A transition as a result of mismatching of its 6-methylguanine product (10). In contrast, no such G to A transition was found in tumors induced by 7,12-dimethylbenz[*a*]anthracene (DMBA) (7). DMBA is a carcinogen that predominantly binds to adenine residues. Dandekar et al. (11) found an A to T transversion at the 61st codon of Ha-*ras* in mammary tumors induced by DMBA. Similarly, DNA from mouse skin papillomas and carcinomas produced by an initiation-promotion protocol had an A to T transversion at the 61st codon of the Ha-*ras* gene only when DMBA or dibenz[*c,h*]acridine were used as initiators (12-14). When benzo[*a*]pyrene or N-methyl-N'-nitro-N-nitrosoguanidine were used as initiators, there was no such mutation (12-14). These results on carcinogen-specific mutagenesis of oncogenes support the usefulness of the mutation assay for the identification of certain carcinogens.

Results from molecular studies of mouse skin carcinogenesis, however, also suggest that mutation is not a sufficient event for carcinogenesis. Although the DNA of tumors produced by initiation-promotion protocols shows initiator-specific activation of oncogenes, initiator application itself is not enough to produce tumors; tumors appear only when mouse skin is subsequently painted with a tumor-promoting agent (14). These results suggest that the cells that have an initiator-induced activated oncogene can stay dormant until they encounter a tumor-promoting stimulus. From the accumulated knowledge of action of tumor-promoting agents, it is becoming clear that these agents act differently from initiating agents (4-6). Because of these facts, the development of short-term tests for tumor promoters requires different approaches from those used for initiating agents.

Currently, there is no single validated assay for predicting the tumor-promoting activity of chemicals. However, two principal approaches are being pursued in this regard: development of in vitro systems in which in vivo multistage carcinogenesis can be mimicked and utilization of cellular and molecular events associated with tumor promotion as end points of short-term tests (15,16). I will present two-stage in vitro cell transformation systems and inhibition of gap-junctional intercellular communication as examples of these two approaches, respectively. First, I would like to define what can and cannot be measured in tumor promotion and my personal view on the need for clear definitions of various terms for multistage carcinogenesis.

CLEAR DEFINITION OF TERMS NEEDED

I believe that the frequent misuse of certain terms in the carcinogenesis literature has generated some confusion. Words used to define different stages of carcinogenesis are often applied to the agents used. Often, also, the stage-related activity of a chemical is confused with its specific activity.

Much of the existing confusion could be avoided if it was realized that the terms that describe the carcinogenic process—initiation, promotion, and progression—are applicable only to the carcinogenic process itself and do not imply any mechanism of action of the chemicals that are involved in these stages. For example, agents involved in the initiation stage of carcinogenesis are often defined as initiators, and those that have tumor-promoting activity in two-stage models are called tumor promoters. These terms are not themselves misleading when used within the correct context, but confusion occurs when the terms initiator and promoter are used independently from the two-stage carcinogenesis concept and it is assumed that tumor-initiating or -promoting activity is the only activity of a chemical. It is important to realize that initiating or promoting activity may be only one characteristic of a chemical and that many carcinogens probably have both activities.

The interchangeable use of the terms stage and agent had led some investigators to conclude that multistage carcinogenesis does not exist. Although no exogenous or endogenous tumor promoter has been identified unequivocally as an agent in human carcinogenesis, there is strong circumstantial evidence for the involvement of such factors in different stages of carcinogenesis (17-20). Phorbol esters are prototypes of tumor-promoting agents for two-stage carcinogenesis in mouse skin, but these agents can also induce tumors in mice not exposed to tumor-initiating agents. This finding has also been used to argue against the two-stage model of carcinogenesis (21). The argument is again based on the misconception that if phorbol esters are tumor-promoting agents they should act only as tumor promoters, whereas tumor promotion is only one of their activities. In practice, it is not important that phorbol esters also have a weak complete carcinogenic activity. What is important is that they can dramatically promote the yield of tumors in mouse skin previously initiated with a low dose of carcinogen (22).

The confusion described above stems from a simplistic extension of initiation-promotion processes to describe the agents that are involved in two-stage carcinogenesis models. However, the stages of carcinogenesis exist, even if pure initiating or promoting agents do not, and chemicals cannot be classified categorically on the basis of their activity in two-stage models of carcinogenesis, as a given agent may have both initiating and promoting activity. These considerations are particularly important in developing an assay system to detect factors involved in the different stages of carcinogenesis.

Another type of confusion derives from a careless extrapolation of results of mechanistic studies of two-stage carcinogenesis to the mechanisms of action of chemicals. Extensive studies with two-stage models of carcinogenesis, particularly in mouse skin and rat liver, provide convincing evidence that the principal mechanism of tumor initiation is a genotoxic one and that nongenotoxic mechanisms may be involved in tumor promotion (4-6). These findings have been interpreted to indicate that chemicals involved in the different stages of carcinogenesis act by those same mechanisms. Thus, it is sometimes suggested that tumor-promoting agents are synonymous with nongenotoxic chemicals. But the fact that a chemical acts by genotoxic or nongenotoxic mechanisms does not restrict its activities. In addition, the terms genotoxic and nongenotoxic are not derived from a stage-related concept of carcinogenesis but from the types of interaction between chemicals and target cells, i.e., whether they act on target DNA or act epigenetically (23-25). The terms genotoxic and nongenotoxic should therefore not be used as synonyms for the stage-related nomenclature of chemicals, such as tumor-initiating or -promoting agents. This distinction should be taken into account when we attempt to establish a test to detect stage-related activity, e.g., tumor-promoting activity of environmental chemicals.

INHIBITED INTERCELLULAR COMMUNICATION IN TUMOR PROMOTION

Inhibition of Gap-Junctional Intercellular Communication by Tumor-Promoting Agents

Phorbol ester tumor-promoting agents were the first compounds among those directly involved in carcinogenesis to have been shown to inhibit gap-junctional intercellular communication (IC) (for reviews, see 26,27). The inhi-

Table 1. Inhibition of Gap-Junctional Intercellular Communication by Tumor-Promoting Stimuli

Method of communication measurement	Promoting stimulus	References
Metabolic cooperation		
[^{3}H]uridine metabolite transfer	Phorbol esters	28
HGPRT$^+$/HGPRT$^-$	Phorbol esters and many other tumor-promoting agents	29, 33, 76
ASS$^-$/ASL$^-$	Phorbol esters	77
AK$^+$/AK$^-$	Phorbol esters	78
Electrical coupling		
	Phorbol esters	30
	Skin wounding	79
Dye transfer		
Microinjection	Phorbol esters and certain other tumor-promoting agents	34, 80, 81
	Partial hepatectomy	82
Photobleaching	TPA, dieldrin	83
Scrape loading	TPA, dieldrin, and other tumor-promoting agents	84
Gap-junction structure analysis		
Electron microscope	Phorbol esters	36, 85
	Phenobarbital, DDT	35
Gel electrophoresis analysis	Phorbol esters	86
Analysis with gap-junction antibody	Partial hepatectomy	87

Abbreviations: HGPRT, hypoxanthine guanine phosphoribosyltransferase; ASS, argininosuccinate synthetase; ASL, argininosuccinate lyase; AK, adenosine kinase; TPA, 12-O-tetradecanoylphorbol-13-acetate; DDT, dichlorodiphenyltrichloroethane.

bition of IC in cultured cells by these phorbol esters was first discovered using metabolic cooperation as an assay to measure gap-junctional communication (28, 29). The finding was soon confirmed by various other investigators and was extended to various tumor promoters in different IC assays (30-34). Examples of tumor-promoter-mediated inhibition of gap-junctional intercellular communication are in Table 1.

It is important to emphasize that not only phorbol esters but also other types of tumor-promoting agents inhibit IC. Moreover, the inhibition of IC by tumor-promoting agents is not limited to cell cultures but has also been observed in vivo. For example, the administration of liver tumor-promoting agents phenobarbital or dichlorodiphenyltrichloroethane (DDT) was shown to reduce the gap-junctional area in rat liver (35), and mouse skin painting of 12-O-tetradecanoylphorbol-13-acetate (TPA) reduced the number of gap junctions in the epidermis

(36). Furthermore, as can be seen from Table 1, not only chemicals but also physical stimuli such as partial hepatectomy and skin wounding resulted in diminished IC. Partial hepatectomy and skin wounding were known to be tumor-promoting stimuli for rat liver (37) and mouse skin (38), respectively.

Evidence described above prompted several investigators to use these phenomena for a possible short-term test to detect tumor-promoting agents. Dr. Trosko's group has pursued this approach intensively and has presented convincing evidence that this approach may be worthwhile to validate as a possible test (39, 40). Meanwhile, as described below, our group and others have provided several lines of evidence that support the idea that blocked intercellular communication may be involved in tumor promotion.

Gap-Junctional Intercellular Communication and Cell Transformation

In order to see whether phorbol ester-mediated inhibition of intercellular communication is related to enhancement of BALB/c 3T3 cell transformation, we measured IC during the promotion phase of cell transformation (41). After tumor initiation with a low dose of 3-methylcholanthrene, BALB/c 3T3 cells were exposed to phorbol esters. When the cells are in exponential growth, phorbol esters can drastically inhibit IC, but the effect is transient; after 1 or 2 days, the communication capacity is recovered even if phorbol esters are repeatedly added (41). However, at culture confluence, repeated addition of phorbol esters resulted in continuous IC inhibition. Moreover, in comparing the effects of TPA and phorbol-12,13-didecanoate, the latter was more effective in decreasing intercellular communication at culture confluence and in enhancing cell transformation (41). These results support the idea that blocked intercellular communication at culture confluence plays an important role in the promotional phase of BALB/c 3T3 cell transformation.

Similar results were obtained with the endogenous functional analogue of phorbol esters, diacylglycerol. When we added diacylglycerol to BALB/c 3T3 cells, IC was inhibited and cell transformation was enhanced (42).

We also obtained evidence that suggests that blocked intercellular communication is not only related to phorbol ester-mediated enhancement of cell transformation but is also intrinsically related to enhancement of the cell transformation process per se, even in the absence of phorbol esters. In such a study, we have compared two variants of BALB/c 3T3 cells that show extremely different degrees of susceptibility to inducers of transformation. When clone A-31-1-13 cells were exposed to chemical carcinogens or ultraviolet light, the extent of induction of cell transformation was 100- to 500-fold higher than that observed with clone A-31-1-8 cells (43,44). In spite of this difference, the extent of DNA damage, DNA repair, and mutation were very similar in the two clones (44, 45). Since DNA damage-related events are considered to be major mechanisms of the initiation phase of cell transformation, we hypothesized that the difference in these cell lines might be found in the later stage of transformation (46). When intercellular communication of these two different cell lines was measured, we found a similar communication capacity in the growth phase. However, at confluence, the transformation-sensitive cells, i.e., A-31-1-13 cells, lost their communication capacity, whereas the transformation-resistant A31-1-8 cells continued to communicate (46). These results indicated that the transformation-sensitive cells can endogenously express a promoter-related effect when they reach confluence. Thus, it appears that although these two cell lines receive the insult from the initiating agent to a similar extent, only transformation-sensitive cells can be easily transformed because of this TPA-like effect during the later stage.

Further evidence for the involvement of IC inhibition in cell transformation came from our studies using inhibitors of tumor promotion. Retinoids, glucocorticoids, and cyclic AMP have been reported to be potent inhibitors of skin tumor-promoting agents (47). We have previously shown that these antipromoters can antagonize the TPA effect on gap-junctional intercellular communication (48). If, then, decreased gap-junctional intercellular communication is indeed involved in cell transformation, we hypothesize that these antipromoters should also inhibit cell transformation. We have indeed found that retinoic acid, dexamethasone, fluocinolone acetonide, and cyclic AMP can inhibit complete or two-step cell transformation of BALB/c 3T3 cells (49).

I have summarized so far only the results that support the hypothesis that inhibited gap-junctional intercellular communication plays a role in cell transformation. However, some evidence does not support this hypothesis. For example, we have recently found that transforming growth factor-beta (TGF-β) is a potent tumor promoter in BALB/c 3T3 cell transformation (50). However, TGF-β had no effect on gap-junctional intercellular communication of BALB/c 3T3 cells during the whole period of transformation (50). In addition, Boreiko's group has shown that 2,3,6,7-tetrachlorodibenzodioxin can enhance transformation of C3H/10T1/2 cells without inhibition of gap-junctional communication (51). It is possible that these compounds affect IC only locally around cells that have undergone initiation, an effect that cannot be examined in the absence of techniques to identify such cells. Nonetheless, it is important to bear in mind such a limitation when we attempt to use gap-junctional intercellular communication as an end point for the detection of tumor-promoting activity of environmental chemicals.

TWO-STAGE IN VITRO CELL TRANSFORMATION

A proposal to use blocked gap-junctional intercellular communication as an end point of an assay for tumor-promoting activity is based on a hypothesis generated from mechanistic studies of tumor promotion. However, mechanisms of tumor promotion are not yet definitively understood, and in spite of a good association between the blockage of intercellular communication and tumor promotion, no direct causal relationship has been documented between them. On the other hand, another possible assay for tumor-promoting activity, namely, the two-stage cell transformation system, is proposed because it was developed to simulate the in vivo process of carcinogenesis. Therefore, regardless of mechanisms involved, the two-stage cell transformation system may be used to detect initiating and promoting activity of chemicals.

There are four two-stage transformation systems reported in the literature, all of which employ rodent fibroblasts: C3H/10T1/2 cells (52), BALB/c 3T3 cells (53), Syrian hamster embryo cells (54), and rat embryo fibroblasts (55). These systems were, however, used mainly for mechanistic studies and have not yet been rigorously exploited as assays to detect tumor-initiating or promoting agents.

Because most adult human cancers are of epithelial cell origin, it is desirable to establish epithelial cell transformation systems. Although various types of epithelial cells have been studied in this regard, there are few systems in which promising progress is being made. In parallel with the advances made in understanding two-stage mouse skin carcinogenesis, there has recently been significant progress in developing in vitro systems for studying multistage mouse epidermal cell transformation (56). The key element in this progress has been the successful culture of primary cells and carcinogen-initiated cells (56-58). Mouse epidermal cells in culture are, however, also presently used for mechanistic purposes more extensively than for screening of chemicals. However, once the behavior of these mouse cells in culture is well characterized, they should serve as a powerful tool to study tumor-initiating and -promoting agents of skin.

One particular mouse epidermal cell line, JB6, has been used extensively to study mechanisms of tumor promotion (59-62). In this cell line, TPA induces irreversible, anchorage-independent growth (59). Other promoting agents active in JB6 cells include certain detergents, cigarette smoke condensate, benzoyl peroxide, di(2-ethylhexyl) phthalate, and epidermal growth factor (61-63).

In studies of multistage rat liver carcinogenesis, efforts have been made to culture the hepatocyte target cells, but because of the difficulty in maintaining differentiated functions of hepatocytes in culture, there are very few studies on tumor promoter effects on these cells (64-65). An interesting approach is the isolation of hepatocytes from rats previously treated by a carcinogen and the subsequent study of tumor promoter effects in culture. Here, some liver-specific tumor-promoting agents have shown positive effects (66). Established lines from rat liver have been frequently used in tumor promoter studies (67); however, the original cell types of these established cell lines are not known.

Other examples of epithelial cells derived from various tissues and used to study the effect of tumor-promoting agents include, of particular importance, the development of techniques to culture human epithelial cells, such as bronchial cells (for review, see ref. 68). One major problem associated with epithelial cell transformation is the lack of phenotypic markers for the assessment of transformation. Nonetheless, it is possible that recent advances in understanding the molecular biology of normal and transformed cells may lead to techniques that will help detect transformed phenotypes in these epithelial cells as well as in fibroblasts.

CONCLUSION

I have briefly reviewed the status of short-term tests for detection of tumor-promoting agents. It is clear that there is as yet no validated test that can be used for routine screening of tumor-promoting agents. Inhibition of gap-junctional intercellular communication and two-stage in vitro cell transformation are discussed as possible end points to be pursued for this purpose (16).

In principle, any biological or biochemical effects related to tumor promotion can be considered as candidate end points for short-term tests. However, it must be always borne in mind that not all promoters operate via the same mechanism. For example, as phorbol esters exert many of their effects through protein kinase C activation, those promoting agents that do not require protein kinase C activation may not be detected if we use these effects as end points of short-term tests. Thus, the Friend erythroleukemia cell adhesion assay can easily quantitate biological potency of phorbol esters, but it failed to detect non-phorbol ester tumor-promoting agents (69). Several non-TPA-type tumor promoters have been identified by Fujiki's group (70), using biochemical assays in intact animals.

Some tumor-promoting agents, mostly phorbol esters, have also been shown to induce sister chromatid exchange (71), aneuploidy in yeast (72), gene amplification (73), DNA strand breaks (74), and clastogenic effects (75). Tests for genetic effects have not been used to identify new promoters, as many tumor promoters exhibit little or no genotoxic activity. Nevertheless, genotoxic assays for possible carcinogenic agents are well established, and any new chemical should be assayed for mutagenic activity to evaluate its potential carcinogenicity; such assays are not designed to detect tumor promoters.

As tumor promotion appears to be a process in which not only interactions between chemicals and cells but also systemic reactions are involved, it may not be possible to develop an in vitro short-term test that can detect all classes of tumor-promoting agents. In view also of the possible tissue specificity of tumor-promoting agents, it would probably be easier to develop in vivo rather than in vitro short-term tests. An in vivo short-term test for tumor-promoting agents should have an end point that can be measured before tumors are produced, e.g., preneoplastic lesions (16). Several attempts have been made to use the production of preneoplastic lesions as a short-term in vivo assay for carcinogens and tumor-promoting agents (16). This kind of assay should be further developed and validated.

ACKNOWLEDGMENTS

Part of the work conducted by the author was supported by National Cancer Institute grant No. RO1 CA40534. I thank Dr. D. J. Fitzgerald for his critical reading of the manuscript and Dr. M. Hollstein for helpful discussion. I also thank C. Fuchez for valuable secretarial help.

OPEN FORUM

Dr. Thomas O'Brien: I think I read a report that the 27-kDa protein involved in gap-junction formation is a substrate of protein kinase C (PKC). Have you confirmed that in your studies? Is that the mechanism for regulation of gap-junction communication by phorbol esters?

Dr. Hiroshi Yamasaki: The gap junction 27-kDa protein could be a substrate for PKC in vitro. I do not know of any experiments that relate such phosphorylation of gap junction with its communication function.

Dr. Allan Balmain: In the experiments with the *myc*-infected 3T3 cells in which you did not see any communication, how do you know which cells had *myc* and which did not, because *myc* does not induce any morphological changes in the 3T3 cells?

Dr. Yamasaki: You are right. We cannot morphologically distinguish *myc*-infected 3T3 cells with control cells. To distinguish them, the *myc* cells were labeled with latex beads by phagocytosis. These beads, and thus *myc* cells, are visible under a fluorescence and phase-contrast microscope.

Dr. Balmain: John Pitts' group in Glasgow has shown that TPA in vivo has no effect on junctional communication between epidermal cells. In fact, it increases communication between epidermal cells and dermal fibroblast cells.

Dr. Yamasaki: We are trying to confirm John Pitts' results, but we could not really show intercellular communication with in vivo systems using micro-injection of Lucifer yellow, which John Pitts is using, because of autofluorescence of skin tissue. Kalimi and Sinsat showed that TPA painting on mouse skin decreases gap-junction protein. I do not want to give the impression that everything is perfectly matched between intercellular communication and tumor promotion. In addition to John Pitt's results, for example, Dr. Boreiko has shown that tetrachlorodibenzodioxin can enhance transformation of C3H/10T 1/2 but does not inhibit intercellular communication. We also have data to show that TGF-beta is a good enhancer of cell transformation; however, we could not see any effect on the cellular communication. It is possible that there may be some surrounding local inhibition that cannot be detected under our experimental conditions. I agree that there is evidence for and against the role of disrupted intercellular communication in carcinogenesis.

Dr. Donald Stevenson: Intercellular communication is very fascinating, but there are some things about it that trouble me. One is that it does not seem to have any organ or species specificity. Recently, Jim Trosko said that it relates to neurotoxicity. That gave me some concern because it suggested that it was a nonspecific toxic phenomenon rather than a specific one for carcinogenicity.

Dr. Yamasaki: It is possible. It is important to realize when we use gap-junctional communication as an assay end point that different mechanistic pathways lead to the same result, i.e., inhibition of the communication. General toxicity is a possible cause, but most of Trosko's studies exclude such a possible artifact.

Dr. Stuart Yuspa: Did you say that your 3T3 clone, which is a high-transforming variant, does not communicate when it reaches confluence? Is that what you think makes it readily transformable?

Dr. Yamasaki: Yes.

Dr. Yuspa: I wonder whether this relates to Dr. Kennedy's findings. Do you know whether protease inhibitors might suppress the transformation in that clone?

Dr. Yamasaki: We have tried antipain and leupeptin on intercellular communication, but we could not see an effect. We have not done any study to see their effects on transformation of these BALB/c3T3 cell variants.

REFERENCES

1. Hollstein M, McCann J, Angelosanto F, Nicols W. Short-term tests for carcinogens and mutagens. Mutat Res 65:133-226, 1979.
2. Purchase IFH. An appraisal of predictive tests for carcinogenicity. Mutat Res 99:53-71, 1982.
3. de Serres FJ, Ashby J (eds). Evaluation for Short-Term Tests for Carcinogens: Report of the International Collaborative Program. New York: Elsevier/North Holland, 1981.
4. Slaga TJ, Sivak A, Boutwell RK (eds). Mechanisms of Tumor Promotion and Cocarcinogenesis. New York: Raven Press, 1978.
5. Hecker E, Fusenig NE, Kunz W, Marks F, Thielmann HW (eds). Cocarcinogenesis and Biological Effects of Tumor Promoters. New York: Raven Press, 1982.
6. Borzsonyi M, Lapis K, Day NE, Yamasaki H (eds). Models, Mechanisms and Etiology of Tumor Promotion. Lyon, France: International Agency for Research on Cancer, 1984. IARC Scientific Publication No. 56.
7. Barbacid M. Oncogenes and human cancer: Cause or consequence? Carcinogenesis 7:1037-1042, 1986.
8. Balmain A, Ramsden M, Bowden GT, Smith J. Activation of the mouse cellular Harvey-ras gene in chemically induced benign skin papillomas. Nature 307:658-660, 1984.
9. Zarbl H, Sukumar S, Arthur AV, Martin-Zanca D, Barbacid M. Direct mutagenesis of Ha-ras-1 oncogenes by N-nitroso-N-methylurea during initiation of mammary carcinogenesis in rats. Nature 315:382-385, 1985.
10. Abbott PJ, Saffhill R. DNA synthesis with methylated poly (dC-dG) templates: Evidence for a competitive nature to miscoding by O^6-methylguanine. Biochim Biophys Acta 562:51-61, 1979.
11. Dandekar S, Sukumar S, Zarbl H, Young LJT, Cardiff RD. Specific activation of the cellular Harvey-ras oncogene in dimethylbenz[a]anthracene-induced mouse mammary tumors. Mol Cell Biol 6:4104-4108, 1986.
12. Quintanilla M, Brown K, Ramsden M, Balmain A. Carcinogen-specific mutation and amplification of Ha-ras during mouse skin carcinogenesis. Nature 322:78-80, 1986.
13. Bizub D, Wood AW, Skalka AM. Mutagenesis of the Ha-ras oncogene in mouse skin tumors induced by polycyclic aromatic hydrocarbons. Proc Natl Acad Sci USA 83:6048-6052, 1986.
14. Yamasaki H, Hollstein M, Martel N, Cabral JRP, Galendo D, Tomatis L. Transplacental induction of a specific mutation in fetal Ha-ras and its critical role in post-

natal carcinogenesis. Int J Cancer 40:818-822, 1987.

15. Yamasaki H. In-vitro approaches to identify tumor-promoting agents: Cell transformation and intercellular communication. Food Addit Contam 1:179-187, 1984.

16. Montesano R, Bartsch H, Vainio H, Wilbourn JD, Yamasaki H (eds). Long-Term and Short-Term Assays for Carcinogens: A Critical Appraisal. Lyon, France: International Agency for Research on Cancer, 1986. IARC Scientific Publication No. 83.

17. Yamasaki H, Weinstein IB. Cellular and molecular mechanisms of tumor promotion and their implication for risk assessment. In Vouk VB, Hoel GC, Peakall DB (eds): Methods for Estimating Risk of Chemical Injury: Human and Non-Human Biota and Ecosystems. New York: John Wiley, 1985, pp 155-180.

18. Day NE. Epidemiological evidence of promoting effects: The example of breast cancer. In Hecker E, Fusenig NE, Kunz W, Marks F, Thielmann HW (eds): Carcinogenesis: A Comprehensive Survey, Vol. 7. Cocarcinogenesis and Biological Effects of Tumor Promoters. New York: Raven Press, 1982, pp 183-199.

19. Doll R. An epidemiological perspective of the biology of cancer. Cancer Res 38:3573-3583, 1978.

20. Weber J, Hecker E. Cocarcinogens of the diterpene ester type from Croton flavens L. and esophageal cancer in Curacao. Experientia 34:679-682, 1978.

21. Iversen OH, Astrup EG. The paradigm of two-stage carcinogenesis: A critical attitude. Cancer Invest 2:51-60, 1984.

22. Schulte-Hermann R. Tumor promotion in the liver. Arch Toxicol 57:147-158, 1985.

23. Druckrey H. Specific carcinogenic and teratogenic effects of "indirect" alkylating methyl and ethyl compounds, and their dependency on stages of ontogenetic developments. Xenobiotica 3:271-303, 1973.

24. Ehrenberg L, Brookes P, Druckrey H, Lagerlof B, Litwin J, Williams G. The relation of cancer induction and genetic damage. In Ramel C (ed): Evaluation of Genetic Risks of Environmental Chemicals. Stockholm: Royal Swedish Academy of Sciences, 1973, pp 15,16.

25. Weisburger JH, Williams GM. Carcinogen testing: Current problems and new approaches. Science 214:401-407, 1981.

26. Trosko JE, Yotti LP, Warren ST, Tsushimoto G, Chang CC. Inhibition of cell-cell communication by tumor promoters. In Hecker E, Fusenig NE, Kunz W, Marks F, Thielman HW (eds): Carcinogenesis: A Comprehensive Survey, Vol. 7. Cocarcinogenesis and Biological Effects of Tumor Promoters. New York: Raven Press, 1982, pp 656-685.

27. Yamasaki H. Aberrant control of intercellular communication and cell differentiation during carcinogenesis. In Maskens AP, Ebbesen P, Burny A (eds): Concepts and Theories in Carcinogenesis. Amsterdam: Elsevier, 1987, pp 117-133.

28. Murray AW, Fitzgerald DJ. Tumor promoters inhibit metabolic cooperation in cocultures of epidermal and 3T3 cells. Biochem Biophys Res Commun 91:395-401, 1979.

29. Yotti LP, Chang CC, Trosko JE. Elimination of metabolic cooperation in Chinese hamster cells by a tumor promoter. Science 206:1089-1091, 1979.

30. Enomoto T, Sasaki Y, Shiba Y, Kanno Y, Yamasaki H. Tumor promoters cause a rapid and reversible inhibition of the formation and maintenance of electrical cell coupling in culture. Proc Natl Acad Sci USA 78:5628-5632, 1981.

31. Umeda M, Noda K, Ono T. Inhibition of metabolic cooperation in Chinese hamster cells by various compounds including tumor promoters. Gann 71:614-620, 1980.

32. Enomoto T, Martel N, Kanno Y, Yamasaki H. Inhibition of cell-cell communication

between BALB/c 3T3 cells by tumor promoters and protection by cAMP. J Cell Physiol 121:323-333, 1984.

33. Williams GM, Telang S, Tong C. Inhibition of intercellular communication between liver cells by the liver tumor promoter 1,1,1-trichloro-2,2-bis(p-chlorophenoyl)ethane. Cancer Lett 11:339-344, 1981.

34. Fitzgerald DJ, Knowles SE, Ballard FJ, Murray AW. Rapid and reversible inhibition of junctional communication by tumour promoters in a mouse cell line. Cancer Res 43:3614-3618, 1983.

35. Sugie S, Mori H, Takahashi M. Effect of in vivo exposure to the liver tumor promoters phenobarbital or DDT on the gap junctions of rat hepatocytes: A qualitative freeze-fracture analysis. Carcinogenesis 8:45-51, 1987.

36. Kalimi GH, Sirsat SM. Phorbol ester tumor promoters affect the mouse epidermal gap junctions. Cancer Lett 22:343-350, 1984.

37. Pound AW, McGuire LJ. Repeated partial hepatectomy as a promoting stimulus for carcinogenic response of liver to nitrosamines in rats. Br J Cancer 37:585-594, 1978.

38. Clarke-Lewis I, Murray AW. Tumor promotion and the induction of epidermal ornithine decarboxylase activity in mechanically stimulated mouse skin. Cancer Res 38:494-497, 1978.

39. Tsushimoto G, Trosko JE, Chang CC, Aust SD. Inhibition of metabolic cooperation in Chinese hamster V79 cells in culture by various polybrominated biphenyl (PBB) congeners. Carcinogenesis 3:181-185, 1982.

40. Trosko JE, Jone C, Chang CC. The use of in-vitro assays to study and to detect tumor promoters. In Borzsonyi M, Lapis K, Day NE, Yamasaki H (eds): Models, Mechanisms and Etiology of Tumor Promotion. Lyon, France: International Agency for Research on Cancer, 1984, pp 239-252. IARC Scientific Publication No. 56.

41. Enomoto T, Yamasaki H. Phorbol ester-mediated inhibition of intercellular communication in BALB/c 3T3 cells: Relationship to enhancement of cell transformation. Cancer Res 45:2681-2688, 1985.

42. Enomoto T, Yamasaki H. Rapid inhibition of intercellular communication by diacylglycerol, a possible endogenous functional analog of phorbol esters. Cancer Res 45:3706-3710, 1985.

43. Kakunaga T, Crow JD. Cell variants showing differential susceptibility to ultraviolet light-induced transformation. Science 209:505-507, 1980.

44. Kakunaga T, Hamada H, Learith J, Crow JD, Hirakawa T, Lo KY. Evidence for both mutational and non-mutational process in chemically induced cell transformation. In Harris CC, Cerutti PA (eds): Mechanisms of Chemical Carcinogenesis. New York: Alan R. Liss, 1982, pp 517-529.

45. Lo KY, Kakunaga T. Similarities in the formation and removal of covalent DNA adduct in benzo[a]pyrene-treated BALB/c 3T3 variant cells with different induced transformation frequencies. Cancer Res 42:2644-2650, 1982.

46. Yamasaki H, Enomoto T, Shiba Y, Kanno Y, Kakunaga T. Intercellular communication capacity as a possible determinant of transformation sensitivity of BALB/c 3T3 clonal cells. Cancer Res 45:637-641, 1985.

47. Slaga TJ. Can tumor promotion be effectively inhibited? In Borzsonyi M, Lapis K, Day DE, Yamasaki H (eds): Models, Mechanisms and Etiology of Tumor Promotion. Lyon, France: International Agency for Research on Cancer, 1984, pp 497-506. IARC Scientific Publication No. 56.

48. Yamasaki H, Enomoto T. Role of intercellular communication in BALB/c 3T3 cell

transformation. In Barrett JC, Tennant RW (eds): Carcinogenesis: A Comprehensive Survey, Vol. 9. Mammalian Cell Transformation: Mechanisms of Carcinogenesis and Assays for Carcinogens. New York: Raven Press, 1985, pp 179-184.

49.   Yamasaki H, Katoh F. Further evidence for the involvement of gap-junctional intercellular communication in induction and maintenance of BALB/c 3T3 cells transformed foci. Cancer Res 48:3490-3495, 1988.

50.   Hamel E, Katoh F, Mueller G, Birchmeier W, Yamasaki H. Transforming growth factor-beta is a potent promoter in two-stage BALB/c 3T3 cell transformation. Cancer Res 48:2832-2836, 1988.

51.   Boreiko CJ, Abernethy DJ, Sanchez JM, Dorman BM. Effect of mouse skin tumor promoters upon [³H]uridine exchange and focus formation in cultures of C3H/10T1/2 mouse fibroblasts. Carcinogenesis 7:1095-1099, 1986.

52.   Mondal S, Heidelberger C. Transformation of C3H/10T1/2 CL8 mouse embryo fibroblasts by ultraviolet irradiation and a phorbol ester. Nature 260:710-711, 1976.

53.   Hirakawa T, Kakunaga T, Fujiki H, Sugimura T. A new tumor-promoting agent, dihydroteleocidin B, markedly enhances chemically induced malignant cell transformation. Science 216:527-529, 1982.

54.   Poiley JA, Raineri R, Pienta RJ. Two-stage malignant transformation in hamster embryo cells. Br J Cancer 39:8-14, 1979.

55.   Lasne C, Gentil A, Chouroulinkov I. Two-stage malignant transformation of rat fibroblasts in tissue culture. Nature 247:490-491, 1974.

56.   Hennings H, Michael D, Cheng C, Steinert P, Holbrook K, Yuspa SH. Calcium regulation of growth and differentiation of mouse epidermal cells in culture. Cell 19:245-254, 1980.

57.   Yuspa SH, Morgan DL. Mouse skin cells resistant to terminal differentiation associated with initiation of carcinogenesis. Nature 293:72-74, 1981.

58.   Miller DR, Viaje A, Aldaz CM, Conti CJ, Slaga TJ. Terminal differentiation-resistant epidermal cells in mice undergoing two-stage carcinogenesis. Cancer Res 47:1935-1940, 1987.

59.   Colburn NH, Former BF, Nelson KA, Yuspa SH. Tumour promoter induces anchorage independence irreversibly. Nature 281:589-591, 1979.

60.   Colburn NH, Koehler BA, Nelson KJ. A cell culture assay for tumor promoter-dependent progression toward neoplastic phenotype: Detection of tumor promoters and promotion inhibitors. Teratogenesis Carcinog Mutagen 1:87-96, 1980.

61.   Diwan BA, Ward JM, Rice JM, Colburn NH, Spangler EF. Tumor promoting effects of di(2-ethylhexyl) phthalate in JB6 mouse epidermal cells and mouse skin. Carcinogenesis 6:343-347, 1985.

62.   Gindhart TD, Srinivas L, Colburn NH. Benzoyl peroxide promotion of transformation of JB6 mouse epidermal cells: Inhibition by ganglioside GT but not by retinoic acid. Carcinogenesis 6:309-311, 1985.

63.   Colburn NH, Wendel E, Srinivas L. Responses of preneoplastic epidermal cells to tumor promoters and growth factors: Use of promoter-resistant variants for mechanism studies. J Cell Biochem 18:261-270, 1982.

64.   Jongen WMF, Hakkert BC, van de Poll MLM. Inhibitory effects of the phorbol ester TPA and cigarette smoke condensate on the mutagenicity of benzo[a]pyrene in a co-cultivation system. Mutat Res 159:133-138, 1986.

65.   Klanning JE, Ruch RJ. Strain and species effects on the inhibition of hepatocyte intercellular communication by liver tumor promoters. Cancer Lett 36:161-168, 1987.

66. Kitagawa T, Watanabe R, Kayano T, Sugano H. In vitro carcinogenesis of hepatocytes obtained from acetylaminofluorene-treated rat liver and promotion of their growth by phenobarbital. Gann 71:747-754, 1980.

67. Mesnil M, Montesano R, Yamasaki H. Intercellular communication of transformed and non-transformed rat liver epithelial cells: Modulation by 12-O-tetradecanoylphorbol 13-acetate. Exp Cell Res 165:391-402, 1986.

68. Harris CC. Human tissues and cells in carcinogenesis research. Cancer Res 47:1-10, 1987.

69. Yamasaki H, Weinstein IB, Van Duuren BL. Induction of erythroleukemia cell adhesion by plant diterpene tumor promoters: A quantitative study and correlation with in vivo activities. Carcinogenesis 2:537-543, 1981.

70. Suganuma M, Fujiki H, Suguri H, Yoshizawa S, Hirota M, Nakayasu M, Ojika M, Wakamatsu K, Yamada K, Sugimura T. Okadaic acid: An additional non-phorbol-12-tetradecanoate-13-acetate-type tumor promoter. Proc Natl Acad Sci USA 85:1768-1771, 1988.

71. Kinsella AR, Radman M. Tumor promoter induces sister chromatid exchanges: Relevance to mechanisms of carcinogenesis. Proc Natl Acad Sci USA 75:6149-6153, 1978.

72. Parry JM, Parry EM, Barrett JC. Tumor promoters induce mitotic aneuploidy in yeast. Nature 294:263-265, 1981.

73. Varshavsky A. Phorbol ester dramatically increases incidence of methotrexate-resistant mouse cells: Possible mechanisms and relevance to tumor promotion. Cell 25:561-572, 1981.

74. Birnboim HC. DNA strand breakage in human leukocytes exposed to a tumor promoter, phorbol myristate acetate. Science 215:1247-1249, 1982.

75. Emerit I, Cerutti PA. Tumor promoter phorbol 12-myristate 13-acetate induces a clastogenic factor in human lymphocytes. Proc Natl Acad Sci USA 79:7509-7513, 1982.

76. Mosser DD, Bols NC. The effect of phorbols on metabolic cooperation between human fibroblasts. Carcinogenesis 3:1207-1212, 1982.

77. Davidson JS, Baumgarten I, Harley EH. Use of a new citrulline incorporation assay to investigate inhibition of intercellular communication by 1,1,1-trichloro-2,2bis-(p-chlorophenyl)ethane in human fibroblasts. Cancer Res 45:515-519, 1985.

78. Gupta RS, Singh B, Stetsko DK. Inhibition of metabolic cooperation by phorbol esters in a cell culture system based on adenosine kinase deficient mutants. Carcinogenesis 6:1359-1366, 1985.

79. Loewenstein WR, Penn RD. Intercellular communication and tissue growth. II. Tissue regeneration. J Cell Biol 33:235-242, 1967.

80. Freidman EA, Steinberg M. Disrupted communication between late-stage premalignant human colon epithelial cells by 12-O-tetradecanoyl-phorbol-13-acetate. Cancer Res 42:5096-5105, 1982.

81. Enomoto T, Martel N, Kanno Y, Yamasaki H. Inhibition of cell-cell communication between BALB/c 3T3 cells by tumor promoters and protection by cAMP. J Cell Physiol 121:323-333, 1984.

82. Meyer DJ, Yancy SB, Revel JP. Intercellular communication in normal and regenerating rat liver: A quantitative analysis. J Cell Biol 91:505-523, 1981.

83. Wade MH, Trosko JE, Schindler M. A fluorescence photobleaching assay of gap junction-mediated communication between human cells. Science 232:525-528, 1986.

84. El-Fouly MH, Trosko JE, Chang CC. Scrape-loading and dye transfer. A rapid and simple technique to study gap junctional intercellular communication. Exp Cell Res 168:422-431, 1987.
85. Yancey SB, Edens JE, Trosko JE, Chang CC, Revel JP. Decreased incidence of gap junctions between Chinese hamster V79 cells upon exposure to the tumor promoter 12-O-tetradecanoylphorbol 13-acetate. Exp Cell Res 139:329-340, 1982.
86. Finbow ME, Shuttleworth J, Hamilton AE, Pitts JD. Analysis of vertebrate gap junction proteins. EMBO J 2:1479-1486, 1983.
87. Traub O, Druge PM, Willecke K. Degradation and resynthesis of gap junction protein in plasma membranes of regenerating liver after partial hepatectomy or cholestasis. Proc Natl Acad Sci USA 80:755-759, 1983.

Skin Carcinogenesis: Mechanisms and Human Relevance, pages 281–291

Diversity in the Chemical Nature and Mechanism of Response to Tumor Promoters

Hirota Fujiki, Masami Suganuma, Hiroko Suguri,
Shigeru Yoshizawa, Mitsuru Hirota, Kanji Takagi,
and Takashi Sugimura

National Cancer Center Research Institute (H.F., M.S., H.S., S.Y., M.H., K.T.)
and National Cancer Center (T.S.), Tokyo 104, Japan

Thus far, 23 new tumor promoters that are structurally different from 12-O-tetradecanoylphorbol-13-acetate (TPA) have been found (1,2). These new tumor promoters are classified into TPA-type and non-TPA-type tumor promoters depending on their ability to bind to phorbol ester receptors in mouse skin. Furthermore, TPA-type tumor promoters activate protein kinase C in vitro, whereas non-TPA types do not. Thus findings with these two types of tumor promoters provide direct evidence for divergent mechanisms of action in two-stage carcinogenesis experiments on mouse skin (3). This chapter deals with four subjects: a screening system for new tumor promoters; TPA-type tumor promoters and their mechanisms of action; non-TPA-type tumor promoters and their unique biological activities, with special reference to the effects of okadaic acid; and common biological activities induced by the two types of tumor promoters.

MATERIALS

Teleocidin, which is a mixture of two teleocidin A isomers and four teleocidin B isomers, was isolated from *Streptomyces mediocidicus* (4). Dihydroteleocidin B is a chemically hydrogenated form of teleocidin B-4 (5). Lyngbyatoxin A was isolated from the blue-green alga *Lyngbya majuscula* (6). Des-O-methylolivoretin C was isolated from *Streptomyces mediocidicus* (7). (–)-Indolactam-V, which is a biosynthetic intermediate of teleocidins, was isolated from *Streptomyces* and *Streptoverticillium* (8). Debromoaplysiatoxin, aplysiatoxin, and anhydrodebromoaplysiatoxin were isolated from another variety of the blue-green alga *Lyngbya majuscula* (9). Bromoaplysiatoxin and oscillatoxin A were isolated from a mixture of *Oscillatoria nigroviridis* and *Shizothrix calcicola* (10). Dibromoaplysiatoxin is a chemically brominated derivative of debromoaplysiatoxin (11). Palytoxin was isolated from the marine coelenterate *Palythoa tuberculosa* (12). Thapsigargin was isolated from the plant *Thapsia garganica* L. (13).

Okadaic acid and dinophysistoxin-1 (35-methylokadaic acid) used for these experiments were isolated from a black sponge, *Halichondria okadai* (14,15). Staurosporine was isolated from *Streptomyces* (16). The structures of these TPA-type and non-TPA-type tumor promoters are shown in Figures 1 and 2.

METHODS

A Short-Term System for Tumor Promoters

The degree of redness of the ears of mice was estimated 24 h after application of test compounds (17), and ornithine decarboxylase (ODC) activity was determined in epidermal extracts prepared 4 h after application of these compounds (18). Their ability to induce HL-60 cell adhesion in vitro was measured by counting the number of HL-60 cells adhering to the bottoms of flasks 48 h after addition of test compounds to culture medium (18). The promoters' ability to inhibit specific binding of [^{3}H]TPA to a particulate fraction of mouse skin was assayed by the cold-acetone filtration method (17). Also, the ability of each agent to activate protein kinase C in vitro was tested using an assay mixture of 20 μM $CaCl_2$, 7.5 μg of phosphatidylserine, and various concentrations of a tumor promoter with 0.05 unit of partially purified enzyme from mouse brain (19).

Two-Stage Carcinogenesis Experiment on Mouse Skin

Tumor-promoting activity was tested by a standard initiation-promotion protocol. Initiation was achieved by a single application of 100 μg 7,12-dimethylbenz[a]anthracene (DMBA) to the skin of the backs of 8-week-old female CD-1 mice (20). From 1 week after initiation, doses of 0.2 nmol to 41.5 nmol of test compounds were applied twice a week until week 30. Groups of 15 mice were used.

RESULTS AND DISCUSSION

Screening System for New Tumor Promoters

Our short-term screening system for tumor promoters consists of three successive tests—an irritant test on the mouse ear, a test of induction of ODC in mouse skin, and a test of induction of HL-60 cell adhesion (17). We examined about 500 materials using the irritant test. These materials included various purified compounds and unpurified preparations such as plant extracts, Japanese and Chinese spices, Chinese medicines, extracts of fungi, and marine natural products that were thought to be irritants. Of these, 96 materials gave positive results in the irritant test, 29 of these 96 compounds induced ODC activity, and 20 of the 29 compounds induced adhesion of HL-60 cells. Seven of these compounds have now been shown to have potent tumor-promoting activity in two-stage carcinogenesis experiments. These 7 are dihydroteleocidin B, teleo-

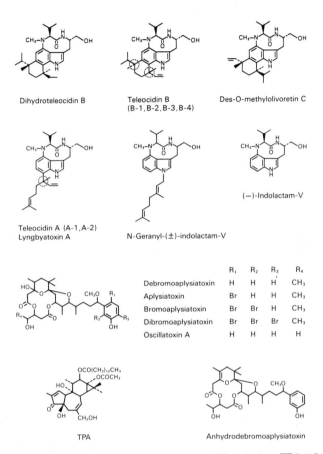

Figure 1. Structures of TPA-type tumor promoters. Abbreviation: TPA, 12-O-tetrade-canoylphorbol-13-acetate.

cidin, lyngbyatoxin A, debromoaplysiatoxin, aplysiatoxin, bromoaplysiatoxin, and oscillatoxin A (Fig. 1). The other 13 compounds have not yet been tested.

In addition, 11 new tumor promoters were obtained as derivatives of the 7 tumor promoters listed above. These additional tumor promoters are 2 teleocidin A isomers (A-1 and A-2), 4 teleocidin B isomers (B-1, B-2, B-3, and B-4), des-O-methylolivoretin C, (–)-indolactam-V, N-geranyl-(±)-indolactam-V, dibromoaplysiatoxin, and anhydrodebromoaplysiatoxin (Fig. 1). All 18 new TPA-type tumor promoters are detectable with this short-term screening system. In addition, the abilities of these compounds to bind to phorbol ester receptors and to activate protein kinase C in vitro were investigated, since these tests are

Table 1. Tumor-Promoting Activities of New Tumor Promoters Compared with That of TPA

	Amount per application (nmol)	Maximal % tumor-bearing mice	Average no. tumors/mouse in week 30
TPA	4.1	100.0	11.0
TPA-type			
Dihydroteleocidin B	5.5	90.0	4.6
Teleocidin	5.7	100.0	4.0
Lyngbyatoxin A	6.9	86.7	3.7
Des-O-methylolivoretin C	5.5	64.3	1.0
N-Geranyl-(±)-indolactam-V	11.4	20.0	0.2
(−)-Indolactam-V	41.5	29.0	0.3
Debromoaplysiatoxin	4.0	73.3	2.9
Aplysiatoxin	4.0	80.0	3.4
Bromoaplysiatoxin	4.0	85.7	3.4
Dibromoaplysiatoxin	4.0	66.7	3.6
Oscillatoxin A	4.0	53.3	1.3
Anhydrodebromoaplysiatoxin	20.0	40.0	0.4
Non-TPA-type			
Palytoxin	0.2	62.5	1.0
Thapsigargin	7.7	53.5	0.7
Okadaic acid	6.2	80.0	3.9
Dinophysistoxin-1	6.1	93.3	4.6
Staurosporine	21.5	33.0	0.5

important for identifying TPA-type tumor promoters (3). The potencies of the tumor-promoting activities of these compounds were tested, and at similar dose ranges, 15 of 18 TPA-type tumor promoters were found to induce tumors at similar rates in mice, while N-geranyl-(±)-indolactam-V, (−)-indolactam-V, and anhydrodebromoaplysiatoxin showed weaker activities. Since all isomers of teleocidins A and B have similar potencies to that of teleocidin, results on individual isomers are not included in Table 1. TPA induced the highest average number of tumors per mouse. The tumor-promoting activities of the new tumor promoters are summarized in Table 1.

In contrast to TPA-type tumor promoters, five non-TPA-type tumor promoters were not found with the short-term screening system, because although they gave positive results in the irritant test, they did not give positive results in one or both of the two further tests, induction of ODC and HL-60 cell adhesion (Table 2). These five non-TPA-type tumor promoters are palytoxin, thapsigargin, okadaic acid, dinophysistoxin-1, and staurosporine (Fig. 2). It is noteworthy that okadaic acid and dinophysistoxin-1 have as high tumor-promoting activities as TPA-type tumor promoters and much higher tumor- promoting activity than the other three non-TPA-type tumor promoters (Table 1).

In summary, all TPA-type tumor promoters give positive results in the

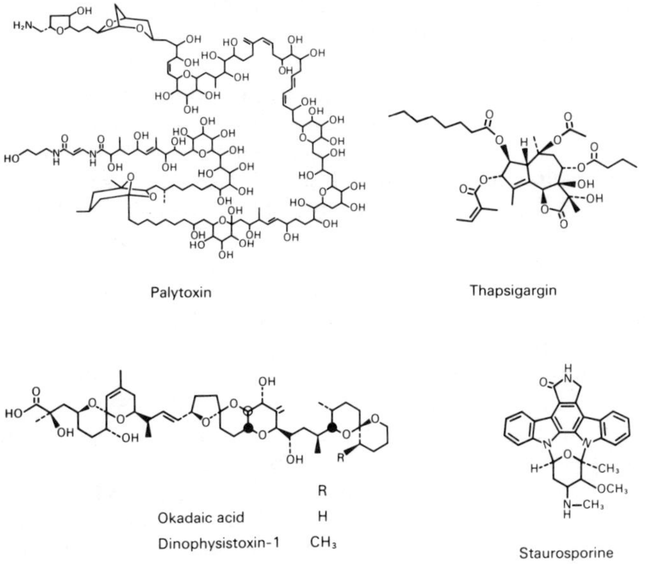

Palytoxin

Thapsigargin

Okadaic acid   H
Dinophysistoxin-1   CH₃

Staurosporine

Figure 2. Structures of non-TPA-type tumor promoters. Abbreviation: TPA, 12-*O*-tetradecanoylphorbol-13-acetate.

three tests in our short-term screening system. But a compound that gives a positive result in the irritant test on mouse ear but negative results in tests on induction of ODC or HL-60 cell adhesion might be a non-TPA-type tumor promoter.

TPA-Type Tumor Promoters

Teleocidin is a mixture of two teleocidin A isomers with a molecular weight of 437 and four teleocidin B isomers with a molecular weight of 451. These isomers were named A-1, A-2, B-1, B-2, B-3, and B-4 in order of their elution on high-performance liquid chromatography (21). Teleocidin A-1 is identical with lyngbyatoxin A, which was isolated from the Hawaiian blue-green alga, *Lyngbya majuscula* (22). The two teleocidin A isomers and four teleocidin B isomers showed similar potencies in tests on irritation of mouse ear, induction of ODC in mouse skin, induction of HL-60 cell adhesion, inhibition of specific binding of [³H]TPA to a particulate fraction of mouse skin, and activation of protein kinase C in vitro. Moreover, the isomers of teleocidins A and B, like dihydroteleocidin B, induced tumors at high rates in mice. Des-*O*-methylolivoretin C is a regio-isomer of teleocidin B-1 in which the isopropyl group and the vinyl group on the cyclohexene ring are reversed. Teleocidin A, teleocidin B, and des-*O*-methylolivoretin C have a common structure, consisting of an indole system and a nine-member lactam ring. The common structure of the teleocidin class of tumor promoters was named (−)-indolactam-V (23) and found to be a biosynthetic intermediate of teleocidins A and B. (−)-Indolactam-V binds to phorbol ester receptors in cell membranes 230 times less strongly than teleocidins A and B and has weaker tumor-promoting activity than teleocidins A and B (Table 1). These results indicate that a hydrophobic domain attached to (−)-indolactam-V increases the biological activity of the latter. N-Geranyl-(±)-indolactam-V was synthesized to study the role of a large hydrophobic domain, but it was found to have weaker tumor-promoting activity than teleocidin A and to be compatible with the low potency of the above biological activities. Later we found that the geranyl group should be attached to C-7 of (−)-indolactam-V to obtain a compound with similar potency to that of teleocidin A (23).

The aplysiatoxin class of tumor promoters was found in blue-green algae during investigations into why more than 200 students in Okinawa had swimmers' itch in 1968 and more than 400 people had swimmers' itch at Kailua Beach on Oahu, Hawaii, in August 1980. Debromoaplysiatoxin and aplysiatoxin were isolated from the blue-green algae as causative agents of swimmers' itch (24,25). Debromoaplysiatoxin, aplysiatoxin, bromoaplysiatoxin, and dibromoaplysiatoxin have the same acetogenic phenolic bis-lactone structure, but have from zero to three bromine atoms (Fig. 1). Debromoaplysiatoxin, aplysiatoxin, and bromoaplysiatoxin showed similar activities in tests of mouse ear irritation, induction of ODC in mouse skin, and inhibition of specific binding of [³H]TPA to a particulate fraction of mouse skin, whereas dibromoaplysiatoxin showed much lower activity in these tests. However, these four aplysiatoxins all showed similar potencies in activating protein kinase C. Thus potency to activate protein kinase C is not related to the other three activities. In two-stage carcinogenesis experiments, these four aplysiatoxins induced similar incidences of tumors in week 30 of tumor promotion protocols (Table 1). Oscillatoxin A, a demethylated form of debromoaplysiatoxin, and anhydrodebromoaplysiatoxin are also included in the aplysiatoxin class of tumor promoters.

TPA-type tumor promoters are known to act through phorbol ester receptors, which are almost identical with protein kinase C (19,26). Activation of protein kinase C induces the phosphorylation of some proteins that act as signals in the cells and consequently promote tumor formation.

Non-TPA-Type Tumor Promoters and Their Unique Biological Activities, with Special Reference to the Effects of Okadaic Acid

Palytoxin, thapsigargin, okadaic acid, dinophysistoxin-1, and staurosporine have fewer biological and biochemical effects than TPA-type tumor promoters (27-29). All five non-TPA-type tumor promoters cause irritation of the mouse ear and stimulate prostaglandin E_2 production but do not induce HL-60 cell adhesion. Okadaic acid induced both ODC and histidine decarboxylase (HDC) activity in mouse skin, whereas thapsigargin and staurosporine induced only HDC activity, and palytoxin did not induce either activity (Table 2). These

Table 2. Effects of Tumor Promoters

Tumor promoters	Irritation	Induction of ODC	HL-60 cell adhesion	Induction of HDC	Prosta-glandin E$_2$ stimulation	Tumor-promoting activity
TPA-type	+	+	+	+	+	+
Non-TPA-type						
Palytoxin	+	−	−	−	+	+
Thapsigargin	+	−	−	+	+	+
Okadaic acid	+	+	−	+	+	+
Staurosporine	+	−	−	+	+	+

results strongly suggest that these non-TPA-type tumor promoters do not act through a common pathway.

Palytoxin is a water-soluble toxin with a molecular weight of 2,700. It is the strongest known inducer of prostaglandins in rat macrophages and rat liver cells. Levine and Fujiki reported that its effect is synergistic with those of TPA-type tumor promoters, epidermal growth factor, and transforming growth factors alpha and beta (30).

Thapsigargin is a sesquiterpene lactone ester with a molecular weight of 650. Although its structure seems to be similar to that of phorbol esters, it did not bind to phorbol ester receptors. It has potent histamine-liberating activity in mast cells (13).

Staurosporine, a microbial alkaloid with a molecular weight of 466, was reported to cause in vitro inhibition of protein kinase C isolated from rat brain (16). It slightly inhibited tumor promotion by teleocidin in mouse skin but had tumor-promoting activity alone in mouse skin. Thus it has dual effects in mouse skin: anti-tumor-promoting activity and tumor-promoting activity.

Okadaic acid is a polyether compound of a C$_{38}$ fatty acid with a molecular weight of 804. Dinophysistoxin-1, or 35-methylokadaic acid, induces the same biological and biochemical effects as okadaic acid. Okadaic acid has as strong tumor-promoting activity as does teleocidin (29). Recently we found that [^{3}H]okadaic acid bound specifically to a particulate fraction of mouse skin. Since this specific binding was not inhibited by TPA, teleocidin, palytoxin, or thapsigargin, we concluded that okadaic acid has a specific receptor. Therefore, okadaic acid has potent tumor-promoting activity through a different pathway from those of TPA-type and the other non-TPA-type tumor promoters.

Common Biological Activities Induced by Two Types of Tumor Promoters

TPA-type tumor promoters such as teleocidins A and B, debromoaplysia-toxin, and aplysiatoxin induce more biological and biochemical effects than do non-TPA-type tumor promoters. Non-TPA-type tumor promoters are thought to act through different pathways, but several effects of five non-TPA-type tumor promoters are the same as those of TPA-type tumor promoters. Therefore, these common effects are thought to be essential for tumor promotion. Besides tumor-promoting activity in mouse skin, the common biological effects of these two types of tumor promoters are irritation of mouse ear and stimulation of prostaglandin E_2 production and arachidonic acid metabolism (3). Both TPA-type tumor promoters and non-TPA-type tumor promoters, such as palytoxin and thapsigargin, also stimulate superoxide anion radical formation (31). Studies are needed on whether okadaic acid, dinophysistoxin-1, and staurosporine also stimulate superoxide anion radical formation. Some of the effects of TPA-type and non-TPA-type tumor promoters, such as stimulation of prostaglandin E_2 production and of superoxide anion radical formation, were found to be synergistic. Such common effects seem to be essential biologically in tumor promotion. Thus these common effects may be the most important in development of a screening system for both TPA-type and non-TPA-type tumor promoters.

ACKNOWLEDGMENTS

This work was supported in part by grants-in-aid for cancer research from the Ministry of Education, Science, and Culture, a grant from the Program for a Comprehensive 10-Year Strategy for Cancer Control from the Ministry of Health and Welfare of Japan, and by grants from the Foundation for Promotion of Cancer Research, the Princess Takamatsu Cancer Research Foundation, and the Smoking Research Foundation.

OPEN FORUM

Question: When you get a negative result for ODC induction by the non-TPA-type tumor promoter, have you done extensive time-course studies and have you looked at chronic application? Dr. DiGiovanni and coworkers have looked at the non-TPA-type tumor promoter chrysarobin, and they have seen quite a different time-course for ODC induction compared with that for TPA. It was much later and shorter.

Dr. Hirota Fujiki: We have not done extensive time-course studies. However, we found that palytoxin and thapsigargin did not induce ODC in mouse skin 4 h after their application. Furthermore, palytoxin did not induce ODC activity within 18 h after application.

Question: Do you think that all tumor-promoting agents have different pathways, or do you think they have a common pathway?

Dr. Fujiki: The TPA-type tumor promoters have a common pathway, whereas non-TPA-type tumor promoters might have different pathways. I think there are some biological effects induced by the two types of tumor promoters.

Dr. Donald Stevenson: I was very intrigued by the large molecular weight of some of your promoters. Do you have any information on the way they penentrate the skin?

Dr. Fujiki: We have not studied their penetration in the skin. But all the tumor promoters that we found are very lipophilic except palytoxin. We suppose that they can penetrate into the skin easily.

Dr. Frederick Cope: Okadaic acid has a transspecies ability to phosphorylate C23-60. This has been demonstrated in humans and in hamster cells in culture. We are not sure yet what this means.

Dr. Fujiki: C23 is a major nucleolar protein and a nonribosomal constituent of nucleolar preribosomal particles. Therefore, we suppose that the hyperphosphorylation of C23-60 is involved in some steps of the proliferative process.

Dr. Cope: It is also induced during the cell cycle, and it appears to have some ability to control the cell cycle in certain types of cells at certain periods of time.

Question: Do you think that the dermatitis you showed is due to aplysiatoxin? If so, do you have any idea what the histology of that reaction is? Is it like that in the mouse? And, finally, is there an increase of tumor incidence in that area?

Dr. Fujiki: Aplysiatoxin produces inflammation on mouse skin. It is a very strong skin irritant. The incidence of skin cancer in that area has not been studied yet.

Question: Is there any hyperplasia of the skin? Is it like the hyperplasia that you see in the mouse? Is there any increase in the tumor incidence among people with that type of dermatitis?

Dr. Fujiki: Aplysiatoxin causes strong inflammation followed by hyperplasia. However, we have no evidence yet showing the relation of tumor incidence of human skin cancer with the exposure of aplysiatoxin.

Dr. R.C. Smart: According to your model with okadaic acid, you show that there is a membrane receptor, but when you measured this, it was found in the cytosol. Have you measured any translocation of the receptor? Do you have any idea what amino acid residues are phosphorylated on this protein?

Dr. Fujiki: We haven't studied whether there is a translocation of a protein kinase. Serine residue was mainly phosphorylated in vitro.

REFERENCES

1. Hecker E. Isolation and characterization of the cocarcinogenic principles from croton oil. Methods in Cancer Research 6:439-484, 1971.
2. Van Duuren BL. Tumor-promoting agents in two-stage carcinogenesis. Prog Exp Tumor Res 11:31-68, 1969.
3. Fujiki H, Sugimura T. New classes of tumor promoters: teleocidin, aplysiatoxin, and palytoxin. Adv Cancer Res 49:223-264, 1987.
4. Fujiki H, Sugimura T. New potent tumour promoters: Teleocidin, lyngbyatoxin A and aplysiatoxin. Cancer Surv 2:539-556, 1983.
5. Fujiki H, Mori M, Nakayasu M, Terada M, Sugimura T, Moore RE. Indole alkaloids: Dihydroteleocidin B, teleocidin, and lyngbyatoxin A as members of a new class of tumor promoters. Proc Natl Acad Sci USA 78:3872-3876, 1981.

6. Cardellina LH II, Marner F-J, Moore RE. Seaweed dermatitis: Structure of lyngbyatoxin A. Science 204:193-195, 1979.

7. Sakai S, Hitotsuyanagi Y, Yamaguchi K, Aimi N, Ogata K, Kuramochi T, Seki H, Hara R, Fujiki H, Suganuma M, Sugimura T, Endo Y, Shudo K, Koyama Y. The structures of additional teleocidin class tumor promoters. Chem Pharm Bull (Tokyo) 34:4883-4886, 1986.

8. Irie K, Hirota M, Hagiwara N, Koshimizu K, Hayashi H, Murao S, Tokuda H, Ito Y. The Epstein-Barr virus early antigen inducing indole alkaloids, (–)-indolactam-V and its related compounds, produced by Actinomycetes. Agricultural and Biological Chemistry 48:1269-1274, 1984.

9. Moore RE, Blackman AJ, Cheuk CE, Mynderse JS, Matsumoto GK, Clardy J, Woodard RW, Craig JC. Absolute stereochemistries of the aplysiatoxins and oscillatoxin A. Journal of Organic Chemistry 49:2484-2489, 1984.

10. Mynderse JS, Moore RE. Toxins from blue-green algae: Structures of oscillatoxin A and three related bromine-containing toxins. Journal of Organic Chemistry 43:2301-2303, 1978.

11. Suganuma M, Fujiki H, Tahira T, Cheuk C, Moore RE, Sugimura T. Estimation of tumor promoting activity and structure-function relationships of aplysiatoxins. Carcinogenesis 5:315-318, 1984.

12. Uemura D, Ueda K, Hirata Y, Naoki H, Iwashita T. Further studies on palytoxin. II. Structure of palytoxin. Tetrahedron Letters 22:2781-2784, 1981.

13. Christensen SB, Rasmussen U, Christophersen C. Thapsigargin, constitution of a sesquiterpene lactone histamine liberator from Thapsia garganica. Tetrahedron Letters 21:3829-3830, 1980.

14. Tachibana Y, Scheuer PJ, Tsukitani Y, Kikuchi H, Van Engen D, Clardy J, Gopichand Y, Schmitz FJ. Okadaic acid, a cytotoxic polyether from two marine sponges of the genus Halichondria. Journal of the American Chemical Society 103:2469-2471, 1981.

15. Yasumoto T, Murata M, Oshima Y, Sano M, Katsumoto GK, Clardy J. Diarrhetic shellfish toxins. Tetrahedron 41:1019-1025, 1985.

16. Tamaoki T, Nomoto H, Takahashi I, Kato Y, Morimoto M, Tomita F. Staurosporine, a potent inhibitor of phospholipid/Ca++ dependent protein kinase. Biochem Biophys Res Commun 135:397-402, 1986.

17. Fujiki H, Sugimura T, Moore RE. New classes of environmental tumor promoters: Indole alkaloids and polyacetates. Environ Health Perspect 50:85-90, 1983.

18. Fujiki H, Mori M, Nakayasu M, Terada M, Sugimura T. A possible naturally occurring tumor promoter, teleocidin B from Streptomyces. Biochem Biophys Res Commun 90:976-983, 1979.

19. Fujiki H, Tanaka Y, Miyake R, Kikkawa U, Nishizuka Y, Sugimura T. Activation of calcium-activated, phospholipid-dependent protein kinase (protein kinase C) by new classes of tumor promoters: Teleocidin and debromoaplysiatoxin. Biochem Biophys Res Commun 120:339-343, 1984.

20. Fujiki H, Suganuma M, Matsukura N, Sugimura T, Takayama S. Teleocidin from Streptomyces is a potent promoter of mouse skin carcinogenesis. Carcinogenesis 3:895-898, 1982.

21. Fujiki H, Suganuma M, Tahira T, Yoshioka A, Nakayasu M, Endo Y, Shudo K, Takayama S, Moore RE, Sugimura T. New classes of tumor promoters: Teleocidin, aplysiatoxin, and palytoxin. Nakahara Memorial Lecture. In Fujiki H, Hecker E, Moore RE, Sugimura T, Weinstein IB (eds): Cellular Interactions by Environ-

mental Tumor Promoters. Tokyo: Japan Scientific Societies Press/Utrecht:VNU Science Press, 1984, pp 37-45.

22. Fujiki H, Suganuma M, Hakii H, Bartolini G, Moore RE, Takayama S, Sugimura T. A two-stage mouse skin carcinogenesis study on lyngbyatoxin A. J Cancer Res Clin Oncol 108:174-176, 1984.

23. Fujiki H, Suganuma M, Hakii H, Nakayasu M, Endo Y, Shudo K, Irie K, Koshimizu K, Sugimura T. Tumor promoting activities of new synthetic analogues of teleocidin. Proceedings of the Japan Academy 61:45-47, 1985.

24. Mynderse JS, Moore RE, Kashiwagi M, Norton TR. Antileukemia activity in the oscillatoriaceae: Isolation of debromoaplysiatoxin from *Lyngbya*. Science 196:538-540, 1977.

25. Fujiki H, Ikegami K, Hakii H, Suganuma M, Yamaizumi Z, Yamazato K, Moore RE, Sugimura T. A blue-green alga from Okinawa contains aplysiatoxins, the third class of tumor promoters. Jpn J Cancer Res (Gann) 76:257-259, 1985.

26. Nishizuka Y. The role of protein kinase C in cell surface signal transduction and tumour promotion. Nature 308:693-697, 1984.

27. Fujiki H, Suganuma M, Nakayasu M, Hakii H, Horiuchi T, Takayama S, Sugimura T. Palytoxin is a non-12-O-tetradecanoylphorbol-13-acetate type tumor promoter in two-stage mouse skin carcinogenesis. Carcinogenesis 7:707-710, 1986.

28. Hakii H, Fujiki H, Suganuma M, Nakayasu M, Tahira T, Sugimura T, Scheuer PJ, Christensen SB. Thapsigargin, a histamine secretagogue, is a non-12-O-tetradecanoylphorbol-13-acetate (TPA) type tumor promoter in two-stage mouse skin carcinogenesis. J Cancer Res Clin Oncol 111:177-181, 1986.

29. Suganuma M, Fujiki H, Suguri H, Yoshizawa S, Hirota M, Nakayasu M, Ojika M, Wakamatsu K, Yamada K, Sugimura T. Okadaic acid: An additional non-phorbol-12-tetradecanoate-13-acetate-type tumor promoter. Proc Natl Acad Sci USA 85:1768-1771, 1988.

30. Levine L, Fujiki H. Stimulation of arachidonic acid metabolism by different types of tumor promoters. Carcinogenesis 6:1631-1634, 1985.

31. Kano S, Iizuka T, Ishimura Y, Fujiki H, Sugimura T. Stimulation of superoxide anion formation by the non-TPA type tumor promoters palytoxin and thapsigargin in porcine and human neutrophils. Biochem Biophys Res Commun 143:672-677, 1987.

APPLICATIONS

Skin Carcinogenesis: Mechanisms and Human Relevance, pages 295–312

Developing Design Standards for Dermal Initiation/Promotion Screening Studies

William C. Eastin Jr.

National Institute of Environmental Health Sciences, Research Triangle Park, North Carolina 27709

Long-term rodent toxicology and carcinogenesis studies are usually done to provide information that can be used to serve common public health concerns. Two-year carcinogenicity studies as conducted by the National Toxicology Program (NTP) continue to be the most definitive method for identifying chemical carcinogens. Chronic studies conducted under conditions that are most relevant to human exposure situations should provide as much information as possible in order to more completely characterize toxicity (1-5).

Carcinogenesis is a multistage process operationally described as initiation, promotion, and progression; each of these stages can be affected by different agents in various ways (4). However, chemical classification by mechanism is not clear since some agents appear to act primarily as initiators and others as promoters, and many carcinogenic compounds appear to affect both activities to some degree. It is not known whether chronic rodent carcinogenesis evaluations would detect all chemicals that act primarily by a promoter mechanism (6). Furthermore, short-term in vitro tests for promoters have not been sufficiently developed to be included in a test battery (7). In its review of the NTP, an ad hoc panel (5) reinforced the importance of developing and validating tests of promoters as a part of either the standard battery or as parallel in vivo testing studies because of the estimated wide extent of human exposure to promoters.

Promotion potential can be evaluated using any one of several test systems. However, only two have been sufficiently developed: the rodent liver and mouse skin systems (8). Of these, the mouse skin tumor initiation/promotion protocol is the most thoroughly studied procedure used to investigate promotion (9-12). In this model, skin tumors are induced by the application of a subthreshold dose of a carcinogen (initiation stage) followed by repetitive treatment with a known or suspected tumor promoter (promotion stage) (10), and tumor development is monitored over time (8). This system can be used not only to determine the tumor-initiating and -promoting activities of a compound but also to determine whether it is a complete carcinogen, i.e., whether it has both tumor-initiating and -promoting activities (8).

The mouse skin protocol is commonly used to study tumorigenesis, and its use as an optional test to obtain additional data would provide a more complete toxicologic characterization of a chemical in testing programs such as those of the NTP. Although the literature provides a basis for designing an appropriate standard tumor initiation/promotion protocol (13), some basic issues need to be addressed. For example, although mice are more sensitive than are rats and hamsters tested in the tumor initiation/promotion protocol (14-16), there are marked differences in sensitivity even among mouse strains (17-19). The outbred Swiss mouse is a responsive strain commonly used in tumor initiation/promotion studies. However, because of the NTP's established use of the B6C3F$_1$ mouse in carcinogenesis evaluations, it was essential to determine whether this strain could serve as a model in initiation/promotion studies as well. And the SENCAR mouse, selectively bred for its sensitivity to 7,12-dimethylbenz[a]anthracene (DMBA)-induced tumor initiation and 12-O-tetradecanoylphorbol-13-acetate (TPA)-induced promotion, was known to be more sensitive than Swiss CD-1 mice to this promoter (19), but the SENCAR mouse's relative sensitivity to other tumor-promoting agents was not well known. In addition, long-term carcinogenesis evaluations usually use both sexes of a strain. However, because group-housed male mice fight, they generally have not been used in tumor-initiation/promotion studies. Thus information on tumors in the male mouse was lacking. In selecting an appropriate model for promotion studies, it would be important to know whether there were gender differences in sensitivity. Therefore, mouse skin tumor initiation/promotion studies were conducted to compare the responses of different strains of mice and of males and females of the same strain and to define the strain and protocol to use in a large-scale program to supplement standard rodent toxicology and carcinogenesis studies.

METHODS

Mouse strain selection was based on an existent toxicology data base and on the initiation/promotion literature. Three mouse strains were selected for this test, the B6C3F$_1$ mouse, which is used in the NTP prechronic and chronic toxicity studies (20,21) as described above, and two established promoter-responsive strains—Swiss CD-1 and SENCAR mice (19). Thirty mice of each sex of each strain per test group were individually housed with food and water available ad libitum. Mice were uniquely identified and randomly assigned to dose groups. Hair was clipped from the back of each animal approximately 24 to 48 h prior to initiator dose application and generally once weekly thereafter, or as needed. Mice were approximately 55 days of age at the time of the first dosing. The number, type, and date of appearance of tumors for each animal were entered weekly into a computer system. Tumor maps were maintained for each animal to record the location and to follow the development of tumors.

To follow the development of tumors, criteria were established to allow calculations of time of appearance and number of tumors per animal. If a tumor was present for 14 days, at least 2 mm in diameter, and not attached to the subcutis, it was recorded as a papilloma. Tumors necrotic in appearance and attached to the subcutis were recorded as carcinomas. The mean time to tumor development was estimated by averaging times of first tumor appearance on individual animals in that group. Animals that did not develop tumors were arbitrarily assigned week 52 for this estimate. To estimate the average number of papillomas per animal in a group, the total number of papillomas was divided by the total number of animals in each group. A final observation and tumor map were made for each animal at necropsy, and skin samples were examined microscopically. Known tumor-initiating and -promoting agents for these studies were selected for possible differences in sensitivity due to strain differences in skin metabolism. N-Methyl-N´-nitro-N-nitrosoguanidine (MNNG) and DMBA were selected as initiators, and the phorbol ester TPA and benzoyl peroxide (BPO) were selected as promoters.

Preliminary studies indicated that 50 µg DMBA followed by 5 µg TPA three times a week produced tumors in B6C3F$_1$ mice (NTP, unpublished data), but lower doses of DMBA or TPA had not been tested in this strain. Initiating doses of 2.5 µg DMBA (10 nmol) followed by twice-weekly applications of 5 µg (~8.5 nmol) TPA had been shown to produce tumors by week 15 of treatment in Swiss CD-1 (60%) and SENCAR (100%) mice (19). Because the number of animals in the current study was limited, we decided to keep the promoter doses constant and vary the initiator doses to best compare the sensitivity of the three strains. However, after several weeks of dosing with 5 µg TPA once a week, the application site on the SENCAR mice showed unexpected signs of extreme irritation, and the SENCAR TPA studies were stopped. A subsequent range-finding study indicated 1 µg was a nonirritating TPA dose level, and the SENCAR TPA studies were restarted. The other two strains did not show signs of irritation after repeated weekly dosing of 5 µg TPA, and these studies were continued as designed. Because of the numbers of animals that would have been required, it was not possible to add Swiss CD-1 and B6C3F$_1$ mice at the 1-µg TPA dose level. Therefore, tumor response comparisons of Swiss CD-1 and B6C3F$_1$ mice with the SENCAR mice need to take into account the difference in TPA dose levels. DMBA, MNNG, and TPA were applied in a volume of 100 µl, and BPO was applied in two 100-µl applications. Chemical applications were conducted once a week for up to 52 weeks as shown in Table 1.

RESULTS

Figure 1 shows the response of male and female mice to initiation with 2.5 µg DMBA followed by TPA promotion for 51 weeks. In males, the response was greatest among Swiss CD-1 mice, then among SENCAR, and then B6C3F$_1$ mice. However, it should be noted that, for the reasons described above, the Swiss and B6C3F$_1$ mice received doses of 5 µg/week TPA, while the SENCAR mice received only 1 µg/week. This strain difference in response was also seen in the average number of tumors per animal per group (Swiss, 3.32; SENCAR, 2.43; B6C3F$_1$, 0.55). Female SENCAR and Swiss CD-1 mice had very similar responses in spite of the fact that the Swiss females received five times as much TPA per week. The B6C3F$_1$ females were much less responsive. Although the percentage of papil-

Table 1. Experimental Design

Group	Chemical application	
	Week 1	Weeks 2–52
Vehicle	Acetone	Acetone
Initiated only	DMBA (0.25, 2.5, 25, or 50 µg)	Acetone
	MNNG (100, 500, or 1000 µg)	Acetone
Complete carcinogen	DMBA (2.5 µg)	DMBA (2.5 µg)
	MNNG (100 µg)	MNNG (100 µg)
	TPA (5 or 1 µg)	TPA (5 or 1 µg)
	BPO (20 mg)	BPO (20 mg)
Initiated/promoted	DMBA (0.25, 2.5, 25, or 50 µg)	TPA (5 or 1 µg)
	DMBA (2.5 or 25 µg)	BPO (20 mg)
	MNNG (100 or 1000 µg)	TPA (5 or 1 µg)
	MNNG (100, 500, or 1000 µg)	BPO (20 mg)

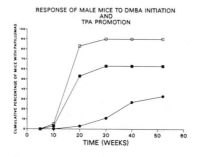

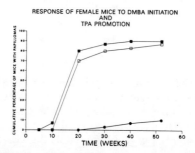

Figure 1. Male (top) and female (bottom) mice underwent initiation with 2.5 µg (10 nmol) of DMBA followed 1 week later by TPA promotion once a week for up to 51 weeks. Swiss CD-1 (□) and B6C3F$_1$ (●) mice received 5 µg (8.1 nmol) TPA, and SENCAR (■) mice received 1 µg (1.6 nmol) TPA/week. Abbreviations: DMBA, 7,12-dimethylbenz[a]anthracene; TPA, 12-O-tetradecanoylphorbol-13-acetate.

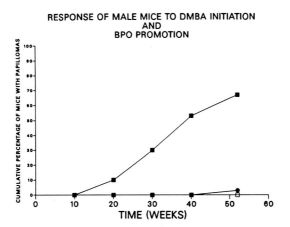

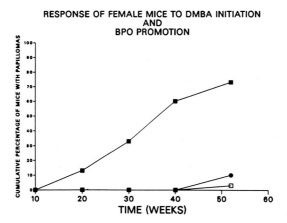

Figure 2. Male (top) and female (bottom) SENCAR (■), Swiss CD-1 (□), and B6C3F$_1$ (●) mice received 0.25 µg (10 nmol) of DMBA followed 1 week later by 20 mg (82.5 µmol) benzoyl peroxide (BPO) promotion once a week for up to 51 weeks.

loma-bearing animals was similar for SENCAR and Swiss CD-1 female mice, the number of tumors per animal per group (3.49 vs. 2.96) suggests that the female SENCAR mice were more sensitive than the female Swiss CD-1 mice.

When BPO was used as the promoter and 2.5 µg DMBA as the initiator, the sensitivity of the SENCAR mice was more striking (Fig. 2). About 70% of the

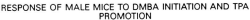

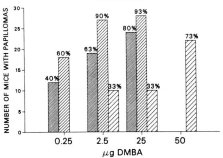

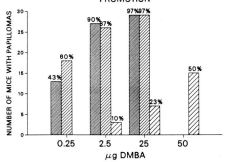

Figure 3. Male (top) and female (bottom) SENCAR (▨), Swiss CD-1 (▨), and B6C3F₁ (▨) mice received 0.25 (1), 2.5 (10), 25 (100), or 50 (200) µg (nmol) of DMBA followed 1 week later by TPA promotion once a week for up to 51 weeks. Swiss CD-1 and B6C3F₁ mice received 5 µg (8.1 nmol) TPA and SENCAR mice received 1 µg (1.6 nmol) TPA/week.

SENCAR males and females had papillomas after 52 weeks. Neither the Swiss CD-1 nor the B6C3F₁ mice were very responsive to this combination of DMBA with BPO.

Figure 3 shows the responses of male and female mice to TPA promotion at different initiating doses of DMBA. Both sexes of all three strains showed an apparent dose response. More male Swiss CD-1 mice developed papillomas than did male SENCAR or B6C3F₁ mice at all DMBA initiating doses. However, the Swiss and B6C3F₁ mice received a fivefold higher promoting dose of TPA than did the SENCAR mice. Female SENCAR and Swiss CD-1 mice had quite similar responses, measured as cumulative percentages of mice with papillomas. The average number of tumors per mouse and mean time to tumor response were also

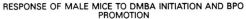

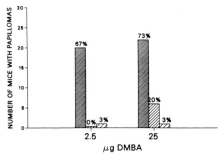

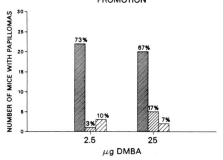

Figure 4. Male (top) and female (bottom) SENCAR (■), Swiss CD-1 (▨), and B6C3F$_1$ (▨) mice received 2.5 (10) or 25 (100) µg (nmol) of DMBA, followed 1 week later by 20 mg (82.6 nmol) BPO once a week for up to 52 weeks.

similar for female SENCAR and Swiss CD-1 mice (data not shown). Both of these strains were more responsive than the B6C3F$_1$ female mice.

However, the degree of responsiveness was quite different when BPO was used as a promoter after DMBA initiation (Fig. 4). At common initiating doses of DMBA (2.5 or 25 µg), both sexes of SENCAR mice were much more responsive than were either the Swiss CD-1 or B6C3F$_1$ mice. Within a strain, sex differences in papilloma response to BPO were small.

The pattern of tumor response of male and female mice to MNNG initiation followed by TPA promotion is shown in Figure 5. With the MNNG/TPA protocol, the percentage of mice with papillomas was similar for SENCAR and Swiss CD-1 mice, and the females of each strain appeared to be slightly more sensitive than did the males (70% vs. 55%). Also, for the SENCAR and Swiss CD-1 strains, the

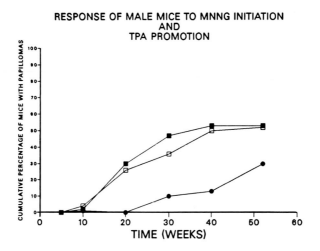

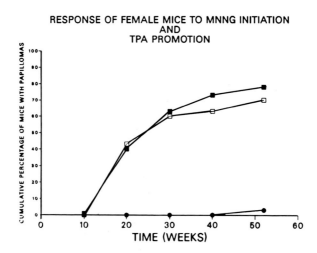

Figure 5. Male (top) and female (bottom) SENCAR (■), Swiss CD-1 (□), and B6C3F₁ (●) mice received a tumor-initiating dose of 100 µg (680 nmol) MNNG followed 1 week later by TPA promotion once a week for up to 51 weeks. Swiss CD-1 and B6C3F₁ mice received 5 µg (8.1 nmol) TPA and SENCAR mice received 1 µg (1.6 nmol) TPA per week. Abbreviation: MNNG, *N*-methyl-*N'*-nitro-*N*-nitrosoguanidine.

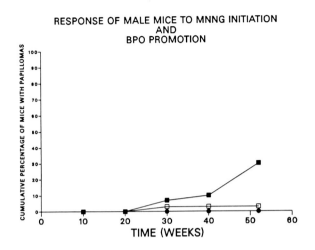

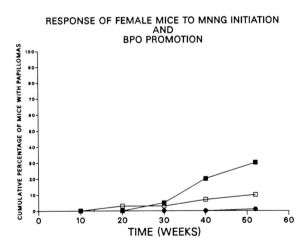

Figure 6. Male (top) and female (bottom) SENCAR (■), Swiss CD-1 (▢), and B6C3F₁ (●) mice received a tumor-initiating dose of 100 μg (680 nmol) MNNG followed 1 week later by 20 mg (82.6 nmol) BPO once a week for up to 51 weeks.

average number of tumors per animal (about 1.30 for males and 1.85 for females) and the mean time to development of the first tumor (about 36 weeks for males and 30 weeks for females) were similar. Fewer B6C3F$_1$ mice developed papillomas, and these papillomas appeared later in the study compared with papillomas in the other strains.

When mice were given tumor-promoting doses of BPO after tumor-initiating treatment with MNNG (Fig. 6), the general response was less than that with TPA as a promoter. Both sexes of SENCAR mice were more sensitive than either the Swiss CD-1 or the B6C3F$_1$ mice. More SENCAR mice developed papillomas, and the papillomas appeared earlier than in the other mice (Fig. 6). In addition, the average number of papillomas per animal was greater for the SENCAR strain (about 0.5 for SENCAR vs. 0.08 for Swiss CD-1 mice).

The responses of the mice to multiple exposures to low doses of initiating carcinogens are shown in Figures 7 and 8. All three strains responded to 2.5 µg DMBA (>65% with papillomas after 52 weeks of exposure) and to 100 µg MNNG (> 50% with papillomas after 52 weeks of exposure). SENCAR mice were slightly more sensitive to DMBA than were Swiss CD-1 or B6C3F$_1$ mice, as determined by the cumulative percentage of mice with tumors (Fig. 7) and the mean time to development of the first tumor (SENCAR, 35.3 weeks; Swiss CD-1, 44.3 weeks; B6C3F$_1$, 46.3 weeks). Although Swiss CD-1 mice got papillomas earlier than did the B6C3F$_1$ mice, after 52 weeks, each strain had equal numbers of tumor-bearing male animals (70%) and there were more tumor-bearing female B6C3F$_1$ than Swiss CD-1 female mice (87% vs. 67%) (Fig. 7).

The response to MNNG as a complete carcinogen also indicates that the SENCAR mice were most sensitive to this initiator (Fig. 8). The mean time to the development of the first tumor (about 32 weeks) for both sexes of this strain was shorter than that observed for the Swiss CD-1 (about 44.1 weeks) or B6C3F$_1$ (39.6 weeks) mice. However, at 52 weeks, there were as many B6C3F$_1$ as SENCAR mice with tumors. In addition, by 52 weeks, the number of SENCAR and B6C3F$_1$ mice of both sexes with tumors was twice the number of Swiss CD-1 (approximately 28 vs. 17).

DISCUSSION

Animal models that display a high degree of responsiveness to carcinogens provide a tool for identifying some of the key steps involved in tumorigenesis. The mouse skin tumor initiation/promotion protocol has been frequently used to distinguish chemicals that are initiators from promoters (22). The present initiation/promotion studies were undertaken to compare tumor responses in males and females of three mouse strains and to define a strain and protocol for use in future studies. The data base on the biology of the B6C3F$_1$ mouse is extensive because of its use in the NTP studies (20,21), and there would be obvious advantages to using the same strain to evaluate chemicals for both initiating and promoting activity. We found no B6C3F$_1$ mouse skin tumor initiation/promotion studies in the literature, and information on skin metabolism of carcinogens in

RESPONSE OF MALE MICE TO WEEKLY DMBA ADMINISTRATION

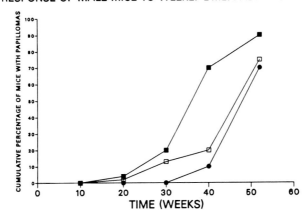

RESPONSE OF FEMALE MICE TO WEEKLY DMBA ADMINISTRATION

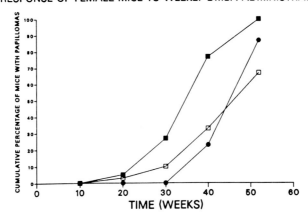

Figure 7. Male (top) and female (bottom) SENCAR (■), Swiss CD-1 (□), and B6C3F₁ (●) mice were treated once a week with 2.5 μg (10 nmol) MNNG for up to 52 weeks.

this strain was lacking. The outbred Swiss albino (CD-1) mouse was selected because of its historical use in the mouse skin protocol (8). The SENCAR mouse, a strain derived by selective breeding for sensitivity to DMBA initiation and TPA promotion (18), was selected because of its reported shortened response time and

RESPONSE OF MALE MICE TO WEEKLY MNNG ADMINISTRATION

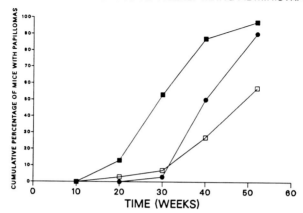

RESPONSE OF FEMALE MICE TO WEEKLY MNNG ADMINISTRATION

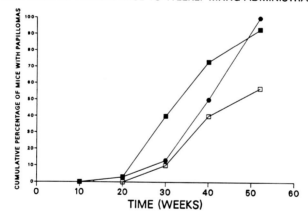

Figure 8. Male (top) and female (bottom) SENCAR (■), Swiss CD-1 (□), and B6C3F$_1$ (●), mice were treated once a week with 100 μg (680 nmol) MNNG for up to 52 weeks.

increased tumor yield compared with those of other strains (19). When we designed our comparative study, it was not known whether this reported increased sensitivity of SENCAR mice was limited to TPA promotion, and thus studies with an additional tumor promoter, BPO, were needed.

The current studies clearly demonstrated that regardless of the combination of tumor initiators and promoters used, B6C3F$_1$ mice were not as sensitive as the SENCAR or the Swiss CD-1 mice. Both the SENCAR and Swiss CD-1 mice responded well to the DMBA/TPA regimen, but it was difficult to quantitatively compare these two strains because of the difference in TPA doses (1 μg for SENCAR vs. 5 μg for Swiss CD-1). Thus, although male Swiss CD-1 mice appeared to be more responsive because more of these animals had tumors, the difference in TPA exposure might account for the higher response of the Swiss CD-1 males. As males are rarely used (because of caging problems), we found no literature to compare with our data. On the other hand, the present studies indicated little difference in papilloma response between female SENCAR and Swiss CD-1 mice in spite of the difference in TPA doses. Slaga and Fischer (19) compared female SENCAR and Swiss CD-1 mice given different initiating doses of DMBA and of benzo[a]pyrene (BaP) and then twice-weekly applications of 8.5 nmol (~5 μg) TPA. Their results showed that SENCAR females were more sensitive to TPA than were the Swiss CD-1 mice at every tumor-initiating dose of DMBA and BaP. And in this study, SENCAR mice were clearly more sensitive to DMBA initiation followed by BPO promotion than were the Swiss CD-1 mice. When MNNG was used as the initiator, the responses of SENCAR and Swiss CD-1 mice to tumor-promoting doses of TPA were similar, again suggesting that SENCAR mice are more sensitive, as they received a lower TPA dose. SENCAR mice were also more sensitive when BPO was used as the promoter after tumor-initiating treatment with MNNG, even though the overall response was not as great as with TPA.

With repeated applications of the direct-acting MNNG or the metabolism-requiring DMBA, at least 70% of the animals in all three strains had papillomas by week 52. This suggests that differences in response among strains are not primarily related to initiation. Furthermore, SENCAR mice developed papillomas earlier than did the other strains, an important consideration in selecting a sensitive mouse strain.

The results of this comparative mouse study are being used to select a mouse strain and to establish standards in protocol design for future initiation/promotion studies. Standardization will provide uniformity in testing procedures and facilitate comparisons between independent studies as well as improve reliability in detecting agents with promotion potential. The two-stage mouse skin tumor protocol is limited in that it will not identify all promoters (22). Other model systems for studying promotion (6) are used in several laboratories, including the National Institute for Environmental Health Sciences. However, the mouse skin model has received the most attention because it offers ease of administration of test agents, a noninvasive measurement of tumor appearance, and direct observation of tumor development. For these reasons, this system has been used in many laboratories to study tumor promoters, cocarcinogens, and tumor inhibitors—with the ultimate goal of better understanding carcinogenesis. Although the term promoter has not been clearly defined, identifying agents that have the potential to complete the carcinogenesis process following initiation is clearly important. Our studies indicate that the B6C3F$_1$ mouse, used in the NTP toxicology and carcinogenesis studies, is not the best strain to use in mouse skin tumor initiation/promotion studies. Recent studies have shown that the SENCAR mouse is one of the most sensitive strains to use in initiation/promotion protocols to study carcinogenesis (for reviews, see refs. 23,24). In this study, the SENCAR mouse was also the most sensitive overall and may thus be the most appropriate strain to use in future NTP initiation/promotion studies aimed at yielding data on mechanisms of carcinogenesis and to aid in the interpretation of the toxicologic effects of chemicals being evaluated by the NTP.

ACKNOWLEDGMENTS

These studies were conducted at Battelle Memorial Institute, Columbus OH, under National Institutes of Health contract N01-ES-55072. Their assistance in preparing the graphs and tables for this presentation is greatly appreciated.

OPEN FORUM

Dr. Steve Lewis: Dr. Eastin, would you recommend that we do histopathological analysis outside the treatment area? How exhaustively would you recommend that we analyze the treated area histopathologically? There is a fair amount of interest in whether any animal model can be developed for systemic carcinogenesis by epicutaneous application. I know that Kettering does an extremely exhaustive necropsy, sectioning not only the lesions in the treated area classified as tumors but also every lesion regardless of whether it appears to be neoplastic. In a pending study, I think they will find a number of tumors that would have been missed if they had done a less exhaustive examination.

Dr. William C. Eastin: At the end of my chapter, I described the initiation-promotion study we had completed. We tried to follow the procedures we use during prechronic and chronic testing for all NTP studies. For future initiation/promotion studies, we would probably only look at skin. For this study, we instructed the pathologists to look at five different tumors or, if all the tumors were the same, to look at five different sizes of tumors. We predicted, based on the literature, what kind of tumors they would be, and we hoped that the description would confirm this. In my experience, you usually do not get as many tumors in initiation-promotion studies with other agents as you do with DMBA and TPA. And we did not expect more than five different kinds of skin tumors. With the standard prechronic and especially the chronic studies, the pathologists are required to look at about 35 tissues. They are also required to look at all gross lesions. That would be true for skin exposure studies. In skin, we look at any tumor that shows up at the application site and any tumor that shows up away from the application site. We also require pathologists to take skin that they consider control samples. If there are no tumors at the application site, they take one section. If there are tumors at the application site, we ask them to take that tumor or tumors and a section of skin without a tumor. We ask them also to section the tumor so that they have apparently unaffected tissue.

Dr. Lewis: You don't necessarily ask them to section lesions that are not classified in vivo—scars, scabs, scratches, pustules, etc.?

Dr. Eastin: We leave it up to the pathologists at the laboratory to identify those. I don't think they look at ones that are obviously from scratching.

Dr. Byron Butterworth: Would it be possible to add a few more animals and measure the extent and duration of hyperplasia, so that you could begin to establish the relationship between that and the carcinogenic response? Perhaps that might aid in some risk assessment evaluations in the future. And would it be possible to look at more biochemical parameters in additional animals?

Dr. Eastin: Are you talking about initiation-promotion studies or exposure of the skin?

Dr. Butterworth: This would be more in the promotion studies. In parallel to promotion studies, you would add a few more animals to obtain the dose-response relationship for the hyperplastic response. Then you could compare that to the tumorigenic response and begin to see if there was a relationship.

Dr. Eastin: Others here might be better able to say how long you would need to expose animals to determine whether they were going to have accomodation or not and whether that would sustain hyperplasia for a length of time. When we expose animals' skin for chronic studies, we have obtained all that information from the prechronic studies. They would have been exposed for 90 days.

Dr. Butterworth: I was thinking that even in the prechronic studies you could gather that additional information. In fact, that might be a rational approach to help you set your dose levels. So often cancer studies come up with a single plus or minus result. It would be nice to get some more scientific information to grapple with these tough issues.

Dr. Eastin: There are five dose levels and controls in the prechronic studies.

Dr. Jerry Smith: Dr. Eastin, I understand you have about 20 compounds that are under percutaneous evaluation. Is that for systemic tumors or both initiation and promotion studies?

Dr. Eastin: That is mostly systemic work. We have about three initiation-promotion studies.

Dr. Smith: What criteria do you use to select a maximum tolerated dose, both for systemic and percutaneous exposure, and how do you use the five dose levels for determining an initiator and a promoter dose level?

Dr. Eastin: For the study that we just completed, the initiator and promoter doses that we selected were based on the literature. For toxicity studies of chemicals on skin it is more difficult. Before we start, we try to obtain information on percutaneous absorption and disposition. This information influences our decision about whether to use the skin as a route of exposure at all. We do repeat dose studies to look for gross toxic effects. These are 2-week studies with five animals per group. We select doses based on the results of the repeat dose study and conduct a 90-day study to establish a dose response. The 90-day studies all include pathological analysis—microscopic evaluation of the tissues and of the skin. Setting doses for the chronic study is difficult.

Dr. Paul Grasso: Dr. Eastin, I think we have learned here that there are two stages in promotion; however, this does not seem to be taken account of in experimental protocols. Is this intended or accidental, and do you intend to do stage 1 and 2 promotion studies later? These might have toxicological implications.

Dr. Eastin: We wanted to establish a standard protocol using a sensitive mouse strain and the capabilities of our contract laboratories that would provide uniformity from lab to lab and study to study. As to when to use an initiation-promotion study, chemical managers currently seem to recommend one for substances that are not genotoxic and that cause sustained hyperplasia. The mouse skin-painting study is not the only one that we use. The liver model is also used, and I don't know what the goals are for those studies.

Dr. Grasso: We had two demonstrations. One was with TPA and mezerein. Mezerein produced a very strong hyperplasia, which later seemed to diminish even though the compound was applied. Yet, when mezerein was applied after an initial dose of TPA, hyperplasia was sustained. Do you take into account these type of compounds? One was called type 2, and the other was called type 1.

Dr. Eastin: I think that is one step beyond where we want to go with this model right now. We carry our compounds through the prechronic and chronic studies and perform a final evaluation, which takes into account clinical observations, toxicity, microscopic evaluations of all the tissues, and comparisons to controls. Some compounds can obviously be categorized as having a clear effect. Now and then a compound produces an increase in a response that cannot be readily classified. We are hoping that these kinds of studies (initiation/promotion) will help to identify promoters. It would be ideal if there were some kind of universal initiator. Then, in one study you could give this tumor initiator to some groups of animals, expose them by any route, and compare the results. If tumors develop in animals that were given initiating agents but not in non-initiated animals, you can say something about the promotion potential of the chemical on the test. Currently, the skin model is well known and has a good-sized data base, and tests for promotion and for systemic carcinogenic effects are performed separately.

Dr. J. Michael Holland: I think we must bear in mind that the labels we use are operational. As our knowledge base increases, so does the complexity of our models. In my mind, the separation between an initiator and a promoter is not distinct in a quantitative sense. Most promoters are weak initiators; some are strong initiators. Initiators are claimed to have promoting activity, but I do not think it has been well defined whether that promoting activity is the same or different from that induced by a pure promoter. That should be considered in the design of protocols to assess these activities.

REFERENCES

1. Rall DP, Hogan MD, Huff JE, Schwetz BA, Tennant RW. Alternatives to using human experience in assessing health risks. Annu Rev Public Health 8:355-385, 1987.
2. Haseman JK, Huff JE, Zeiger E, McConnell EE. Comparative results of 327 chemical carcinogenicity studies. Environ Health Perspect 74:229-235, 1987.
3. Huff JE, McConnell EE, Haseman JK, Boorman GA, Eustis SL, Schwetz BA, Rao GN, Jameson CW, Hart LG, Rall DP. Carcinogenesis studies: Results of 398 experiments on 104 chemicals from the U. S. National Toxicology Program. Ann NY Acad Sci 534:1-30, 1988.
4. International Agency for Research on Cancer. Long-term and short-term screening assays for carcinogens: A critical appraisal. Suppl. 2. Lyon, France: IARC Monographs, 1980.
5. National Toxicology Program. Report of the NTP ad hoc panel on chemical carcinogenesis testing and evaluation. Prepared for the National Toxicology Program Board of Scientific Counselors, August 17, 1984.
6. Langenbach R, Elmore E, Barrett C (eds). Tumor Promoters: Biological Approaches for Mechanistic Studies and Assay Systems. Progress in Cancer Research and Therapy, Vol. 34. New York: Raven Press, 1988.
7. International Agency for Research on Cancer. Approaches to classifying chemical carcinogens according to mechanism of action. Technical Report No. 83/001. Lyon, France: IARC Monographs, 1983.
8. Slaga TJ. Mechanisms involved in two-stage carcinogenesis in mouse skin. In Slaga TJ (ed): Mechanisms of Tumor Promotion, Vol II. Tumor Promotion and Skin Carcinogenesis. Boca Raton, FL: CRC Press, 1984, pp 1-16.
9. Berenblum I, Shubik P. A new, quantitative approach to the study of the stages of chemical carcinogenesis in mouse skin. Br J Cancer 1:383-391, 1947.
10. Boutwell RK. Some biological aspects of skin carcinogenesis. Prog Exp Tumor Res 4:207-250, 1964.
11. Boutwell RK. The function and mechanism of promoters of carcinogenesis. CRC Crit Rev Toxicol 2:419-443, 1974.
12. Van Duuren BL. Tumor-promoting agents in two-stage carcinogenesis. Prog Exp Tumor Res 11:31-68, 1969.
13. Van Duuren BL, Melchionne S. Mouse skin application in chemical carcinogenesis. Prog Exp Tumor Res 26:154-168, 1983.
14. Barrett JC, Sisskin EE. Studies on why 12-O-tetradecanoyl-phorbol-13-acetate (TPA) does not promote epidermal carcinogenesis of hamsters. In Pullman B, Ts'o POP, Gelboin H (eds): Carcinogenesis: Fundamental Mechanisms and Environmental Effects. Hingham, MA: D. Reidel Publishing, 1980, pp 427-439.
15. Slaga TJ, Fischer SM, Triplett LL, Nesnow S. Comparison of complete carcinogenesis and tumor initiation and promotion in mouse skin: The induction of papillomas by tumor initiation-promotion: A reliable short term assay. J Environ Pathol Toxicol 4:1025-1041, 1981.
16. Stenback F. Skin carcinogenesis as a model system: Observations on species, strain and tissue sensitivity to 7,12-dimethylbenz[a]anthracene with and without promo-

tion from croton oil. Acta Pharmacol Toxicol 46:89-97, 1980.

17. DiGiovanni J, Masashi N, Chenicek KJ. Genetic factors controlling susceptibility to skin tumor promotion in mice. In Langenbach R, Elmore E, Barrett C (eds): Tumor Promoters: Biological Approaches for Mechanistic Studies and Assay Systems. Progress in Cancer Research and Therapy, Vol. 34. New York: Raven Press, 1988, pp 51-69.

18. Slaga TJ. SENCAR mouse skin tumorigenesis model versus other strains and stocks of mice. Environ Health Perspect 68:27-32, 1986.

19. Slaga TJ, Fischer SM. Strain differences and solvent effects in mouse skin carcinogenesis experiments using carcinogens, tumor initiators and promoters. Prog Exp Tumor Res 26:85-109, 1983.

20. Haseman JK, Huff J, Boorman GA. Use of historical control data in carcinogenicity studies in rodents. Toxicol Pathol 12:126-133, 1984.

21. Haseman JK, Huff JE, Rao GN, Arnold JE, Boorman GA, McConnell EE. Neoplasms observed in untreated and corn oil gavage control groups of F344/N rats and (C57BL/6N X C3H/HeN)F$_1$ (B6C3F$_1$) mice. JNCI 75:975-983, 1985.

22. Pereira MA. Mouse skin bioassay for chemical carcinogens. Journal of the American College of Toxicology 1:47-82, 1982.

23. The SENCAR mouse in toxicological testing. (Conference report, May 1-2, 1985, Cincinnati, OH) Environ Health Perspect 68:1-151, 1986.

24. Bull RJ, Robinson M, Laurie RD. Association of tumor yield with early papilloma development in SENCAR mice. Environ Health Perspect 68:11-17, 1986.

Skin Carcinogenesis: Mechanisms and Human Relevance, pages 313–329

Prospective Assessment of Human Carcinogens: The Determination of Genotoxic Action in Human Skin

A.S. Wright and W.P. Watson

Shell Research Limited, Sittingbourne Research Centre, Sittingbourne, Kent, U.K.

Epidemiological evidence indicates that a high proportion of human cancer is caused by exposure to environmental factors (1) and is, therefore, preventable. The basic causative agents include ultraviolet (UV) light, penetrating ionizing radiation, and chemicals of both natural and industrial origin. Radiation hazards are relatively easy to detect and monitor. Furthermore, cancer risks (i.e., quantitative human dose-response relationships) associated with exposures to ionizing radiation are reasonably well defined. The position with chemicals is less clear. Retrospective epidemiological analyses of tumor incidence in cigarette smokers and in populations with high dietary exposures to mycotoxins have revealed the impact that chemical exposures can have on human cancer. However, few individual chemicals have been identified as contributing to overall cancer incidence. Thus, except in cases of specific, localized, and high exposures to chemicals such as 2-naphthylamine, vinyl chloride, and diethylstilbestrol, current epidemiological methods employed to investigate the causes of human cancer lack the sensitivity and resolving power needed to identify specific chemical hazards. However, even when the specific hazard has been identified, it is difficult to estimate the carcinogenic impact of low exposures in human populations. Thus, information on the potency (dose-response relationships) of chemical carcinogens is almost completely lacking in man—particularly on that of low doses. The problem of assessing the carcinogenic impact of chemicals is compounded by the complex interactive effects by which chemicals variously exacerbate or reduce the tumorigenic action of other chemical or physical agents.

These considerations suggest that, in seeking approaches to reduce human cancer, it is essential to develop methods to detect, identify, and evaluate the specific chemical hazards in the environment. Furthermore, it is clear that the methods should be prospective for man. Thus, the methods should be sensitive and should aim to determine early events, so as to be as predictive as possible and provide an early warning of biological hazards (see refs. 2-4). Of course, cancer prevention also requires effective prescreening of new products: such screening must obviously be prospective in terms of predicting human hazards.

PROSPECTIVE RISK MODELS

Long-Term Cancer Studies

Until the mid-1970s, prospective methods for the detection and identification of human carcinogens and estimation of risks to man were based almost exclusively on the results of long-term cancer studies in laboratory animals. There were three main problems with this approach.

First, the detection limits of experimental cancer studies do not permit the detection of risk at a level that would be considered acceptable from a sociopolitical standpoint, i.e., 10^{-6}/year (5). The detection limit in such studies rarely approaches 10^{-2}, suggesting that conventional cancer bioassays may fail to detect some significant carcinogens. In some instances the possibility of testing at high doses may compensate for the poor resolving power of the assay. However, the application of high doses may often confound the issue by introducing nonspecific mechanisms, e.g., tissue injury, that are not relevant to an assessment of hazards posed by low doses/exposures. Conversely, the high-dose strategy may fail because of a threshold limit on net bioactivation.

Second, when a positive result is obtained in a conventional cancer bioassay, it may be necessary to evaluate the risks posed by low concentrations encountered in the environment or workplace. The evaluation of low-level risks necessitates extrapolation from risk data determined at the high doses needed to produce measurable effects. Such extrapolation is subject to uncertainty and error.

Third, additional uncertainty and error arises when seeking to extrapolate from the experimental model to man. Thus, the frequent occurrence of marked quantitative and apparent qualitative species differences in response to chemical carcinogens caution against direct extrapolation. The onus should therefore be on establishing the qualitative and quantitative relevance of the model for the prediction and estimation of the human hazard.

Solutions to these interpretative problems are dependent upon knowledge of the mechanisms of chemical carcinogenesis. Fortunately, research during the past 20 years has provided some important insights and basic tenets that are now being applied to develop improved procedures for detecting human carcinogens, monitoring human exposure to these agents, and evaluating the risks to man. In particular, it is now accepted that mutagenic action, i.e., the induction of transmissible alterations in DNA structure, is fundamental to the operation of most chemical carcinogens. Such agents are classified as genotoxic (6). DNA is regarded as the primary and critical target of genotoxic carcinogens, although primary DNA damage and mutation can also be induced by indirect genotoxic mechanisms (7). Furthermore, many chemicals classified as genotoxic are precursors that require metabolic conversion into reactive forms (electrophiles) in order to undergo chemical reaction with DNA. The primary products of these reactions with DNA are generally promutagenic or lethal. These products include DNA base adducts, which have been accorded special attention not only because of their mutagenic propensity but also because of the sensitivity and specificity of the techniques available for their analysis (for a review, see ref. 8).

Short-Term Tests

The evidence that a sequential mechanism links electrophilic reactivity of chemicals or their metabolites with the induction of primary chemical damage in DNA, leading to mutation and cancer (Fig. 1), provided the theoretical justification for the development and application of rapid genotoxicity assays—mainly in vitro assays—to predict carcinogenic activity. The relative simplicity and low cost of these in vitro assays has permitted widespread screening for environmental and occupational mutagens and carcinogens and also prescreening of new products, e.g., drugs and agrochemicals. However, just as conventional carcinogenicity assays are, at best, qualitative in terms of predicting human hazard, the in vitro genotoxicity assays are considered to be only qualitative in terms of their capacity to predict carcinogenic activity. It may be argued that qualitative procedures would provide entirely satisfactory screens for human carcinogens. Thus, it is generally accepted that human contact with carcinogens should be minimized irrespective of potency. However, numerous

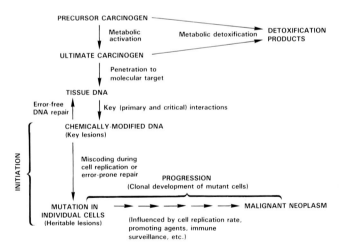

Figure 1. Principal stages and determinants of chemical carcinogenesis. From F. K. Silbergeld et al. In: Fowler, BA (ed): Mechanisms of Cell Injury: Implications for Human Health, pp 405-429, Copyright 1987 John Wiley & Sons, Ltd., Chichester, U.K. Reprinted by permission of John Wiley & Sons, Ltd.

qualitative discrepancies have been reported between the results of in vitro mutation assays and conventional cancer bioassays (9). These discrepancies have led to concern about the value of in vitro genotoxicity tests as qualitative indicators of carcinogenic hazards. Nevertheless, the evidence that genotoxic action is critical to the initiation of chemical carcinogenesis is overwhelming. It is therefore important to consider the limitations of genotoxicity assays in predicting carcinogenic activity and vice versa (see ref. 10). There are three main reasons for discrepancies in the correlation between genotoxic action in vitro and carcinogenic action in vivo (7). First, except for cell transformation assays, in vitro genotoxicity assays are not designed to respond to nongenotoxic carcinogens or to tumor-promoting agents. Second, the expression of genotoxic potential is strongly influenced by toxicokinetic and toxicodynamic factors whose operation can vary markedly between species and in vivo/in vitro (11,12). Interpretative problems arising because of differences in the operation of these systemic determinants can be minimized by developing in vitro systems that are more representative of the species and tissue at risk, e.g., human skin. The third reason hinges on the relative resolving powers of in vitro and in vivo studies and is likely to have the most far-reaching consequences. Thus, it is important to recognize that the resolving power of experimental cancer studies does not permit carcinogenic effects to be detected or measured at a level of risk that would be acceptable for man. The difference between the limits of detection and the required sensitivity invariably exceeds a factor of 10^4. In vitro genotoxicity assays often have resolving powers that permit the detection of genotoxic action at exposures or doses below the limits of detection of in vivo cancer studies. This higher resolving power may, therefore, lead to apparent false-positive results in vitro. However, when these false positives are considered in the context of the poor sensitivity of carcinogenicity bioassays and in the light of evidence that genotoxic action precedes and, in a stochastic sense, predicts carcinogenic action, then it is clear that such false-positive results should not be lightly dismissed. This interpretative dilemma is likely to become more severe as new and increasingly precise and sensitive genotoxicity assays, e.g., postlabeling assays (13) are introduced. The introduction of these assays will undoubtedly lead to increases in the occurrence of so-called false-positive results in the future.

STRATEGIES TO IMPROVE HAZARD ASSESSMENT

By the mid-1970s, in vitro genotoxicity assays were becoming widely used as qualitative tests for the prediction of carcinogenic activity. In vivo carcinogenicity studies continued to be applied as the reference standard and for the quantitative estimation of risks to man. However, as previously noted, the short-term tests may, in certain respects, be more reliable qualitative indicators of carcinogenic hazards than the long-term studies conventionally employed as reference standards to gauge the performance of the short-term tests (see ref. 10). Indeed, it is clear that the interpretation of both classes of assay is subject to major uncertainties and errors.

Several groups, most notably Ehrenberg and his colleagues at the University of Stockholm, have recognized these deficiencies in the available risk models and developed strategies to improve the quality of procedures to detect human carcinogens and assess cancer risks (3,14-20). In the main, these strategies focus on the need to correct or compensate for differences between experimental models and man in the operation of systemic factors that influence or determine the critical stages or critical events in the carcinogenic process (Fig. 1). Some of these factors, such as enzyme-mediated activation and detoxification pathways and DNA repair processes, are reasonably well defined. In other instances such as fidelity of DNA repair processes, factors controlling DNA/cell replication, and status of immunological defense systems, our understanding of both the nature of the factors and their impact on the carcinogenic process is much less well defined and is, therefore, an important focus of current research. Nevertheless, qualitative and/or quantitative differences in the operation of these factors are responsible for differences in susceptibility and response at the level of the cell, tissue, individual, strain, and species. In seeking to reduce the errors incurred when extrapolating experimental risk data to man, it is essential to correct for the influence of these systemic factors and general extrinsic factors, e.g., exogenous promoters, at each stage of the process.

THE TARGET DOSE CONCEPT

Ehrenberg et al. (15) were the first to propose that, as an initial step in seeking to improve the quality of prospective risk assessment, a new dose concept should be developed to measure the amount of ultimate genotoxic agents penetrating to the DNA in the tissues of cells. Such measurements would compensate for species differences in metabolism and related factors that determine the qualitative and quantitative relationships between exposure dose and dose of the ultimate toxicant(s) delivered to the target molecule (Fig. 1).

Assessment of Target (DNA) Dose in Man

Measurements of DNA adducts probably provide the most satisfactory basis for determining tissue or target doses of genotoxic chemicals. DNA adducts can be directly determined in the cells or tissues of laboratory species using radiochemical techniques. Such direct methods cannot be used in man, and Ehrenberg suggested that indirect dose monitors could be developed to determine the doses of genotoxic chemicals delivered to the DNA in inaccessible tissues in humans who may be exposed to chemical mutagens or carcinogens (15-17). For example, DNA adducts could be monitored in accessible tissues or body fluids, e.g., white blood cells, sperm, or placentas. Alternatively, the corresponding protein adducts could be determined in plasma proteins or hemoglobin.

Hemoglobin tends to be favored as a tissue dose monitor largely because of its ready availability and relative abundance, coupled with the stability of hemoglobin adducts (18,21) and the longevity of red blood cells, which permit integrated dose measurements over a period of about 4 months (22). To date, all genotoxic agents that react with DNA have been found to react with hemoglobin. Furthermore, the rates of formation of hemoglobin adducts are quantitatively related to the formation of DNA adducts in the tissues. However, the proportional relationships between the doses delivered to the dose monitor (blood proteins or "accessible" DNA) and to target tissue DNA will usually differ for every chemical. The fact that these relationships cannot normally be directly determined in man is a further complication. Reliance must, therefore, be placed on experimentally determined coefficients relating these doses. In order to justify the use of such experimentally determined coefficients to estimate human target (DNA) doses, it is necessary to ensure that, for any given chemical, the dose coefficients, e.g., skin DNA/hemoglobin; liver DNA/hemoglobin, are not subject to significant species variations.

Hemoglobin has been validated for use as an indirect tissue DNA dose monitor for ethylene oxide (15,20,21), methyl methanesulfonate (23,24), and ethyl methanesulfonate (25). Validation data have been obtained for vinyl chloride and certain aromatic amines (for reviews, see refs. 16,26,27). Furthermore, the reported correlation between the dose of benzo[a]pyrene (BaP) applied to mouse skin and the amounts of BaP adducts formed in hemoglobin (28,29) suggests that the determination of hemoglobin adducts may have direct applications in estimating dermal cancer risks as well as providing a biomonitoring technique for determining dermal exposure to carcinogens in man.

Analytical Methods

Powerful analytical techniques have been developed for the analysis of hemoglobin adducts (for a review, see ref. 27). In particular, rapid and sensitive GC/MS (4,30,31) and immunochemical techniques (32) are available for routine application. The sensitivity and scope of these analytical procedures became clear when background alkylations (methyl, ethyl, 2-hydroxypropyl, and 2-hydroxyethyl groups) were discovered in the hemoglobin of rodents and humans who had not knowingly been exposed to genotoxic chemicals or their precursors (17,20,32-34). Current methods focus on the determination of alkylation of the amino function of the N-terminal valine residues of the α- and β-chains of hemoglobin (30,31). These N-terminal alkyl groups are undoubtedly introduced by exposures to alkylating chemicals of endogenous or exogenous origin. Methods with a sensitivity sufficient to permit the detection of the corresponding adducts at the level of DNA are being developed. ^{32}P-Postlabeling techniques have already detected background alkylations in the DNA of human and rodent tissues (for a review, see ref. 8). These postlabeling techniques are particularly suited to the determination of higher molecular weight adducts in DNA, e.g., adducts formed during exposure to polycyclic aromatic hydrocarbons. Some modifications are required to obtain satisfactory levels of sensitivity with low-molecular-weight adducts. Thus, at this stage, the techniques for the determination of protein adducts and DNA adducts are largely complementary (15).

QUALITATIVE DETERMINANTS OF CARCINOGENESIS

In the main, the impact of species differences in the operation of systemic determinants of carcinogenesis (Fig. 1) is quantitative. Of course, quantitative differences, either singly or in combination, can be of such magnitude as to create the impression of a qualitative species difference in response. Absolute differences between risk models and man in the operation of qualitative systemic determinants of carcinogenesis are far less common but could arise, for example, as a consequence of a species difference in the bioactivation of precursor genotoxic agents. A qualitative difference in bioactivation could lead to the formation of a unique genotoxic agent in man or the model. Such a difference could, if undetected, confound risk assessment and invalidate the use of the model for the qualitative detection of human carcinogens. It is therefore important to check on possible qualitative differences in bioactivation, particularly when alternative bioactivation reactions are possible, as is the case with polycyclic aromatic hydrocarbons.

Comparative analysis of the chromatographic profiles of DNA adducts formed from reactions of genotoxic metabolites with DNA in target tissues provides a powerful and selective approach to detect qualitative differences in bioactivation products formed in vitro and in vivo and in different species. Of course, information on the corresponding DNA adduct profiles formed in human tissues in vivo is required as the reference standard to gauge the appropriateness of bioactivation pathways in model systems. This requirement necessitates the development of in vitro preparations of human tissues that qualitatively mimic human bioactivation pathways in vivo. Human in vitro systems are not amenable to direct validation. However, it is possible to achieve an indirect validation by demonstrating that the DNA adducts formed in analogous tissue preparations from laboratory animals are identical to the adducts formed in these tissues in vivo.

Genotoxic Metabolism in Mouse and Human Skin

We have applied this approach to compare the bioactivation of polycyclic aromatic hydrocarbons and the subsequent formation of DNA adducts in the skin of humans and various prospective risk models, using BaP as a model. In the initial studies, the profiles of DNA adducts, formed in the dorsal epidermis and dermis of CD-1 mice treated topically with [^{14}C]BaP, were determined as the corresponding deoxyribonucleosides by high-performance liquid chromatography. Typically, chromatographic profiles showed a single major peak of radioactivity and five minor components (Fig. 2). The major component was (+)-$N2$-(7R,8S,9R-trihydroxy-7,8,9,10-tetrahydrobenzo[a]pyrene-10S-yl)-2'deoxyguanosine ((+)-7R-$trans$-($anti$)-BPDE-dGuo). The assignments of the minor components are given in Fig. 2. Qualitatively similar profiles were obtained using CF-1 mice and athymic nude mice. Furthermore, essentially identical results were obtained with CD-1 mice treated with [^{3}H]BaP or [^{14}C]BaP. In each case the

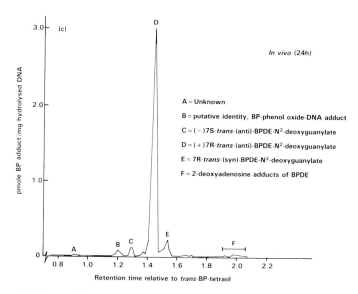

Figure 2. [³H]Benzo[a]pyrene metabolite deoxyribonucleoside adduct profiles formed in the epidermis of CD-1 mice. Abbreviations: BP, benzo[a]pyrene; BPDE, 7R,8S,9R-trihydroxy-7,8,9,10-tetrahydrobenzo[a]pyrene-10S-yl.

amount of DNA adducts in the epidermis exceeded that in the dermis by a factor of about 10.

Explant cultures of CD-1 mouse skin were developed in an attempt to mimic the bioactivation of BaP in mouse skin in vivo. The system comprised discs of skin resting on filter paper discs and maintained under aseptic conditions in culture medium (35). Each skin explant was treated with [³H]BaP in acetone applied to the epidermal surface of the disc and incubated at 37°C for up to 24 h. After incubation, the explants were immersed in liquid nitrogen, and the culture fluid was checked for microbial contamination. Some of the initial experiments included antibiotics. However, this practice was discontinued when inhibitory effects on adduct formation were observed. The epidermal layer of each disc was removed, and the DNA was isolated for analysis of the adducts. The yields of adducts after 24 h were approximately 50% of those obtained in vivo. Qualitative agreement between the high-performance liquid chromatography (HPLC) profiles obtained in vivo and in vitro was excellent (Figs. 3a,b). In each case, the major adduct accounted for more than 70% of the total adduct fraction. Furthermore, the relative proportions of individual adducts showed good agreement in vivo and in vitro.

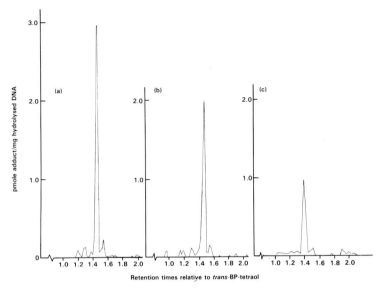

Figure 3. High-performance liquid chromotography profiles of [³H]benzo[a]pyrene-deoxyribonucleoside adducts obtained from epidermal DNA of (a) CD-1 mouse in vivo, (b) CD-1 mouse skin explant, and (c) human skin explant. Abbreviations: BP, benzo[a]pyrene.

The excellent qualitative and consistent quantitative correlations be-tween BaP-DNA adducts formed in mouse skin in vivo and in vitro suggested that the corresponding human explants would be acceptable models for deter-mining both the qualitative and quantitative aspects of genotoxic metabolism in human tissue in vivo. Accordingly, exactly analogous explants were prepared from five mastectomy patients. Excellent qualitative agreement was observed between the HPLC profiles of [³H]BaP-DNA adducts formed in the epidermal tissue of explants from each patient. In each case, the major adduct was (+)-7R-*trans*-(*anti*)-BPDE-dGuo, and the relative proportions of the minor adducts were similar to those observed in mouse skin in vivo and in vitro (Fig. 3c). Cochroma-tography showed that the minor peaks were the same as those formed in mouse skin in vivo.

The amounts of the major adduct formed in human and mouse skin explants were of the same order (Table 1). However, interindividual differences were larger in the human explants than in those from mice. The more marked individual variations observed among the human samples would be anticipated on the basis of known variations in the activities of monooxygenases, detoxifica-tion enzymes, and DNA repair functions in human populations (36). Such variations underline the importance of dosimetry techniques to evaluate DNA dose not only as a means of compensating for species differences in toxicokinetic

Table 1. Amounts of (+)-7R-*trans*-(*anti*)-BPDE-dGuo Formed in Mouse and Human Epidermis Treated In Vitro with [³H]BaP

Source of skin		Dose of [³H]BaP (μg/cm^{-2})	(+)-7R-*trans*-(*anti*)-BPDE-dGuo (pmol/mg hydrolyzed DNA)
Mouse	CD-1	8.5	3.3 (1.8–4.2)
Human*	a	17.0	3.8
	b	17.0	8.5
	c	8.5	1.7
	d	8.5	1.9
	e	8.5	8.0

*Individual's age, smoking habits, and medication were as follows: (a) 60, smoker (30 cigarettes/day), tamoxifen; (b) 66, nonsmoker, diazepam; (c) 65, nonsmoker; (d) 66, nonsmoker; and (e) 73, nonsmoker.

and toxicodynamic determinants of the relationships between exposure and target dose but also in evaluating risks to individuals.

Determination of Genotoxic Action in Human Skin

The results obtained with [³H]BaP suggested that the human skin explant system could provide the basis of a direct model for the prospective detection of human genotoxic agents. However, practical applications were limited by a requirement for radiolabeled test chemicals. A variety of approaches may be used to overcome this problem. For example, the analysis of protein adducts in skin explants using techniques analogous to those developed for the assay of hemoglobin adducts would provide the basis of a sensitive general procedure. However, confirmatory studies may be necessary to establish the relationships between the protein adducts and DNA adducts. We, therefore, chose a more direct approach by coupling the skin explant model with the ³²P-postlabeling method that was developed by Randerath et al. (13) for the determination of DNA adducts.

In initial experiments, the ³²P-postlabeling approach was applied to analyze DNA adducts formed in the epidermis of mice treated topically with unlabeled BaP in vivo or in vitro. An essentially identical pattern of adducts was obtained in vivo and in vitro. The principal adduct (adduct 1, Figs. 4a,b) was the 3'-5'bisphosphate corresponding to the principal adduct, (+)-7R-*trans*-(*anti*)-BPDE-dGuo, determined using prelabeling methods. This assignment was confirmed by postlabeling calf thymus DNA that had been derived by reaction with (+)-*anti*-BPDE and was known to contain (+)-7R-*trans*-(*anti*)-BPDE-dGuo as the principal adduct. Interestingly, the postlabeling method revealed a second major adduct (adduct 2, Figs. 4a,b). This finding contrasted with the results of the earlier prelabeling experiments, which revealed only a single major component. The second adduct has not yet been characterized, although an adduct pos-

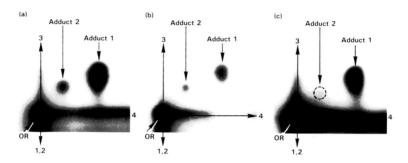

Figure 4. ^{32}P-Postlabeling maps of benzo[a]pyrene-modified epidermal DNA from (a) CD-1 mouse skin in vivo, (b) CD-1 mouse skin explant, and (c) human skin explant.

sessing similar chromatographic properties was observed in a ^{32}P-postlabeling study in which the skin of BALB/c mice was treated with BaP in vivo (37).

[32]P-Postlabeling studies also revealed the presence of both of the bisphosphate adducts (1 and 2, Figs. 4a,b) in human skin explants treated with BaP. (+)-7R-*trans*-(*anti*)-BPDE-dGuo was readily detected (Fig. 4c). Interestingly, however, the amounts of adduct 2 in DNA from human skin explants were much smaller than those from mouse skin treated with BaP in vivo or in vitro, and in some instances this adduct was difficult to detect (Fig. 4c). The ^{32}P-postlabeling approach appears, therefore, to have revealed a quantitative difference between the genotoxic metabolism of BaP in mouse and human skin that was not observed by direct labeling studies. Thus, adduct 2 does not appear to correspond to any of those adducts detected using [^{3}H]- or [^{14}C]BaP. There is little doubt that adduct 2 is a product of BaP toxicity. Thus control experiments showed that adduct 2 was neither present in DNA from untreated mouse skin nor an artifact of the postlabeling procedure. Studies are in progress to determine whether this adduct is formed by a direct genotoxic mechanism, i.e., by reaction of a BaP metabolite with DNA, or by an indirect mechanism occasioned by a disturbance of normal metabolic processes.

Applications to Assess Human Risks

The coupled human skin explant-postlabeling system provides a reference standard for validating the bioactivation systems of potential risk models and a basis for the study of human polymorphism without the use of radiolabeled test chemicals. Additionally, the coupled system provides a powerful direct approach to detect human genotoxic agents. Theoretically, this approach can be applied to any human tissue. Most of the advantages are inherent in the ^{32}P-postlabeling method and include high sensitivity and resolving power, which permit the detection of individual genotoxic components in complex mixtures and also provide a basis for the identification of these components (7). These postlabeling approaches are currently being applied in mouse and human models in studies seeking to identify individual genotoxic components of mineral oils.

The main value of the human model resides in the improvements it brings to interpretation by avoiding a need for species extrapolation and by providing human reference data. On the premise that a sequential mechanism has been established in which primary DNA damage leads to mutation and to cancer, then the detection of DNA adducts in the coupled system provides qualitative evidence of carcinogenic action toward human tissues. Of course, not all DNA adducts are equally promutagenic (procarcinogenic). However, since no intrinsically reactive electrophile displays absolute specificity for any particular nucleophile, the detection of even a weakly promutagenic adduct signals the formation of more strongly promutagenic adducts.

Whereas the detection of DNA adducts in human tissue explant systems provides unequivocal evidence of genotoxic activity toward those tissues, the detection of such adducts in man in vivo provides qualitative evidence of exposure to a carcinogenic hazard. Insofar as the measurement of protein adducts reflects the formation of the corresponding DNA adducts, the detection of protein adducts may also signify exposure to a carcinogenic hazard (38,39).

The new analytical techniques for the determination of DNA and protein adducts represent the first generation of methods that possess sufficient sensitivity and resolving power to warrant systematic application to detect and, subsequently, to identify the specific chemical initiators of human cancer. These procedures are already finding applications in molecular epidemiology studies (40) to detect and monitor human exposures to genotoxic chemicals. The initial promise of these approaches appears to have been borne out by the detection of background exposures (17,20,32-34). Indeed, it seems clear that the sensitivities of these methods will exceed that required for the determination of acceptable risks (10^{-6}/year). In this respect, the determination of DNA or protein adducts in vitro or in vivo would satisfy the criteria for a test to detect human carcinogens. However, it is also clear, as we progress toward increasingly precise and sensitive indicators of genotoxic (carcinogenic) action, that risk measurement is essential and that a purely qualitative judgment that a substance is carcinogenic has little or no significance. Of course, negative results obtained in a sensitive human genotoxicity assay could lead to some relaxation of controls (see ref. 5).

Extension of the Target Dose Approach

The great sensitivity of the new procedures to determine DNA and protein adducts permits the assessment of tissue or target DNA doses of genotoxic chemicals at low environmental or occupational exposures in man and laboratory animals. By compensating for differences between test species and man in factors that determine the formation of the primary and critical lesions in DNA (Fig. 1), the determination of target dose improves the translation of experimental risk data to man and provides a better definition of individual risks. However, in order to further improve the quality of prospective risk assessment, it is necessary to develop procedures to correct for differences between experimental models and man in factors that determine the progression, first, of key lesions into mutations and, second, of the affected cells into malignant neoplasms (Fig. 1). In an extension of his target dose approach, Ehrenberg has proposed that the determination of rad-equivalence values for the induction of forward mutation by genotoxic chemicals may be of value in achieving these objectives (3).

A rad-equivalent dose is defined as the dose of low-linear energy transfer radiation producing the same response as the unit target dose (mMh) of an alkylating agent in the low dose region of the dose-response curve in forward mutation systems (38). There are sound theoretical reasons and a substantive experimental basis, developed with chemicals of widely differing structures and reactivity (e.g., ethylene oxide and BaP) to support the view that the rad-equivalent value for the induction of mutation (and transformation) in a wide range of test systems and species by a given chemical is approximately constant. Since there is no a priori reason to suppose that a different value would be obtained for man, such rad-equivalent values may therefore be applied to correct for differences between man and test species in factors (e.g., rates and fidelity of DNA repair) that determine the progression of primary DNA damage to mutation (7). In the cited instances, it is clear that the measurement of target dose must have provided a reliable proportional measure of reaction at the sites within the target molecule (DNA) that are critical for the induction of the mutagenic event or transformation. However, it is easy to envision selective interactions in which the measurement of target dose may underestimate or overestimate the primary damage. Such precise measurements of target interactions, i.e., at the level of a specific base within DNA, cannot be made routinely. It is important, therefore, to select mutagenic end points that reflect random, preferably multi-hit, interactions with the target gene or gene complex rather than specific mutagenic events that arise through interactions with a specific base.

In considering the application of rad-equivalent values for mutation to assess cancer risks, it may be anticipated that at low doses any intrinsic promoting activity of genotoxic chemicals would be of a low order. Contingent, therefore, on the essentially random nature of the genotoxic action of chemicals and of radiation and on a common basis for initiation, i.e., mutation in a specific set or family of genes or their regulators (proto-oncogenes), it seems probable that at low doses, cells that have been exposed to either radiation or genotoxic chemicals would be subject to the same general tumor-promoting and -modulating influences acting within an individual. On this basis, Ehrenberg proposes that experimentally determined rad-equivalent values (for mutation) may be used to assess human cancer risks by reference to human risk coefficients established for radiation. Of course, the rad-equivalent approach cannot be applied to evaluate cancer risks posed by high exposures to genotoxic chemicals that also exert a significant promoting action on tumor development. Thus, it is unlikely that this procedure can be applied in the case of carcinogenic mineral oils in which genotoxicity is often of a very low order and promoting action (in a broad sense) is likely to exert a major influence on carcinogenic potency (41). In such instances, it is important to evaluate the impact of tumor-promoting activity on the development of cells that have undergone initiation either by exposure to genotoxic elements in the oil or by previous or concomitant exposures to genotoxic chemicals.

OPEN FORUM

Dr. Paul Grasso: Dr. Wright, my impression is that genotoxic carcinogens seem to alkylate practically every cell in the body, or at least every organ, and yet cancer actually appears in only one or two target organs. Did you do your adduct studies in the target organ or on cells easily available for such studies?

Dr. A. S. Wright: Both our direct-labeling and postlabeling studies were performed in skin, which is a target for benzo[a]pyrene-induced carcinogenesis. Although genotoxic carcinogens can react with DNA in any tissue, constraints are imposed by factors such as instability and selective transportation. In general, therefore, alkylating species do not react uniformly with tissue DNA. Ethylene oxide is an exception, being relatively stable and freely diffusible. However, the more reactive alkylating agents show a degree of tissue specificity that is usually dependent upon the route of exposure or the site of bioactivation.

Dr. Donald Stevenson: Just one word of caution on the use of the adduct approach. Even using agents such as cisplatin, a chemotherapeutic agent with a defined dose, the range of adducts found in people varies from undetectable to a fairly high level. So I think we must talk about this in terms of populations and not of individuals.

REFERENCES

1. Higginson J. Present trends in cancer epidemiology. Canadian Cancer Conference 8:40-75, 1969.
2. Miller EC, Miller JA. Biochemical mechanisms of chemical carcinogenesis. In Busch H (ed): The Molecular Biology of Cancer. New York and London: Academic Press, 1974, pp 377-402.
3. Ehrenberg L. Genotoxicity of environmental chemicals. Acta Biologica Yugoslavia, Ser. F, Genetika 6:367-398, 1974.
4. Mowrer J, Tornqvist M, Jensen S, Ehrenberg L. Modified Edman degradation applied to haemoglobin for monitoring occupational exposure to alkylating agents. Toxicol Environ Chem 11:215-231, 1986.
5. Silbergeld EK, Ehrenberg LG, Hemminki K, Hutton M, Laib RJ, Lauwerys RR, Neuman H-G, Nordberg GF, Piotrowski J, Thilly WG, Wright AS. Exposures: Uptake, tissue and target dose. In Fowler BA (ed): Mechanisms of Cell Injury: Implications for Human Health. London: John Wiley and Sons, Ltd., 1987, pp 405-429.
6. Ehrenberg L, Brookes P, Druckrey H, Lagerlorf B, Litwin J, Williams G. The relation of cancer induction and genetic damage. In Ramel C (ed): Evaluation of Genetic Risks of Environmental Chemicals, Ambio, Special Report No. 3. Royal

Swedish Academy of Sciences/Universitetforlarget, 1973, pp 15-16.

7. Wright AS, Bradshaw TK, Watson WP. Prospective detection and assessment of genotoxic hazards: A critical appreciation of the contribution of L.G. Ehrenberg. In Bartsch H, Hemminki K, O'Neill IK (eds): Methods for Detecting DNA Damaging Agents in Humans: Applications in Cancer Epidemiology and Prevention. Lyon, France: IARC, 1988, pp 237-247 (IARC Scientific Publication No. 89).

8. Watson WP. Post-radiolabelling for detecting DNA damage. Mutagenesis 2:319-331, 1987.

9. Tennant RW, Margolin BH, Shelby MD, Zeiger E, Hazeman JK, Spalding J, Caspary W, Resnick M, Stasiewitz S, Anderson B, Minor R. Predictions of chemical carcinogenicity in rodents from in vitro genetic toxicity assays. Science 236:933-941, 1987.

10. Bridges BA. Genetic toxicology at the crossroads: A personal overview of the development of short-term tests. In Montesano R, Bartsch H, Vaino H, Wilbourne J, Yamasaki H (eds): Long-Term and Short-Term Assays for Carcinogens: A Critical Appraisal. Lyon, France: IARC, 1986, pp 519-527. (IARC Scientific Publication No. 83).

11. International Commission for Protection against Environmental Mutagens and Carcinogens. Committee 2 Report. Mutagenesis testing as an approach to carcinogenesis. Mutat Res 99:73-91, 1982.

12. Watson WP, Brooks TM, Huckle KR, Hutson DH, Lang KL, Smith RJ, Wright AS. Microbial mutagenicity studies with (Z)-1,3-dichloropropene. Chem Biol Interact 61:17-30, 1987.

13. Randerath K, Reddy MV, Gupta RC. ^{32}P-labelling test for DNA damage. Proc Natl Acad Sci USA 78:6126-6129, 1981.

14. Ehrenberg L. Risk assessment of ethylene oxide and other compounds. In Elheny VK, Abrahamson S (eds): Banbury Report 1: Assessing Chemical Mutagens. The Risk to Humans. Cold Spring Harbor, NY: Cold Spring Harbor Laboratory, 1979, pp 157-190.

15. Ehrenberg L, Hiesche KD, Osterman-Golkar S, Wennberg I. Evaluation of genetic risks of alkylation agents: Tissue doses in the mouse from air contaminated with ethylene oxide. Mutat Res 24:83-103, 1974.

16. Ehrenberg L, Moustacchi E, Osterman-Golkar S, Ekman G. Dosimetry of genotoxic agents and dose-response relationships of their effects. Mutat Res 123:121-182, 1983.

17. Calleman CJ, Ehrenberg L, Jansson B, Osterman-Golkar S, Segerback D, Svensson D, Wachtmeister CA. Monitoring and risk assessment by means of alkyl groups in hemoglobin in persons occupationally exposed to ethylene oxide. J Environ Pathol Toxicol 2:427-442, 1978.

18. Osterman-Golkar S, Ehrenberg L, Segerback D, Hallstrom I. Evaluation of genetic risks of alkylating agents. II. Hemoglobin as a dose monitor. Mutat Res 34:1-10, 1976.

19. Wright AS. New strategies in biochemical studies for pesticide toxicity. In Bandall SK, Marco GJ, Goldberg L, Leng ML (eds): The Pesticide Chemist and Modern Toxicology. ACS Symposium Series 160. Washington DC: American Chemical Society, 1981, pp 285-304.

20. Wright AS. Molecular dosimetry techniques in human risk assessment: An industrial perspective. In Hayes AW, Schnell RC, Miya TS (eds): Developments in the Science and Practice of Toxicology. Amsterdam, New York, Oxford: Elsevier Science Publishers, 1983, pp 311-318.

21. Segerback D, Calleman CJ, Ehrenberg L, Lofroth G, Osterman-Golkar S. Evaluation of genetic risks of alkylating agents. IV. Quantitative determination of alkylated amino acids in haemoglobin as a measure of the dose after treatment of mice with methyl methanesulfonate. Mutat Res 49:71, 1978.

22. Mollinson PL. Blood Transfusion in Clinical Medicine. Oxford: Blackwell Scientific Publications, 1983, p 108.

23. Frei JV, Lawley PD. Tissue distribution and mode of DNA methylation in mice by methyl methanesulphonate a ıd N-methyl-N'-nitro-N-nitrosoguanidine: Lack of thymic lymphoma induction and low extent of methylation of target tissue DNA at 0^6 of guanine. Chem Biol Interact 13:215-222, 1976.

24. Van Sittert NJ, Wooder MF, Dean BJ, Wright AS, Stevenson DE. Molecular studies on thresholds for the induction of mutagenic effects in mammals by a model alkylating agent, MMS (abstract). Proceedings of the First International Congress on Toxicology, 1977, p 15.

25. Murthy MSS, Calleman CJ, Osterman-Golkar S, Segerback D, Svensson K. Relationships between ethylation of haemoglobin, ethylation of DNA and administered amount of ethyl methanesulfate in the mouse. Mutat Res 127:1-8, 1984.

26. Farmer PB, Neumann H-G, Henschler D. Estimation of exposure of man to substances reacting covalently with macromolecules. Arch Toxicol 60:251-260, 1987.

27. Neumann H-G. Analysis of hemoglobin as a dose monitor for alkylating and arylating agents. Arch Toxicol 56:1-6, 1984.

28. Shugart L. Quantitating exposure to chemical carcinogens: In vivo alkylation of haemoglobin by benzo[a]pyrene. Toxicology 34:211-220, 1985.

29. Shugart L. Quantifying adductive modification of haemoglobin from mice exposed to benzo[a]pyrene. Anal Biochem 152:365-369, 1986.

30. Tornqvist M, Mowrer J, Jensen S, Ehrenberg L. Monitoring of environmental cancer initiators through hemoglobin adducts by a modified Edman degradation method. Anal Biochem 154:255-266, 1986.

31. Tornqvist M, Osterman-Golkar S, Kautianinen A, Jensen S, Farmer PB, Ehrenberg L. Tissue doses of ethylene oxide in cigarette smokers determined from adduct levels in haemoglobin. Carcinogenesis 7:1519-1521, 1986.

32. Wraith MJ, Watson WP, Eadsforth CV, van Sittert NJ, Wright AS. An immunoassay for monitoring human exposure to ethylene oxide. In Bartsch H, Hemminki K, O'Neill IK (eds): Methods for Detecting DNA Damaging Agents in Humans: Applications in Cancer Epidemiology and Prevention. Lyon, France: IARC, 1988, pp 271-274 (IARC Scientific Publication No. 89).

33. Osterman-Golkar S, Farmer PB, Segerback D, Bailey E, Calleman CJ, Svensson K, Ehrenberg L. Dosimetry of ethylene oxide in the rat by quantitation of alkylated histidine in haemoglobin. Teratogenesis Carcinog Mutagen 3:395-405, 1983.

34. Van Sittert NJ, De Jong G, Clare MG, Davies R, Wren LJ, Wright AS. Cytogenetic, immunological and haematological effects in workers in an ethylene oxide manufacturing plant. Br J Ind Med 42:19-26, 1985.

35. Huckle KR, Smith RJ, Watson WP, Wright AS. Comparison of hydrocarbon-DNA adducts formed in mouse skin in vivo and in organ culture in vitro following treatment with benzo[a]pyrene. Carcinogenesis 7:965-970, 1986.

36. Wright AS. The role of metabolism in chemical mutagenesis and chemical carcinogenesis. Mutat Res 75:215-241, 1980.

37. Randerath E, Agrawal MP, Reddy MV, Randerath K. Highly persistent polycyclic hydrocarbon-DNA adducts in mouse skin: Detection by ^{32}P-postlabelling analysis. Cancer Lett 20:109-114, 1983.

38. Ehrenberg L. Methods of comparing risks of radiation and chemicals. In Fowler BA (ed): Radiobiological Equivalents of Chemical Pollutants. Vienna: IAEA, 1980, pp 11-21.

39. Hemminki K, Randerath K. Detection of genetic interaction of chemicals by biochemical methods: Determination of DNA and protein adducts. In Fowler BA (ed): Mechanisms of Cell Injury: Implications for Human Health. London: John Wiley and Sons, Ltd., 1987, pp 209-227.

40. Perera FP. Molecular cancer epidemiology: A new tool in cancer prevention. JNCI 78:887-898, 1987.

41. Watson WP, Brooks TM, Meyer AL, Wright AS. Determinants of the potencies of carcinogenic mineral oils. In Cooke M, Dennis AJ (eds): Polynuclear Aromatic Hydrocarbons: Chemistry, Characterisation and Carcinogenesis. 9th International Symposium. Columbus, OH: Battelle Press, 1986, pp 971-983.

Skin Carcinogenesis: Mechanisms and Human Relevance, pages 331–345

Mechanistic Studies of Tobacco Carcinogenesis in Mouse Epidermis and Lung Tissues

Assieh A. Melikian, Stephen S. Hecht, and Dietrich Hoffmann

Naylor Dana Institute for Disease Prevention, American Health Foundation, Valhalla, New York 10595

Epidemiological studies have established a causal relationship of cigarette smoking with cancer of the respiratory tract, the upper digestive tract, pancreas, renal pelvis and bladder, and possibly cancer of the cervix. Cigar and pipe smoking are also causally related to cancer of the lung, oral cavity, and esophagus—although, in the case of lung cancer, not to the same extent as cigarette smoking (1-8). Tobacco chewing and snuff dipping have been associated with cancer of the mouth (9). The exposure to tobacco sidestream smoke as an indoor air pollutant has recently been incriminated as a possible risk factor in lung cancer among nonsmokers (8,10,11).

All of these observations support the concept that tobacco smoke is a complete carcinogen. Long-term inhalation studies with Syrian golden hamsters have shown that whole cigarette smoke can induce benign and malignant tumors in the larynxes of the animals (12-15). The inability to induce significant numbers of tumors in the trachea and lungs of the smoke-exposed hamsters may result from the fact that the shallow breathing of the hamsters in the exposure tubes prevents smoke particulates from reaching these parts of their respiratory systems. This was evident from model studies of smoke deposition with markers in the inhalant (12,15,16). However, significant tar deposition was measured in the upper larynx. A number of bioassays show a significant incidence of benign and malignant tumors at this site in smoke-exposed hamsters.

For laboratory studies, tobacco smoke is arbitrarily divided into gaseous and particulate phases by means of filtration through a glass fiber filter. The gaseous phase of the smoke does not by itself induce tumors of the respiratory tract in laboratory animals (13,17). Thus, it may be deduced that the major carcinogenic activity of tobacco smoke resides in the particulate phase, commonly known as tar. Tobacco tar has induced benign and malignant tumors in the skin and ear of rabbits, the connective tissue of rats, and, after intratracheal instillation, in the bronchi of rats. Topical applications of tar solutions have led to both papillomas and carcinoma of the skin in various strains of mice (18-22).

FRACTIONATION OF CIGARETTE SMOKE PARTICULATES FOR ISOLATION AND IDENTIFICATION OF CARCINOGENS, COCARCINOGENS, AND PROMOTERS

Since 1957, a large number of studies in the United States, the United Kingdom, France, West Germany, and other countries have utilized mouse skin bioassays in attempts to identify the tumor initiators, tumor promoters, and cocarcinogens in cigarette tars (14,19-26). Results of our fractionation studies have been confirmed by many others showing that complete tumorigenic activity is exhibited only by those fractions and subfractions that contain the bulk of polynuclear aromatic hydrocarbons (PAHs) (Fig. 1). The neutral subfraction B1 amounts to about 0.6% of the dry tar and contains the PAHs and aza-arenes. When all fractions and subfractions were recombined, mouse skin assays reflected that 80%–90% of the tumorigenic activity was recovered. As expected, the fractionation procedure caused some loss of activity (26,27).

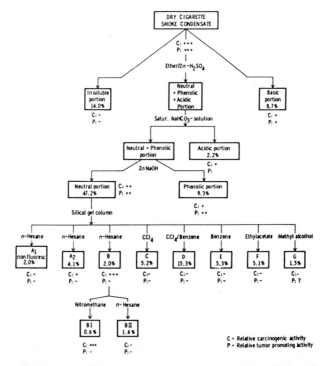

Figure 1. Fractionation of tobacco smoke particulates and relative carcinogenic and promoter activities of major fractions. Reprinted with permission from Wynder EL, Hoffmann D. Tobacco and Tobacco Smoke: Studies in Experimental Carcinogenesis. New York: Academic Press, 1967.

When fraction B1 was set aside, the recombined material from all other fractions and subfractions had only low tumorigenic activity. B1 alone accounts for less than 10% of the tumorigenic activity and appears to be largely responsible for the tumor-initiating potential of the whole tar, as measured on mouse skin (23-26).

We must realize that the mouse skin screening test is limited to the evaluation of certain classes of carcinogens and responds particularly well to PAHs. The carcinogenic activities of compounds such as N-nitrosamines, aromatic amines, and inorganic carcinogens are not readily detected in mouse skin assays. These compounds may be associated with the cigarette smokers' increased risk for cancer of the pancreas, kidney, and urinary bladder, as well as the esophagus and lung (8). Nevertheless, mouse skin assays of cigarette smoke condensates have served as valuable indicators of the tumorigenic potential of tobacco smoke in epithelial tissues.

TOBACCO SMOKE AS A PROMOTER AND/OR COCARCINOGEN IN HUMANS AND LABORATORY ANIMALS

In humans, tobacco smoke may be a tumor promoter and/or cocarcinogen, as indicated by its role as a cause of cancer in uranium miners and asbestos workers. Occupational exposure to alpha particles from radon and radon daughters represents a causative factor for increased lung cancer risk among uranium miners (8,28,29). This is documented by an annual lung cancer incidence rate of 71 per 100,000 nonsmoking uranium miners in the United States. The lung cancer incidence rates per year for individuals who are not subjected to occupational uranium exposure are 11 per 100,000 for nonsmokers and 44 per 100,000 for heavy cigarette smokers. This contrasts sharply with the rate of 422 per 100,000 for lung cancer among cigarette-smoking uranium miners (30). In asbestos workers and among workers in industries utilizing asbestos, tobacco smoking has been shown to elevate the lung cancer risk that is inherent in occupational exposure (31,32).

In bioassays with hamsters, application of 7,12-dimethylbenz[a]anthracene (DMBA) to the larynx or intratracheal instillation of this tumor initiator, followed by exposure to air-diluted cigarette smoke, has demonstrated the tumor-promoting potential of cigarette smoke (17).

Constituents of the weakly acidic fraction of tobacco tar have been shown to act as tumor promoters or as cocarcinogens on mouse skin (14,23,33,34). When this weakly acidic portion was combined with the neutral fraction and bioassayed on mouse skin, the tumorigenic activity observed approximated 60% of the activity of the whole tar. The weakly acidic portion by itself was inactive as a carcinogen but clearly showed cocarcinogenic potential on mouse skin when applied together with benzo[a]pyrene (BaP) and other tumor-initiating PAHs.

Bioassays of subfractions of the weakly acidic portion demonstrated that the major cocarcinogenic activity was concentrated in subfractions that contained 1,2-dihydroxybenzene (catechol) and substituted catechols, such as coni-

COCARCINOGENIC SUBFRACTIONS OF THE WEAKLY ACIDIC FRACTION

FRACTION	% WAF	% TBA	CHARACTERISTIC COMPONENTS
A	2.5	63*	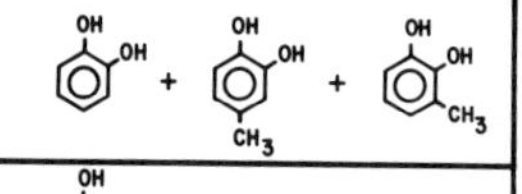 (catechol) + (methylcatechol, CH3) + (methylcatechol, CH3)
B	1.6	45	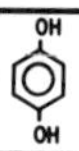 (hydroquinone, OH/OH)
C	0.14	38	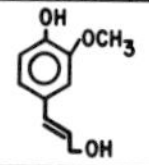 (OH, OCH3, OH substituted benzene)
D	0.14	18	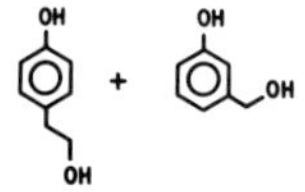 (OH/OH) + (OH, CH2OH)
E	1.6	12	UNKNOWN

FRACTION	% WAF	% TBA	CHARACTERISTIC COMPONENTS
F	12	83*	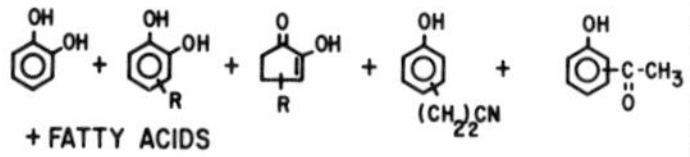 (OH/OH) + (OH/OH, R) + (O, OH, R) + (OH, (CH2)22CN) + (OH, C-CH3, O) + FATTY ACIDS
G	2.5	24	UNKNOWN
H	3.6	73*	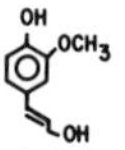 (OH, OCH3, OH) + RELATED COMPOUNDS
I	1.9	46	UNKNOWN
J	5.1	28	UNKNOWN
BaP (0.003%)		7	

Figure 2. Major constituents of the weakly acidic subfractions (from ref. 34). Abbreviations: WAF, weight of acidic fraction; TBA, tumor-bearing animals.

feryl alcohol (34,35) (Fig. 2). Van Duuren et al. have demonstrated that catechol is a strong cocarcinogen on mouse skin when applied together with BaP (33,36).

It is our aim to elucidate the mechanisms by which PAHs and their methylated derivatives act together with tobacco smoke cocarcinogens to exert their biological activities in epithelial tissues. Two of these studies are presented in this chapter.

STUDIES ON THE MECHANISM OF COCARCINOGENESIS OF CATECHOL WITH BaP IN MOUSE SKIN

Catechol is formed in the degradation and metabolism of many synthetic and naturally occurring organic compounds (37-39). It is present in certain foods (40-42), coffee (0.42–0.74 mg/6-oz cup) (S.G. Carmella and S.S. Hecht, unpublished data), hair dyes (43), and petroleum products (44). Catechol is the most abundant phenol in tobacco mainstream smoke (0.09–0.28 mg/cigarette) and sidestream smoke (0.09–0.2 mg/cigarette). Conjugates of catechol are found in human urine (1.3 mg/24 h) primarily as a consequence of dietary intake (including coffee consumption) and tobacco smoking. A high degree of exposure to catechol may constitute a risk factor in view of the compound's biological activities.

To discover how catechol acts as a cocarcinogen in mouse skin, we have studied the effects of catechol on the metabolism of [^{3}H]BaP and of (+)- and (–)-[^{3}H]trans-7,8-dihydroxy-7,8-dihydrobenzo[a]pyrene (BaP-7,8-diol) in mouse epidermis. We have also studied the binding of [^{3}H]BaP metabolites to epidermal DNA at intervals of from 30 min to 24 h (44).

Effects of catechol on the metabolism of BaP are illustrated in Figure 3. Several effects of catechol were important. Catechol suppressed the formation of H_2O-soluble BaP metabolites such as glucuronide and sulfate conjugates, especially 30 min posttreatment, as seen in Figures 3 I and J. Catechol reduced the formation of quinones and 7,8,9,10-tetrahydroxy-7,8,9,10-tetrahydrobenzo[a]-pyrene (BaP-tetraol) but doubled the levels of unconjugated 3-hydroxy-BaP at all measured intervals after treatment. Catechol also caused a small increase in the levels of BaP-7,8-diol and BaP-9,10-diol. Two hours after treatment, the levels of these metabolites had subsided to those of the controls (Figs. 3 C and E). Catechol elevated the ratio of anti-/syn-7,8-dihydroxy-9,10-epoxy-7,8,9,10-tetra-hydrobenzo[a]pyrene (BPDE) adducts with DNA 1.6- to 2.9-fold (Table 1). These observations suggest that catechol affects the oxidation of BaP-7,8-diol in mouse skin. Indeed, cocarcinogenicity bioassays of catechol in mouse skin indicate that catechol is a more potent cocarcinogen when applied together with BaP-7,8-diol than with BaP (unpublished data). These observations led us to study the effects of catechol on the metabolism of (+)- and (–)-BaP-7,8-diol in mouse epidermis. There were no qualitative changes in the metabolism of BaP-7,8-diol in the presence of catechol. The major metabolites of the BaP-7,8-diol were BaP-tetraols formed by hydrolysis of syn- or anti-BPDE. But there were quantitative changes. Catechol slowed down the oxidation of BaP-7,8-diols. Metabolism of (+)-BaP-7,8-diol was decreased to a greater extent than metabolism of (–)-BaP-7,8-diol. Catechol suppressed the formation of H_2O-soluble derivatives of both enantiomers, but did not significantly affect the levels of BaP-tetraols derived from syn-BPDE. On the other hand, catechol decreased the levels of BaP-tetraols when it was co-applied with (+)-BaP-7,8-diol (Fig. 4A), but when coadministered with (–)-BaP-7,8-diol, it caused no significant changes in the level of BaP-tetraols except 30 min after treatment (Fig. 4B).

Our study results suggest that catechol has an impact on the secondary

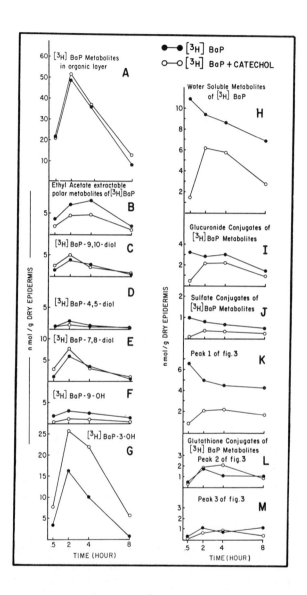

Figure 3. Levels of various metabolites of [³H]BaP in mouse epidermis at various times after topical treatment of [³H]BaP in the absence (•) and presence (o) of catechol. (From Melikian et al. Carcinogenesis 7:9-15, 1986.)

Table 1. Binding of [³H]BaP metabolites to DNA of mouse epidermis*

Treatment protocol 0.015 mg [³H]BaP/Mouse		pmol/mg DNA	
Survival time (h)	Catechol/ mouse (mg)	[³H]BPDE- DNA adducts	Ratio of anti/syn BPDE-DNA adducts
2	0	2.5	4.0
2	0.5	3.1	6.7
8	0	3.3	2.6
8	0.5	6.1	7.8
24	0	3.1	3.3
24	0.5	4.7	8.4

*Ten mice/group were treated with either [³H]BaP or [³H]BaP plus catechol and killed at the times indicated. The treated area of skin was removed and analyzed as described in ref. 45.

metabolism of BaP. It affects the level of epoxidation of (+) and (−) enantiomers of BaP-7,8-diol to different extents, which, in turn, changes the ratio of *anti-/syn*-BPDE and the ratio of the corresponding DNA adducts of the epoxides. This alteration in DNA adducts in catechol-treated mice could partially account for the increase in tumorigenic activity seen when BaP or BaP-7,8-diol was coadministered with catechol.

COMPARATIVE STUDIES ON THE MECHANISM OF CARCINOGENESIS OF BaP AND *ANTI*-BPDE IN MOUSE SKIN AND IN THE LUNGS OF NEWBORN MICE

Whereas extensive evidence indicates that *anti*-BPDE is a major ultimate carcinogen of BaP in mouse skin, tumorigenicity studies have consistently shown that *anti*-BPDE is less active than BaP in this model system (46-51). In the newborn mouse, *anti*-BPDE is 40-fold more active than BaP in producing pulmonary adenoma (52). In order to investigate this difference, we have studied the disposition and metabolism of BaP and (±)-*anti*-BPDE in mouse skin and in the lungs of mice on the first, eighth, and fifteenth days of life. Differences in the activation, detoxification, and transportation of BaP and *anti*-BPDE and their metabolites in the two systems have been noted. The biological half-life of (±)-*anti*-BPDE in mouse epidermis and mouse lung was determined by trapping the unhydrolyzed (±)-*anti*-BPDE with mercaptoethanol (53).

The total radioactivity recovered from mouse epidermis at various times after topical application of [³H]BaP and (±)-[³H]BaP is shown in Figure 5. [³H]*anti*-BPDE and its metabolites are removed from mouse epidermis gradu-

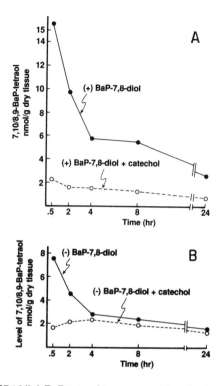

Figure 4. Levels of 7,10/8,9-BaP-tetraol in mouse epidermis at various times after treatment with (+)-BaP-7,8-diol (A) and (-)-BaP-7,8-diol (B) in the presence (o) and absence (•) of catechol.

ally. Some of the (±)-[³H]*anti*-BPDE is removed immediately, but the remaining radioactive material becomes immobilized in the epidermis and is removed very slowly.

The newly developed technique of trapping unhydrolyzed (±)-[³H]*anti*-BPDE with mercaptoethanol in various tissues allowed us to estimate the half-life of the diol epoxide in various organs. Figure 6 shows the percentage of radioactive material present as unhydrolyzed (±)-[³H]*anti*-BPDE in the organic extracts obtained from mouse epidermis or from the lungs of mice on the first day of life. The calculated half-life of (±)-[³H]*anti*-BPDE in the lungs of mice is about 10 min, whereas in mouse epidermis its initial half-life is 6 min. In epidermis the [³H]*anti*-BPDE is hydrolyzed only for the first few minutes. Then it becomes trapped and protected from hydrolysis, and its half-life is extended beyond 2 h.

Qualitatively, the patterns of BaP metabolites in mouse epidermis and in the lungs of newborn mice in all three experimental series were similar. However, the proportion of BaP metabolites varies in the different tissues. A

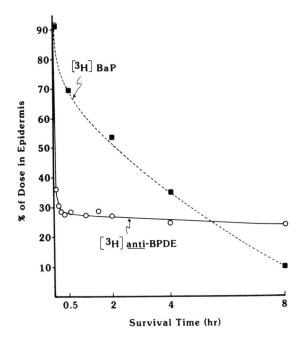

Figure 5. Time course of disappearance of radioactivity from mouse epidermis following topical application of [³H]BaP (■) and [³H](±)anti-BPDE (o). Points, mean of three experiments using 5 mice per time point. (From Melikian et al. Cancer Res 47:5354-5360, 1987.)

notable difference in the BaP metabolism pattern lies in the greater extent of formation of BaP-quinones and H_2O-soluble metabolites in the lungs of newborn mice than in mouse epidermis.

The profiles of organic soluble (±)-[³H]anti-BPDE metabolites in newborn mouse lung in all three experimental series were similar to those obtained in mouse skin (53) and in vitro (54-57). anti-BPDE spontaneously hydrolyzes to BaP-tetraols, predominantly to the tetraol formed from trans-ring opening. Quantitatively, major differences were observed in the kinetics of penetration and absorption of BaP and (±)-anti-BPDE in mouse epidermis and in regard to the stability of anti-BPDE in mouse epidermis and mouse lung. Comparison of the total radioactivity recovered at various times after topical application of [³H]BaP and (±)-[³H]anti-BPDE (see Fig. 5) clearly demonstrates that BaP and anti-BPDE are removed from mouse epidermis by different mechanisms. The disappearance of BaP and its metabolites is monophasic, with a half-life of about 2.5 h. In contrast, a fraction of anti-BPDE disappeared from the epidermis within a few minutes, and the remaining compound became sequestered and immobilized. Development of a method for quantifying the unhydrolyzed (±)-anti-BPDE

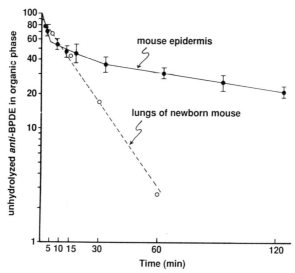

Figure 6. Comparison of concentration of unhydrolyzed (±)-[³H]*anti*-BPDE in organic phases, extracted from mouse epidermis (•) and from the lungs of newborn mice (o) at various times after application of (±)-[³H]*anti*-BPDE.

in tissues by trapping with mercaptoethanol allowed us to estimate the stability of (±)-*anti*-BPDE in mouse epidermis as well as in the lungs of newborn mice. The initial half-life of *anti*-BPDE in mouse epidermis was estimated to be about 6 min, similar to that observed in the lungs of mice and at pH 7.4 in vitro (58,59). However, after the initial rapid penetration of *anti*-BPDE, the remaining material became sequestered in the mouse epidermis and was thus protected from hydrolysis. As shown in Figure 6, its half-life then extended beyond 2 h, whereas the half-life of *anti*-BPDE in the lungs was about 9 or 10 min in one-day-old pups. The highest concentration of *anti*-BPDE detected in the lungs was equal to the highest level of its corresponding tetraols. These observations suggest that transportation of intraperitoneally injected (±)-*anti*-BPDE to the lungs is fast and that a significant fraction of the dose that reaches the lungs is probably structurally intact. In mouse skin, on the other hand, there is only a brief initial hydrolysis of topically applied (±)-*anti*-BPDE at a rate similar to this reaction in vitro. Thereafter, entrapment of the compound in the epidermis prevents further hydrolysis and reaction with cellular nucleophiles, including DNA. We believe that these differences may in part be responsible for the higher tumorigenic activity of (±)-*anti*-BPDE in the lungs of newborn mice than in mouse skin.

SUMMARY

The particulate matter of tobacco smoke induces benign and malignant tumors in various animal tissues and species. The most widely used bioassay system for evaluating the carcinogenicity of tobacco tars is mouse skin. Mouse skin bioassays have led to the identification of the PAHs as the major tumor initiators, while showing that catechols are important cocarcinogens in tobacco smoke. Mechanistic studies suggest that catechol affects BaP metabolism and especially secondary oxidation reactions of this carcinogen and thus changes the proportion of BPDE–DNA adducts.

Comparison of the disposition and metabolism of BaP and its ultimate carcinogenic derivative, *anti*-BPDE, in mouse epidermis demonstrates that the lower activity of BPDE relative to BaP in mouse skin is partially due to differences in penetration and trapping of BPDE within the epidermis, where it is protected from hydrolysis and reaction with intracellular macromolecules. Although screening for tumorigenicity on mouse skin is limited to the detection of certain classes of carcinogens and is not helpful for the evaluation of organ-specific carcinogens, mouse skin assays of cigarette smoke condensates have nevertheless served as valuable indicators of the tumorigenic potential of tobacco smoke for epithelial tissues.

ACKNOWLEDGMENT

The studies described in this chapter were supported by research grants ES 03278 from the National Institute of Environmental Health Sciences and CA 43910 from the National Cancer Institute.

OPEN FORUM

Question: Which enzyme is responsible for hydroperoxide-dependent oxidation of BaP-7,8-diol to *anti*-BaP-diol-epoxide in mouse epidermis?

Dr. Assieh Melikian: To my knowledge, it is not known. Dix and Marnett have discovered that hematin, the prosthetic group of prostaglandin synthase, catalyzes BaP-7,8-diol epoxidation by unsaturated fatty acid hydroperoxides. Eling and Marnett and their coworkers have also shown that BaP-7,8-diol is epoxidized to BaP-diol-epoxide by peroxyl radical dependent oxidation in the presence of mouse keratinocytes in vitro.

REFERENCES

1. National Clearinghouse for Smoking and Health. The Health Consequences of Smoking: A Public Health Service Review, 1967. Washington, DC: U.S. Public Health Service, 1967. (Publication no. 1696.)
2. National Clearinghouse for Smoking and Health. The Health Consequences of Smoking: 1968 Supplement to the 1967 Public Health Service Review. Washington, DC: Public Health Service, 1968. (Publication no. 1696-1.)
3. National Clearinghouse for Smoking and Health. The Health Consequences of Smoking: 1969 Supplement to the 1967 Public Health Service Review. Washington, DC: U.S. Department of Health, Education, and Welfare, 1969. (Public Health Service publication no. 1696-2.)
4. U.S. Public Health Service. The Health Consequences of Smoking: A Report of the Surgeon General: 1971. Washington, DC: U.S. Public Health Service, 1971. (Department of Health, Education, and Welfare publication no. [HSM] 71-7513.)
5. U.S. Health Services and Mental Health Administration. The Health Consequences of Smoking: A Report of the Surgeon General: 1972. Washington, DC: U.S. Public Health Service, 1972. (Department of Health, Education, and Welfare publication no. [HSM] 72-7516.)
6. U.S. Department of Health, Education, and Welfare. The Health Consequences of Smoking: A Public Health Service Review, 1973. Washington, DC: Public Health Service, 1973. (Department of Health, Education, and Welfare publication no. [HSM] 73-8704.)
7. U.S. Public Health Service. The Health Consequences of Smoking: January 1974. Washington, DC: Public Health Service, 1974. (Department of Health, Education, and Welfare publication no. [CDC] 74-8704.)
8. Office of Smoking and Health. Smoking and Health: A Report of the Surgeon General, 1979. Rockville, MD: Department of Health, Education, and Welfare. (Department of Health, Education, and Welfare publication no. [PHS] 79-50066.)
9. Winn DM, Blot WJ, Shy MC, Pickle LW, Toledo MA, Fraumeni JF Jr. Snuff dipping and oral cancer among women in the Southern United States. N Engl J Med 304:745-749, 1981.
10. Hirayama T. Non-smoking wives of heavy smokers have higher risk of lung cancer: A study from Japan. Br Med J 282:183-185, 1981.
11. Brunnemann KD, Hoffmann D. Chemical studies on tobacco smoke. LIX. Analysis of volatile nitrosamines in tobacco smoke and polluted indoor environments. In Walker EA, Castegnaro M, Griciute L, Lyle RE (eds): Environmental Aspects of N-Nitroso Compounds. Lyon, France: IARC, 1978, pp 343-356. (IARC Scientific Publication No. 19).
12. Bernfeld P, Homburger F, Soto E, Pai KJ. Cigarette smoke inhalation studies in inbred Syrian golden hamsters. JNCI 63:675-689, 1979.
13. Dontenwill W, Chevalier HJ, Harke HP, Lafrenz U, Reckzeh G, Schneider B. Investigations on the effects of chronic cigarette smoke inhalation in Syrian golden hamsters. JNCI 51:1781-1832, 1973.
14. Hoffmann D, Schmeltz I, Hecht SS, Wynder EL. Chemical studies on tobacco smoke. XXXIX. On the identification of carcinogens, tumor promoters and cocarcinogens in tobacco smoke. In Wynder EL, Hoffmann D, Gori GB. Smoking and Health, Vol I. Modifying the Risk for the Smoker. Washington, DC: U.S. Department of Health, Education, and Welfare, 1976, pp 125-146. DHEW publication no. (NIH)-76-1221.

15. Mohr U, Reznik G. Tobacco carcinogenesis. In Harris CC (ed): Pathogenesis and Therapy in Lung Cancer, Vol 10. Lung Biology in Health and Disease. New York: Dekker, 1978, pp 263-367.

16. Hoffmann D, Rivenson A, Hecht SS, Hilfrich J, Kobayashi N, Wynder EL. Model studies in tobacco carcinogenesis with the Syrian golden hamster. Prog Exp Tumor Res 24:370-390, 1979.

17. Kobayashi N, Hoffmann D, Wynder EL. A study of tobacco carcinogenesis. XII. Epithelial changes induced in the upper respiratory tracts of Syrian golden hamsters by cigarette smoke. JNCI 53:1085-1089, 1974.

18. Day TD. Carcinogenic action of cigarette smoke condensate on mouse skin. An attempt at a quantitative study. Br J Cancer 21:56-81, 1967.

19. Graham EA, Croninger AB, Wynder EL. Experimental production of carcinoma with cigarette tar. IV. Successful experiments with rabbits. Cancer Res 17:1058-1066, 1957.

20. Lee PN, Rothwell K, Whitehead KJ. Fractionation of mouse skin carcinogens in cigarette smoke condensate. Br J Cancer 35:730-742, 1977.

21. Wynder EL, Graham EA, Croninger AB. Experimental production of carcinoma with cigarette tar. Cancer Res 13:855-864, 1953.

22. Wynder EL, Hecht SS. Lung cancer. Workshops in the Biology of Human Cancer. Union Internationale Contra le Cancer Technical Report Series 25:170, 1976.

23. Wynder EL, Hoffmann D. Tobacco and tobacco smoke. Studies in experimental carcinogenesis. New York: Academic Press, 1967, p 730.

24. Bock FG, Swain AP, Stedman RL. Bioassays of major fractions of cigarette smoke condensate by an accelerated technique. Cancer Res 29:584-587, 1969.

25. Dontenwill W, Wiebecke B. Tracheal and pulmonary alterations following the inhalation of cigarette smoke by golden hamsters. In Severi L (ed): Lung tumours in Animals: Proceedings of the Third Quadrennial Conference on Cancer, June 24th to 29th, 1965, University of Perugia. Perugia, Italy: University of Perugia, 1966, pp 519-526.

26. Hoffmann D, Wynder EL. A study of tobacco carcinogenesis. XI. Tumor initiators, tumor accelerators and tumor-promoting activity of condensate fractions. Cancer 27:848-864, 1971.

27. Dontenwill W, Elmenhorst H, Harke HP, Reckzeh G, Weber KH, Misfeld J, Timm J. Experimentelle Untersuchungen über die tumorerzeugende Wirkung von Zigarettenrauch-Kondensaten an der Mäusehaut. Zeitschrift für Krebsforschung 73:264-314, 1970.

28. Hoffmann D, Wynder EL. Smoking and occupational cancers. Prev Med 5:245-261, 1976.

29. Donaldson AW. The epidemiology of lung cancer among uranium miners. Health Phys 16:563-569, 1969.

30. Archer VE, Wagoner JK, Lundin FE Jr. Uranium mining and cigarette smoking effects on man. J Occup Med 15:204-211, 1973.

31. Saracci R. Asbestos and lung cancer. An analysis of the epidemiological evidence on the asbestos-smoking interaction. Int J Cancer 20:323-331, 1977.

32. Selikoff IJ. Cancer risk of asbestos exposure. In Hiatt HH, Watson JD, Winston JA (eds): Origins of Human Cancer. Cold Spring Harbor, NY: Cold Spring Harbor Laboratory, 1977, pp 1765-1784.

33. Van Duuren BC, Goldschmidt BM. Cocarcinogenic and tumor promoting agents in tobacco carcinogenesis. JNCI 56:1237-1242, 1976.

34. Hecht SS, Carmella S, Mori H, Hoffmann D. A study of tobacco carcinogenesis. XX.

Role of catechol as major cocarcinogen in the weakly acidic fraction of smoke condensate. JNCI 66:163-169, 1981.

35. Brunnemann KD, Lee HC, Hoffmann D. Chemical studies on tobacco smoke. XLVII. On the quantitative analysis of catechols and their reduction. Analytical Letters 9:939-955, 1976.

36. Van Duuren BC, Katz C, Goldschmidt BM. Cocarcinogenic agents in tobacco carcinogenesis. JNCI 51:703-705, 1973.

37. Snook ME, Fortson PJ. Gel chromatographic isolation of catechols and hydroquinones. Anal Chem 51:1814-1819, 1979.

38. Irons RD, Dent JG, Baker TS, Rickert DE. Benzene is metabolized and covalently bound in bone marrow in situ. Chem Biol Interact 30:241-245, 1980.

39. Roshmore T, Snyder R, Kalf G. Covalent binding of benzene and its metabolites to DNA in rabbit bone marrow mitochondria in vitro. Chem Biol Interact 49:133-153, 1984.

40. Luh BS, Hsu ET, Stachowicz K. Polyphenolic compounds in canned cling peaches. Journal of Food Science 32:251-258, 1967.

41. Tolstikova IK. Phenolic compounds of fermented apple juices. Vinodel Vinograd SSSR 3:61-63, 1981.

42. DelValle JC, Vasquez RA. A study of the polar compounds in olive by gas chromatography. Grasas y Aceites 31:309-316, 1980.

43. Konrad E, Mager H. (Wella AG) German Offenlegungsschrift [Patent Document] 806, 603(Cl.A61K7/13), 23 Aug. 1979, Appl. 16 Feb 1978.

44. Van Der Linden AC, Thijesse JE. The mechanisms of microbiol oxidations of petroleum hydrocarbons. Adv Enzymol 27:469-546, 1965.

45. Melikian AA, Leszczynska JM, Hecht SS, Hoffmann D. Effects of the co-carcinogen catechol on benzo[a]pyrene metabolism and DNA adduct formation in mouse skin. Carcinogenesis 7:9-15, 1986.

46. Conney AH. Induction of microsomal enzymes by foreign chemicals and carcinogenesis by polycyclic aromatic hydrocarbons: G.H.A. Clowes memorial lecture. Cancer Res 42:4875-4917, 1982.

47. Levin W, Wood AW, Chang RL, Slaga TJ, Yagi H, Jerina DM, Conney AH. Marked differences in the tumor-initiating activity of optically pure (+) and (−) trans-7,8-dihydroxy-7,8-dihydrobenzo[a]pyrene on mouse skin. Cancer Res 37:2721-2725, 1977.

48. Chouroulinkov J, Gentil A, Grover PL, Sims P. Tumour-initiating activities on mouse skin of dihydrodiols derived from benzo[a]pyrene. Br J Cancer 34:523-532, 1976.

49. Slaga TJ, Bracken WJ, Levin W, Yagi H, Jerina DM, Conney AH. Comparison of tumor-initiating activities of benzo[a]pyrene arene oxides and diol-epoxides. Cancer Res 37:4130-4133, 1977.

50. Slaga TJ, Bracken WJ, Gleason G, Levin W, Yagi H, Jerina DM, Conney AH. Marked differences in skin tumor-initiating activities of the optical enantiomers of the diastereomeric benzo[a]pyrene-7,8-diol-9,10-epoxides. Cancer Res 39:67-71, 1979.

51. Slaga TJ, Viage A, Bracken WM, Berry DL, Fischer SM, Miller DR, Leclerc SM. Skin tumor-initiating ability of benzo[a]pyrene-7,8-diol-9,10-epoxide (anti) when applied topically in tetrahydrofuran. Cancer Lett 3:23-30, 1977.

52. Kapitulnik J, Wislocki PG, Levin W, Yagi H, Jerina DM, Conney AH. Tumorigenicity studies with diol-epoxides of benzo[a]pyrene which indicate that (±) *trans*-7β,8α-dihydroxy-9α,10α-epoxy-7,8,9,10-tetrahydrobenzo[a]pyrene is an ultimate carcinogen in newborn mice. Cancer Res 38:354-358, 1978.

53. Melikian AA, Bagheri K, Hecht SS. Contrasting disposition and metabolism of topically applied benzo[a]pyrene, *trans*-7,8-dihydroxy-7,8-dihydrobenzo[a]pyrene, and 7β,8α-dihydroxy-9α,10α-epoxy-7,8,9,10-tetrahydrobenzo[a]pyrene in mouse epidermis in vivo. Cancer Res 47:5354-5360, 1987.

54. Jernstrom B, Martinez M, Svenssen SA, Dock L. Metabolism of benzo[a]pyrene-7,8-dihydrodiol and benzo[a]pyrene-7,8-dihydrodiol-9,10-epoxide to protein-binding products and glutathione conjugates in isolated rat hepatocytes. Carcinogenesis 5:1079-1085, 1984.

55. Jernstrom B, Dock L, Martinez M. Metabolic activation of benzo[a]pyrene-7,8-dihydrodiol and benzo[a]pyrene-7,8-dihydrodiol-9,10-epoxide to protein-binding products and the inhibitory effect of glutathione and cysteine. Carcinogenesis 5:199-204, 1984.

56. Yang SK, McCourt DW, Roller PP, Gelboin HV. Enzymatic conversion of benzo[a]pyrene leading predominantly to the diol-epoxide *r*-7,*t*-8-dihydroxy-*t*-9,10-oxy-7,8,9,10-tetrahydrobenzo[a]pyrene through a single enantiomer of *r*-7,*t*-8-dihydroxy-7,8-dihydrobenzo[a]pyrene. Proc Natl Acad Sci USA 73:2594-2598, 1976.

57. Thakker DR, Yagi H, Akagi H, Koreeda M, Lu AH, Levin W, Wood AW, Conney AH, Jerina DM. Metabolism of benzo[a]pyrene. VI. Stereoselective metabolism of benzo[a]pyrene 7,8-dihydrodiol to diol epoxides. Chem Biol Interact 16:281-300, 1977.

58. Wood AW, Wislocki PG, Chang RL, Levin W, Lu AYH, Yagi H, Hernandez O, Jerina DM, Conney AM. Mutagenicity and cytotoxicity of benzo[a]pyrene benzo-ring epoxides. Cancer Res 36:3358-3366, 1976.

59. MacLeod MC, Selkirk JK. Physical interactions of isomeric benzo[a]pyrene diol epoxides with DNA. Carcinogenesis 3:287-292, 1982.

Skin Carcinogenesis: Mechanisms and Human Relevance, pages 347–361
© 1989 Alan R. Liss, Inc.

Mouse Skin Tumors as Predictors of Human Lung Cancer for Complex Emissions: An Overview*

Stephen Nesnow

Carcinogenesis and Metabolism Branch, Health Effects Research Laboratory, U.S. Environmental Protection Agency, Research Triangle Park, North Carolina 27711

In the late 1970s, the U.S. Environmental Protection Agency (EPA) was faced with having to assess the impact of the introduction of the diesel-powered passenger automobile into the current fleet of gasoline-powered vehicles. The expected 25% penetration into the U.S. automobile market was based on the lower cost of diesel fuel, the improved operating characteristics of diesel engines, and projected lower vehicle costs (1).

At that time, little was known about the toxicological effects of exposure to diesel emissions, the components of diesel exhaust, or their physical characteristics. Although a number of epidemiological studies had been completed, none showed a causal relationship between exposure to diesel exhaust and an increased incidence of lung cancer (2). In addition, no well-conducted studies in experimental animals indicated a cancer hazard by any route of administration.

Given this background, a broad research program was initiated to study the mutagenic and carcinogenic effects of diesel engine emissions and other related complex mixture samples. These studies featured a combined approach of analytical chemistry, genetic toxicity bioassay, and tumor bioassay to fully characterize both the complex mixtures themselves and individual components that might be responsible for biological activities (3).

The approach selected for a preliminary risk assessment of diesel emissions had to take into account several factors: that diesel exhaust, like other products of incomplete combustion, contained classes of chemicals (e.g., polycyclic aromatic hydrocarbons) known to induce tumors in experimental animals, that exposed populations studied did not exhibit an increased incidence of respiratory cancer, and that there were no experimental studies in rodents that showed an association between diesel exposure and lung cancer.

---

*The research described in this paper has been reviewed by the Health Effects Research Laboratory, U.S. Environmental Protection Agency, and approved for publication. Approval does not signify that the contents necessarily reflect the views and policies of the Agency nor does mention of trade names or commercial products constitute endorsement or recommendation for use.

The risk assessment method selected was based on the constant relative potency assumption as applied to human respiratory cancer (4,5). Under this assumption, the relationship between the potency of inducing respiratory cancer in man for two human carcinogens, X and Y, is proportional to the relationship between the potency of X and Y in a surrogate bioassay system, in this case, mouse skin tumorigenesis, such that

$$\frac{\text{Potency (Lung cancer in man) of X}}{\text{Potency (Lung cancer in man) of Y}} = K \left(\frac{\text{Potency (Mouse skin) of X}}{\text{Potency (Mouse skin) of Y}} \right). \quad (1)$$

The proportionality constant K can be measured experimentally by data from pairs of human respiratory carcinogens. The more similar the K values for pairs of respiratory carcinogens, the more credence can be put in this extrapolation approach. Human respiratory cancer risk for diesel exposure can be calculated from the following equation, where HRC is a human respiratory carcinogen:

$$\frac{\text{Potency (Lung cancer in man) of diesel}}{\text{Potency (Lung cancer in man) of HRC}} = \frac{\text{Potency (Mouse skin) of diesel}}{\text{Potency (Mouse skin) of HRC}}. \quad (2)$$

Therefore, a series of human respiratory carcinogens previously identified by epidemiological studies were selected for this analysis, and samples of these materials were collected and bioassayed using mouse skin as the target bioassay system. In addition, samples were collected from diesel-powered automobiles and also subjected to mouse skin bioassay.

This chapter briefly summarizes previously published data and presents some of our current research efforts.

RESULTS AND DISCUSSION

The choice of mouse skin as a target for the tumorigenic effects of complex mixtures associated with combustion and related emissions was predicated on the previously demonstrated sensitivity of this organ (Table 1). Skin has been used as a target system since the finding of Percival Pott that young male chimney sweeps had an unusually high incidence of scrotal tumors (6). The etiological factor identified in this rare tumor type was chimney soot, which, in combination with a lack of personal hygiene, resulted in this preventable cancer. In 1915, rabbit ear skin was used by Yamagawa and Ichikawa (7) as a target system to study the role of hyperplasia in the cancer process, and coal tar was used to induce tumors. Complete carcinogenesis in mouse skin was used as early as 1922 to identify carcinogens in organic extracts of organic particulate samples and to try to link these materials to the etiology of human cancer, when Passey found that ether extracts of coal chimney soot produced both warts (papillomas) and cancers (carcinomas) when applied repetitively to the depilated backs of mice (8). Campbell (9,10) confirmed these results with soot and also reported the carcinogenic activity on mouse skin of road dust extracts. Kotin and coworkers

Table 1. Skin Carcinogenesis by Organic Extracts of Particulates: Historical Summary

Particulate source	Mouse strain	Tumor type	Reference
Ambient	Swiss ICR	Carcinoma; papilloma	Wynder and Hoffmann (12)
	C57 Black	Carcinoma; papilloma	Kotin et al. (11)
Coal chimney soot	White	Carcinoma; papilloma	Passey (8) Campbell (9)
Diesel engine	C57 Black	—	Kotin et al. (15)
	A	Carcinoma; papilloma	Kotin et al. (15)
Gasoline engine	C57 Black	Carcinoma; papilloma	Kotin et al. (13)
	Swiss	Carcinoma; papilloma	Wynder and Hoffmann (14)
Industrial carbon black	Swiss	Carcinoma; papilloma	Von Haam and Mallette (16)
Oil shale soot	White	Carcinoma; papilloma	Vosamae (17)
Road dust	—	Carcinoma; papilloma	Campbell (9,10)

examined the carcinogenic effects of organic extracts of air particulate samples from the Los Angeles area (11). These extracts produced both malignant and benign tumors when applied repeatedly to the backs of C57BL/6 mice. Wynder and Hoffmann reported studies on the administration of air particulate extracts from the Detroit area to Swiss ICR mice (12). Both groups concluded that benzo[a]pyrene (BaP) alone could not account for all the carcinogenic activity observed. Kotin et al. (13) and Wynder and Hoffmann (14) also studied the carcinogenic effects of organic extracts of particulate emissions from gasoline engines; both concluded that these extracts produce tumors in mice. Kotin et al. (15) studied extracts from particulates isolated from a diesel engine. In contrast to the positive results reported for air particulate and gasoline engine emissions, these investigators found C57BL/6 mice to be refractory to the diesel extracts. However, tumors were produced in strain A mice treated repetitively with the diesel mixtures. Von Haam and Mallette (16) and Vosamae (17) were able to induce tumors in mice by applying extracts of industrial carbon black and oil shale soot, respectively.

We initiated a series of studies to explore the tumorigenic effects of complex environmental mixtures using mouse skin as a target and using standardized protocols. This protocol used male and female SENCAR mice, a mouse strain bred for increased sensitivity toward the tumor-initiating effects of 7,12-dimethylbenz[a]anthracene (DMBA) with 12-O-tetradecanoylphorbol-

13-acetate (TPA) promotion (18). Also featured were the use of a five-dose exposure scheme, 40 mice of each sex per dose, and four administration protocols: tumor initiation, tumor promotion, cocarcinogenesis, and complete carcinogenesis.

Three complex environmental mixtures were selected for bioassay on SENCAR mouse skin: coke oven emissions, roofing tar emissions, and cigarette smoke condensate. These three emissions have previously been shown to be highly associated with the induction of respiratory cancer in exposed populations.

Coke Oven Emissions

Coke oven emissions had been previously studied by Mazumdar et al. (19) in populations of exposed workers. A representative sample of coke oven emissions was obtained from particulates (1.7 μm) collected from the top of a coke oven battery with the use of a massive air volume sampler. The coke oven particulates were extracted with a Soxhlet apparatus using dichloromethane as the extraction solvent, and the dichloromethane was removed by evaporation.

Roofing Tar Emissions

Emissions from roofing tar pots have been causally associated with respiratory cancer in exposed populations as shown by Hammond et al. (20). A sample of roofing tar emissions was collected by means of a conventional tar pot with an external propane burner. Tar was heated to 182°C–193°C, and particulate emissions were collected from a 1.8-m stack extension. A Teflon-coated aluminum pipe led from the hood to a small bag house containing a Teflon sock. Roofing tar emission samples were extracted with dichloromethane using a Soxhlet extraction apparatus, and the dichloromethane was removed by evaporation.

Cigarette Smoke

Several epidemiological studies have related cigarette smoking and respiratory cancer in humans, the most notable a study by Doll and Peto (21). An acetone-water condensate of cigarette smoke was collected by the method of Patel (22) using a reference Kentucky R21 cigarette (85 mm) in a cigarette smoking machine.

Mouse Skin Studies

Each of these materials was evaluated on SENCAR mouse skin using both the tumor initiation and complete carcinogenesis protocols. In the tumor initiation protocol, the organic extract sample was administered to the shaved backs of SENCAR mice during the first week of treatment. Tumor promotion followed with twice-weekly applications of TPA (4.0 μg/week) for 26 weeks. In the complete carcinogenesis protocol, SENCAR mice were treated twice weekly with the organic extract for 52 weeks. We previously reported the tumor initiation data for these samples (18,23).

Two statistical procedures were developed to analyze mouse skin tumor data. The first analysis was based on tumor incidence data and used a probit model (18,23,24). This model was fitted with the use of log dose as the regression and also included the assumption that some tumors occur in the TPA controls. The probit formula used is:

$$P = \beta_0 + (1 - \beta_0) \, \phi \, (\beta_1 + \beta_2 \ln x), \tag{3}$$

where P is the probit proportion, x is the dose applied, and ϕ is the standard normal cumulative distribution function. The model parameters β_0, β_1, and β_2 were estimated from the raw data by maximum likelihood methods. The TD_{50} was then directly estimated as a function of these fitted parameters, and 95% confidence intervals were constructed using the asymptotic variance of these parameter estimates. The second statistical model employed tumor multiplicity data (18,23) and featured a nonlinear Poisson model with a background correction term:

$$\lambda = \beta_0 + e^{\beta_1} + \beta_2 \ln x, \tag{4}$$

where λ is the number of papillomas per mouse, x is the dose, β_0 is the background activity, and β_1 and β_2 are the model parameters that jointly determine the increase in tumor multiplicity with increasing dose. Using maximum likelihood methods, the model parameters were estimated from the raw data and then used to calculate the number of excess papillomas per mouse over background at a dose of 1 mg organic extract. Asymptotic 95% confidence intervals for these activities were obtained by means of the variance-covariance matrix estimated during the model-fitting process.

A summary of the nonlinear Poisson and probit model estimates, based on the papilloma data after 6 months of TPA promotion, indicated the following relative order of potency: BaP > coke oven > roofing tar (Table 2). Both the papilloma multiplicity and papilloma incidence data supported this ranking. Ninety-five percent confidence intervals were generally tightly clustered around the potency estimates (23).

To compare the potency estimates between samples, the results from the two sexes for each sample were averaged (because no sex differences were observed) (Table 3). Based on mouse skin tumor initiation data, the coke oven sample was approximately 5 times more active than the roofing tar sample, which was approximately 200 times more active than the cigarette smoke condensate. The relative ranking (coke oven = 1.0) based on tumor multiplicity data was coke oven: roofing tar: cigarette smoke condensate, 1.0: 0.2: 0.0011 (4).

When comparing the tumor incidence data, a new standard had to be devised, the TD_{25}. This was done in order to account for the low maximal tumor incidence observed with the cigarette smoke condensate sample. The relative ranking based on tumor incidence data was coke oven: roofing tar: cigarette smoke condensate, 1.0: 0.22: 0.0017 (4).

Table 2. SENCAR Mouse Skin Tumor Initiation: Incidence and Tumor Multiplicity Analyses by Statistical Models*

Sample	Sex	Nonlinear Poisson		Probit	
		Papillomas/ mouse at 1 mg	95% Confidence interval	Dose for 50% papilloma incidence (TD_{50}) (mg)	95% Confidence interval
BaP	M	NC†		0.0036	0.0021–0.0062
	F	NC†		0.0091	0.0057–0.015
Coke oven	M	2.2‡	2.0–2.4	0.30	0.22–0.4
	F	2.0‡	1.9–2.2	0.42	0.31–0.58
Roofing tar	M	0.38‡	0.30–0.49	1.8	1.2–2.7
	F	0.44‡	0.35–0.55	2.1	1.5–2.8

*Reprinted from Nesnow S et al. Environ Health Perspect 47:255-268, 1983.
†Not calculated because data were obtained at a lower dose range.
‡The distribution of tumors at some dose levels were not Poisson, as the variances exceeded the means.
Abbreviations: BaP, benzo[a]pyrene.

Table 3. SENCAR Mouse Skin Tumor Initiation by Human Respiratory Carcinogens*

Sample	Tumor multiplicity (Papillomas/mouse at 1 mg)		Tumor incidence (Dose in mg yielding 25% mice with papillomas)	
Coke oven	2.1†	(1.0)‡	0.16§	(1.0)‡
Roofing tar	0.4†	(0.20)‡	0.71§	(0.22)‡
Cigarette smoke	0.0024¶	(0.0011)‡	92¶	(0.0017)‡

*Reproduced with permission from Albert RE, et al. Risk Anal 3:101-117, 1983. Copyright Plenum Publishing Corp., New York.
†Values based on statistical analyses of the papilloma incidence data by a log-probit model with background correction.
‡Values in parentheses are normalized to the coke oven sample.
§Values based on statistical analyses of the papilloma multiplicity data by a Poisson model with background correction.
¶Values based directly on papilloma multiplicity data at 1 mg.

Human Cancer Studies

The basis for comparing human cancer risks was the unit risk, defined as the lifetime probability of respiratory cancer death due to a constant lifetime exposure to 1 µg/m³ benzene-soluble organic (BSO)-equivalent emissions in the inhaled air (4). The unit risk estimates for coke oven emissions, roofing tar emissions, and cigarette smoke were based on a linear nonthreshold extrapola-

Table 4. Summary of Results for Human Lung Cancer Unit Risks*†

Emission source	Lower limit	Best estimate (Relative ranking)		Upper limit
Coke oven‡	5.0×10^{-4}	9.3×10^{-4}	(1.0)	15.0×10^{-4}
Roofing tar‡	1.0×10^{-4}	3.6×10^{-4}	(0.39)	7.2×10^{-4}
Cigarette smoke§	1.3×10^{-6}	2.2×10^{-6}¶	(0.0024)	3.7×10^{-6}

*Reproduced with permission from Albert RE, et al. Risk Anal 3:101-117, 1983. Copyright Plenum Publishing Corp., New York.
†Lifetime risk/mg organics/m³.
‡95% confidence intervals for linear model.
§Bounds from linear and quadratic model.
¶Geometric mean of the limits.

Table 5. Proportionality Constants (K) for Pairs of Human Respiratory Carcinogens*

	Coke oven	Roofing tar
Roofing tar	2.03	—
Cigarette smoke	2.07	1.0

*Calculated from each unique pair of human respiratory carcinogen according to equation 1. By convention, the more active agent was placed in the numerator.

tion model (4). This method requires an age-specific lung cancer rate function. This function is transformed into a probability of cancer death equation by the method of Gail (25).

Specific changes in this approach for coke oven emissions required the use of BSO as a surrogate for coke oven emission exposure. The unit risk was, therefore, estimated to be 9.3×10^{-4} (Table 4) (4).

The roofing tar study of Hammond et al. (20) was used to calculate the risk for roofing tar exposure. This method and its associated assumptions are described by Albert et al. (4). The unit risk calculated for roofing tar emissions was 3.6×10^{-4}.

Two statistical models were used to calculate the unit risk based on cigarette smoking, the quadratic and linear models. Using these procedures, with some additional assumptions, the unit risk for cigarette smoking was estimated as the geometric mean of the two model estimates and was calculated to be 2.2×10^{-6} (Table 5) (4). The relative potency of these three human respiratory carcinogens was coke oven: roofing tar: cigarette smoke, 1.0: 3.9: 0.0024 (4).

To test the comparative potency—relative constant potency hypothesis, a series of K values were calculated based on the mouse skin tumor initiation and tumor multiplicity data and the unit lung cancer risk estimates for coke oven emission, roofing tar emission, and cigarette smoke condensate (Table 5). Using a 2 x 2 pairwise comparison, the K values ranged from 1.0-2.0, with a mean of 1.7.

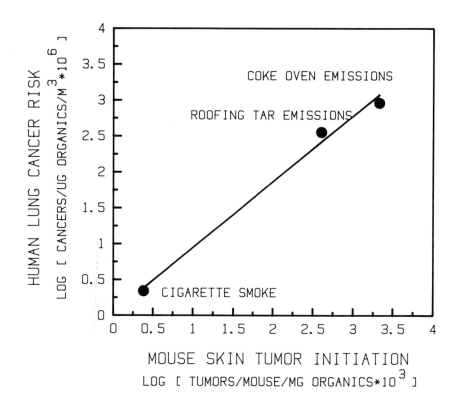

Figure 1. Correlation of mouse skin tumor initiation activity and human lung cancer activity for three human carcinogens. The line represents the least-squares linear regression for the three data points.

The correlation between the mouse skin tumor initiation–tumor multiplicity data and the unit risk estimates was quite good, with a correlation constant of 0.99 and a slope value of 0.92 (Fig. 1).

The close similarity between the K values for the three pairwise comparisons provided a strong rationale for using this approach for the comparative risk assessment of diesel engine emissions.

Estimate of Human Lung Cancer Risk for Diesel Emissions

To estimate the unit risk to humans for exposure to diesel engine emissions, a series of diesel engine particulate emissions was collected. Diesel-equipped vehicles were mounted on a chassis dynamometer and driven in a repeated highway fuel economy test cycle using No. 2 diesel fuel (see ref. 18 for details). Particulate samples were collected with the dilution tunnel in which the hot exhaust was diluted, cooled, and filtered through Pallflex Teflon-coated fiberglass filters. Dichloromethane extracts of these emissions were prepared as previously described. Three samples were evaluated: a 1973 preproduction Nissan-Datsun 220C (Nissan), a 1976 prototype Volkswagen TurboRabbit (VW Rabbit), and an Oldsmobile Diesel 350 (Olds).

Following the standard protocol, we evaluated these three diesel emission particulate extracts for their activity as tumor initiators on SENCAR mouse skin. Using the tumor multiplicity data, we found that the samples ranged in activity approximately twofold in the following order: Nissan > VW Rabbit > Olds (Table 6) (23). The tumor initiation data for the Nissan sample is described in Figure 2. A strong dose-response relationship is evident, with the highest response obtained at 10 mg/mouse. At that dose, almost 100% of the mice had developed tumors.

The measurement of the activity of the diesel samples as mouse skin tumor initiators on SENCAR mice provided the data needed for the estimation of the human lung cancer risks based on equation 2. The unit risk of exposure to Nissan diesel exhaust particulate extracts was calculated for each of the human lung carcinogens. This was done using the unit risk data from Table 4, the mouse skin tumor initiation data for the human respiratory carcinogens from Table 3, and the mouse skin tumor initiation data for the Nissan sample in Table 6 (Table 7). The unit risk values for the Nissan sample ranged from 2.6 to 5.4×10^{-4}, with a mean of 4.4×10^{-4}, lifetime risk/µg organics/m³. When represented in particulate concentration, this value was 3.5×10^{-5} lifetime risk/µg particulates/m³ (4).

Table 6. SENCAR Mouse Skin Tumor Initiation by Diesel Emission Samples*

Sample	Tumor multiplicity (Papillomas/mouse at 1 mg)		Tumor incidence (Dose in mg yielding 25% mice with papillomas)	
Nissan	0.59†	(0.28)‡	0.61§	(0.26)‡
Volkswagen Rabbit	0.24¶	(0.11)‡	ND	
Oldsmobile	0.31¶	(0.15)‡	ND	

*Data are from ref. 18.
†Value based on statistical analyses of the papilloma incidence data by a log-probit model with background correction.
‡Values in parentheses are normalized to the coke oven sample.
§Values based on statistical analyses of the papilloma multiplicity data by a Poisson model with background correction.
¶Values based directly on papilloma multiplicity data at 1 mg.

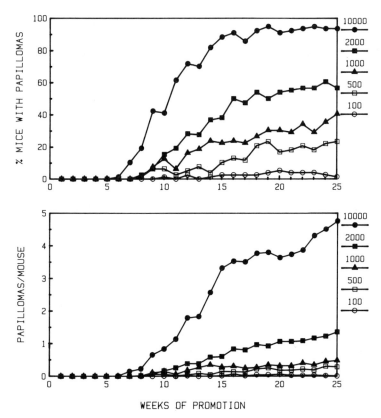

Figure 2. Nissan extract-induced tumor initiation in SENCAR mice. Tumors were initiated with an extract of Nissan emissions at the mg/mouse doses indicated and promoted twice weekly with 12-O-tetradecanoylphorbol-13-acetate.

Table 7. Unit Lung Cancer Estimates for the Nissan Diesel Particulate Emissions*†

Basis for estimate	Nissan unit risk estimate (Lifetime risk/µg organics/m³)
Coke oven	2.6×10^{-4}
Roofing tar	5.3×10^{-4}
Cigarette smoke	5.4×10^{-4}
Mean	4.4×10^{-4}

*Reproduced with permission from Albert RE, et al. Risk Anal 3:101-117, 1983. Copyright Plenum Publishing Corp., New York.
†Based on mouse skin tumor multiplicity data from Tables 3 and 6 and the best estimate unit risks from Table 4 using equation 2.

Table 8. Unit Lung Cancer Risk Estimates from Diesel Engine Exhaust Based on the Lovelace Inhalation Toxicology Research Institute Diesel Exhaust Inhalation Study in F344 Rats*

| Particulate exposure level (mg/m³) | Number of rats | Number of animals with lung tumors | | |
		All types including squamous cysts	All types except squamous cysts	Carcinoma only
0	220	2	2	2
0.35	216	3	3	3
3.5	213	8	6	1
7.1	221	29	18	17
Unit cancer risk (lifetime risk/µg particulates/m³)†		1.6×10^{-5}	1.2×10^{-5}	3×10^{-6}

*From Albert RE and Chen C, In: Ishinishi et al. (eds): Carcinogenic and Mutagenic Effects of Diesel Engine Exhaust. New York: Elsevier Science Publishers, 1986, pp 411-419.
†Calculated by the use of the linearized multistage extrapolation model.

Since the publication of the estimates for human lung cancer risk based on exposure to diesel engine emissions in 1983 (4), several chronic lifetime inhalation studies on diesel emissions have been reported (26). All of these studies confirmed that diesel exhaust was indeed a rodent lung carcinogen, as it was a mouse skin carcinogen. These inhalation studies indicated positive results in rats, whereas two indicated negative results in mice.

One of these diesel inhalation studies in F344 rats, that of Mauderly et al. (27), has been used by Albert and Chen (28) to calculate a unit risk for human lung cancer due to diesel exposure using a linearized multistage extrapolation model (Table 8). Using all types of rat lung tumors observed in the exposed animals (except squamous cysts), Albert and Chen (28) estimated the risk to be 1.2×10^{-5} lifetime risk/µg particulates/m³. This value agrees quite well with the value predicted by the comparative potency approach for the Nissan diesel vehicle (3.5×10^{-5}) and even better with the average of the individual unit risk values of 2.6×10^{-5} based on the Nissan, VW Rabbit and Olds diesel automobiles.

The close agreement between the two predictions, which use completely different scientific bases, assumptions, tumor incidences, and target tissues, confirms the confidence in the estimated unit risks. In addition, because the method of extrapolation of rodent lung cancer to human lung cancer is well established, its agreement with the comparative potency method serves to strengthen the argument for the comparative potency method in risk assessment.

Given these predicted unit risks, an important question is why no epidemiological study of ambient-exposed populations has identified diesel engine exhaust as a causative factor in human respiratory cancer. McClellan (26) calculated the excess lung cancer deaths to be 100, based on the Nissan unit risk and

Table 9. Annual Lung Cancer Mortality Rates in China and the United States from 1973–1979*

Place	Age-adjusted to 1964 China population		Age-adjusted to 1970 U.S. population	
	Males	Females	Males	Females
China†	6.8	3.2	12.3	5.7
United States‡	30.0	6.3	53.7	12.0
Yunnan Province	4.3	1.5	6.9	2.5
Xuan Wei County	27.7	25.3	43.2	38.7
Three high-mortality Xuan Wei communes	118.0	125.6	186.8	193.4
Three low-mortality Xuan Wei communes	4.3	3.1	5.8	4.3

*From Mumford et al. Science 235:217-220, 1987. Copyright 1987 by the AAAS.
†During the period 1973–1975.
‡Based on 1970 data.

a population of 230×10^6 exposed to 1 µg diesel emission particulate/m³. Obviously, this small number would be difficult to detect using epidemiological methods. For occupationally exposed populations, exposures to diesel exhaust would be greater; recently Garshick et al. (29) reported a causal association between exposure to diesel exhaust and lung cancer in railroad workers.

Although the rat inhalation data provide a method to test the adequacy of the comparative potency method, a more stringent test would be to predict the unit risk of lung cancer of a potential human respiratory carcinogen by use of mouse skin data and then to determine the unit risk from epidemiological studies. Such an approach is part of an EPA–People's Republic of China Cooperative Research Program (30). A recent survey of China's population for cancer incidence identified Xuan Wei County in Yunnan Province as a high lung cancer mortality area (Table 9) (30). The rates for Xuan Wei County are six times the mortality rates for Yunnan Province for males and 16 times those for females.

Within Xuan Wei County, there are 20 communes, and lung cancer mortality rates vary by commune. A remarkable difference (30- to 40-fold) exists between the lung cancer mortality rates for the three high-mortality communes and the three low-mortality communes. The etiological factor that is associated with lung cancer incidence and that correlates with commune practices is the burning of fuel in unvented houses. The fuel most commonly used in high-mortality communes is a smoky coal mined in the county. This fuel-burning for heat and cooking purposes creates a very high level of pollutants, both particulate and gaseous. The concentration of airborne particles (PM10) within the homes burning smoky coal ranged from 9.5–24.4 mg/m³, values that are approximately 100 times the proposed U.S. ambient air standard (30).

Xuan Wei County thereby provides another test for the comparative potency model for complex emissions. Particulate samples have been collected and extracted, and the extracts subjected to evaluation on SENCAR mouse skin as tumor initiators and complete carcinogens. Preliminary results suggest that an extract of particulates collected from homes burning smoky coal is a potent mouse skin tumor initiator and also induces squamous cell carcinomas as a complete carcinogen.

When all the data from the mouse skin studies are analyzed, the unit lung cancer risk of exposure to smoky coal can be predicted by use of the comparative potency model. This predicted unit risk can then be compared with the unit lung cancer risk calculated from the epidemiological studies.

In conclusion, the comparative potency approach shows great promise as a method of estimating the potential risks for man from his exposure to complex environmental mixtures. Continued testing and evaluation of this approach is necessary to reinforce its utility and accuracy.

OPEN FORUM

Dr. Paul Grasso: According to one calculation, about 60,000 people in the United States are dying from cancer as a result of diesel exhaust. This may be an overestimate when you consider two factors. First, I think the reason tumors developed in the rat is that the particles remained trapped in the lung at that level of administration. The concentration was so high that the normal clearance levels were grossly exceeded. At the low levels, this was not so, and therefore the tumors did not develop. Second, the concentration that produced the tumors in rats is approximately 1,000 times greater than the so-called curbside exposure. Do you have any comment on that, Dr. Nesnow?

Dr. Stephen Nesnow: With regard to your first comment, I think you are off by a factor of close to 1,000. McClellan has reported the range of excess cancer deaths due to exposure to 1 µg diesel emission particulates/m^3 to be 40–230, based on the rat inhalation and comparative potency data. The human risk estimate depends totally on the exposure model. Various exposure models can be used to estimate the average human lifetime exposure. With respect to your second question, there is some evidence that the induction of lung cancer in rodents depends on the particulate burden. In fact, I believe that the reason that the early inhalation studies did not show any activity is because the particulate level is not that high. That brings up an interesting question. How do you extrapolate from the rodent cancer inhalation study to man, in whom the exposure is much lower and other processes affect carcinogenesis? We cannot answer this yet. But there may be a secondary process involving particulates that is related to cancer.

REFERENCES

1. Springer KJ. Diesel emissions: A worldwide concern. In Lewtas J (ed): Toxicological Effects of Emissions from Diesel Engines. New York: Elsevier-North Holland, 1982, pp 3-14.

2. National Research Council, National Academy of Science. Health effects of exposure to diesel exhaust. Report of the Health Effects Panel Diesel Impacts Study Committee, Washington, DC: National Academy of Science Press, 1981.

3. Lewtas J (ed). Developments in Toxicology and Environmental Science, Vol. 10. Toxicological Effects of Emissions from Diesel Engines. New York: Elsevier Biomedical, 1982.

4. Albert RE, Lewtas J, Nesnow S, Thorslund TW, Anderson E. Comparative potency method for cancer risk assessment: Application to diesel particulate emissions. Risk Anal 3:101-117, 1983.

5. Lewtas J, Nesnow S, Albert RE. A comparative potency method for cancer risk assessment: Clarification of the rationale, theoretical basis, and application to diesel particulate emissions. Risk Anal 3:133-137, 1983.

6. Pott P. Chirurgical observations relative to the cataract, the polypus of the nose, the cancer of the scrotum, the different kinds of ruptures, and the mortifications of the toes and feet. The Chirurgical Works of Percival Pott, Vol. 5. London: L Hawes, W Clarke, R Collins, 1775.

7. Yamagawa K, Ichikawa K. Experimentelle studies uber die pathogenese der epithelialgeschwulste. Mitt Med Fak Tokyo 15:295-344, 1915.

8. Passey RD. Experimental soot cancer. Br Med J 2:1112-1113, 1922.

9. Campbell JA. Carcinogenic agents present in the atmosphere and incidence of primary lung tumours in mice. Br J Exp Pathol 20:122-132, 1939.

10. Campbell JA. Cancer of skin and increase in incidence of primary tumours of lung in mice exposed to dust obtained from tarred roads. Br J Exp Pathol 15:287-294, 1934.

11. Kotin P, Falk HL, Mader MP, Thomas M. Aromatic hydrocarbons. I. Presence in the Los Angeles atmosphere and the carcinogenicity of atmospheric extracts. AMA Arch Ind Hyg Occup Med 9:153-163, 1954.

12. Wynder EL, Hoffmann D. Some laboratory and epidemiological aspects of air pollution carcinogenesis. J Air Pollut Control Assoc 15:155-159, 1965.

13. Kotin P, Falk HL, Thomas M. Aromatic hydrocarbons. II. Presence in the particulate phase of gasoline-engine exhausts and the carcinogenicity of exhaust extracts. AMA Arch Ind Hyg Occup Med 9:164-177, 1954.

14. Wynder EL, Hoffmann D. A study of air pollution carcinogenesis. III. Carcinogenic activity of gasoline engine exhaust condensate. Cancer 15:103-108, 1962.

15. Kotin P, Falk HL, Thomas M. Aromatic hydrocarbons. III. Presence in the particulate phase of diesel-engine exhausts and the carcinogenicity of exhaust extracts. AMA Arch Ind Health 11:113-120, 1955.

16. Von Haam E, Mallette FS. Studies on the toxicity and skin effects of compounds used in the rubber and plastics industries. III. Carcinogenicity of carbon black extracts. AMA Arch Ind Hyg Occup Med 6:237-242, 1952.

17. Vosamae AI. Carcinogenicity studies of Estonian oil shale soots. Environ Health Perspect 30:173-176, 1979.

18. Nesnow S, Triplett LL, Slaga TJ. Comparative tumor-initiating activity of complex mixtures from environmental particulate emissions on SENCAR mouse skin. JNCI 68:829-834, 1982.

19. Mazumdar S, Redmond CK, Sollecito W, Sussman N. An epidemiological study of exposure to coal tar pitch volatiles among coke oven workers. J Air Pollut Control Assoc 25:382-389, 1975.

20. Hammond EC, Selikoff IJ, Lawther PL, Seidman H. Inhalation of benzpyrene and cancer in man. Ann NY Acad Sci 271:116-124, 1976.

21. Doll R, Peto R. Cigarette smoking and bronchial carcinoma: Dose and time relationships among regular smokers and lifelong non-smokers. J Epidemiol Community Health 32:303-313, 1978.
22. Patel AR. Preparation and monitoring of cigarette smoke condensate samples. In Gori GB (ed): Report No. 3. Toward Less Hazardous Cigarettes: The Third Set of Experimental Cigarettes. Washington, DC: Department of Health, Education, and Welfare, 1977, pp 67-80.
23. Nesnow S, Triplett LL, Slaga TJ. Mouse skin tumor initiation-promotion and complete carcinogenesis bioassays: Mechanisms and biological activity of emission samples. Environ Health Perspect 47:255-268, 1983.
24. Hasselblad V, Stead AG, Creason JP. Multiple probit analysis with a nonzero background. Biometrics 36:659-663, 1980.
25. Gail M. Measuring the benefit of reduced exposure to environmental carcinogens. J Chron Dis 28:135-147, 1975.
26. McClellan RO. Health effects of exposure to diesel exhaust particles. Annu Rev Pharmacol Toxicol 27:279-300, 1987.
27. Mauderly JL, Jones RK, Griffith WC, Henderson RF, McClellan RO. Diesel exhaust is a pulmonary carcinogen in rats exposed chronically by inhalation. Fundam Appl Toxicol 9:208-221, 1987.
28. Albert RE, Chen C. U.S. EPA diesel studies on inhalation hazards. In Ishinishi N, Koizumi A, McClellan RO, Stober W (eds): Carcinogenic and Mutagenic Effects of Diesel Engine Exhaust. New York: Elsevier Science Publishers, 1986, pp 411-419.
29. Garshick E, Schenker MB, Munoz A, Segal M, Smith TJ, Woskie SR, Hammond SK, Speizer FE. A retrospective cohort study of lung cancer and diesel exhaust exposure in railroad workers. Am Rev Respir Dis 137:820-825, 1988.
30. Mumford JL, He XZ, Chapman RS, Cao SR, Harris DB, Li XM, Xian YL, Jiang WZ, Xu CW, Chuang JC, Wilson WE, Cooke M. Lung cancer and indoor air pollution in Xuan Wei, China. Science 235:217-220, 1987.

Skin Carcinogenesis: Mechanisms and Human Relevance, pages 363–379
© 1989 Alan R. Liss, Inc.

Experience Gained by the Petroleum Industry in the Conduct of Dermal Carcinogenesis Bioassays

R. H. McKee, S. C. Lewis, and G. F. Egan

Exxon Biomedical Sciences, Inc., East Millstone, New Jersey 08875

HISTORICAL PERSPECTIVE

Model Development Based on Oil Industry Applications

Experimental dermal carcinogenesis in rabbits was first reported in 1915 (1). This finding was extended to mice 3 years later (2). The development of the mouse skin model resulted in experimental confirmation that a number of materials were occupational carcinogens (e.g., coal tar, coal tar pitch, shale oil, and soot) (reviewed in ref. 3). Further studies by Kennaway and coworkers (4,5) and later by Cook et al. (6) led to the hypothesis that the dermal carcinogenic activity of these materials was related to the presence of polycyclic aromatic hydrocarbons (PAHs).

Of particular interest to petroleum companies was the association of exposure to certain lubricating oils formulated from unrefined base oils and the production of scrotal cancer. A cancer excess was first documented in the British textile industry, i.e., "mule-spinners' cancer" (7), and subsequent studies also associated cancer with exposure to complex metalworking oils such as cutting fluids (8-10). Experimental studies in mice also confirmed that unrefined vacuum distillates that boiled above ~370°C and contained PAHs were dermal carcinogens (11-15). Similarly, it was found that lubricating oils and other industrial oils formulated from unrefined vacuum distillates also induced tumors in mouse skin (16).

A predecessor of Exxon, Standard Oil of New Jersey, first initiated dermal carcinogenesis studies in 1945. The specific objectives of the early studies were to develop and validate a model for experimental skin cancer studies and to then evaluate industrial processes that appeared to be excessively hazardous.

The first group of studies used high-boiling-point liquids from a fluid catalytic-cracking unit for methods development. Catalytic cracking converts the large, complex hydrocarbon molecules that are constituents of petroleum residuum (i.e., high-boiling-point catalytically cracked oil, or CCO, cat slurry oil, and heavy clarified oil) into smaller molecules suitable for blending as fuels. It was recognized that catalytic cracking produced polycyclic aromatic material and that this material was then concentrated in the residuum. It was suspected

Table 1. Comparison of Various Animal Species/Strains to Tumor Induction Following Treatment with Catalytically Cracked Oils*

Species	Strain	Weekly dose	First tumor	Tumor response
Mouse	White (Rockland)	45 mg/week (Back)	Day 29	51/63 survivors were tumor-bearing by day 141
Mouse	C57BL	45 mg/week (Back)	Day 71	11/13 survivors were tumor-bearing by day 130
Rabbit	Not specified	1.5 mg/week (Ear)	Not specified	13/21 rabbits were tumor-bearing by day 42; 21/21 by day 100†
Rat	Not specified	300 mg/week (Back & ear)	None found	No animals developed tumors (final killing at day 1069)
Hamster	Not specified	300 mg/week (Back & ear)	None found	Reduced survival due to oil toxicity
Monkey	Not specified	(Several)	Day 317	After 5 years, 6/6 monkeys had papillomas and 3/6 had carcinomas‡

*Reproduced from Sugiura et al., Cancer Res 10:951-955, 1956 with permission.
†Progression to malignancy slow in rabbits as compared to mice. At study termination (2 years), three rabbits had carcinomas.
‡Preliminary data: studies continued for approximately 5 additional years, but final data have never been reported.

that high-boiling-point cracked oils might present a greater cancer hazard than other process streams in the refineries (3).

Influence of species. Initial studies of CCO were conducted in several different animal species, including the mouse, hamster, rat, rabbit, and monkey (Table 1) (17). The test material was applied to the backs of rodents, ears of rabbits, and various sites including the back, stomach, forearm, and scrotum of monkeys. The mouse appeared to be the most sensitive species. Treated mice developed benign tumors in a matter of weeks, and in many cases the tumors then became malignant. These cancers, identified as squamous cell carcinomas, were histologically similar to those seen in humans. Rabbits also were a sensitive species as measured by time to appearance of papillomas; however, progression to carcinoma was not observed until near the end of the 2-year study. The monkeys eventually developed tumors, but were much less sensitive than either mice or rabbits. No papillomas appeared before the end of the first year of the study, and development of carcinomas required 4 or 5 years. Rats and hamsters did not develop tumors. Thus the mouse was selected as the species of choice for further investigations.

Comparable results were obtained by other investigators. Berenblum (18) was successful in inducing skin tumors in rats and hamsters with dimethylbenz[a]-anthracene (DMBA), but mice and rabbits were much more sensitive. In other laboratories (reviewed in ref. 18), the rat and hamster were found to be either less sensitive than the mouse to a range of chemical carcinogens or totally refractory to skin tumor induction. It was concluded both by Berenblum (18) and by Sugiura et al. (17) that the rat, hamster, and rabbit provided no obvious advantage over the mouse.

Influence of strain and sex. Another Standard Oil of New Jersey–sponsored study compared the carcinogenic response in white mice (obtained from Rockland Farms) and black mice (C57BL). The white mice appeared to be more sensitive, as determined by time to tumor appearance (i.e., latency); however, with continued treatment, similar numbers of mice eventually developed tumors (19). Early studies also compared responses in male and female mice; significant sex differences were not reported. As a result, the American Petroleum Institute (API, an organization that sponsors toxicological testing on behalf of the entire petroleum industry) and various individual petroleum companies in the United States have used male white mice for testing purposes. Studies conducted by U.S. National Laboratories have tended to use mice of both sexes. There is no compelling evidence that testing in both sexes is advantageous; however, the question has not been systematically examined.

Protocol design. The remainder of the early Standard Oil of New Jersey–sponsored studies were carried out with a fixed protocol derived from the experience gained in the validation program. Approximately 15 mg of test sample was applied three times weekly to the interscapular area. The study groups contained 30 mice, and each test material was evaluated at a single concentration—usually undiluted. At autopsy, sections were taken for microscopic examination of representative tumors and any internal organs of interest. Through the years, this protocol has undergone some modification, but the basic study parameters have been preserved.

Among the protocol features that have been modified by various petroleum companies including Exxon are mouse strain, application volume and frequency, number of animals per group, length of study, and extent of pathology. The C3H mouse is the strain most commonly used for dermal carcinogenesis assays in the United States. Studies of petroleum-derived materials that were conducted in the Kettering Laboratories on behalf of the API used the C3H mouse because it was commercially available and docile. It was found that, because it was an inbred strain, it tended to yield fairly reproducible data (20). In other studies conducted at about the same time, it was found that the C3H mouse was relatively hardy and tolerated repeated dermal application of petroleum-derived materials better than the Swiss mouse (unpublished Exxon data). For these reasons the C3H mouse is currently used by Exxon and other U.S. petroleum companies (see refs. 21,22), the API (23), and various national laboratories (see refs. 24-26).

Frequency of dosing. Mice are commonly treated either two or three times weekly with 25 or 50 μl of a chemical, although other doses have been reported. Daily application of petroleum-derived materials is not advisable because repeated exposure to these materials may produce dermatitis and even frank necrosis. In one study of coal liquids that contained relatively high levels of phenolic compounds, it was found that limiting the number of applications reduced the extent of skin injury and increased the sensitivity of the assay (27). For materials that are not highly irritating, tumor response does not appear to

Table 2. Carcinogenic Response Data Following Application of Raw Vacuum Distillate at Differing Frequencies*

Test concentration	Tumor response†		Median latency‡	Statistical comparison
	Malignant	Benign		
25 µl, 3 x/week	8	3	95 (86–107) weeks	Tumor frequency not significantly different
75 µl, 1 x/week	7	1	105 (91–118) weeks	Median latencies not significantly different

*Unpublished Exxon data.
†Animals were classified on the basis of the most advanced tumor type in the treatment area. The number shown is the total number of mice in each category from a test group initially consisting of 50 animals.
‡The brackets define the 95% confidence interval around the median latency, as estimated by the Weibull method.

be substantially influenced by application frequency (Table 2). Thus, for dermal carcinogenesis studies, the critical feature appears to be the total weekly dose rather than the number of applications (28,29).

Group size. Initial studies used 30 animals per group. In subsequent studies, the number was increased to 40 and then 50 animals. A comparison of studies using 40 or 50 animals per group indicated that these were equally reliable as a means of detecting weak carcinogens (Exxon unpublished data). We currently believe that study groups should contain at least 40 animals, but we have no reason to believe that utilization of 50 mice per group provides substantially greater sensitivity.

Length of study. Because a common objective of the early studies was to detect relatively potent dermal carcinogens, the studies were often terminated within 6 to 12 months. As attention shifted to less potent materials, the length of studies was increased. Early studies sponsored by the API and conducted in the Kettering Laboratories were terminated at 18 months because that was felt to be the approximate life span of the mice. As animal husbandry has improved, life span has lengthened. If C3H mice are individually housed and cared for in accordance with current guidelines (30), survival is normally adequate for a 20-24 month study. Although some mice may live longer, it seems neither humane nor experimentally sound to continue studies for more than 24 months.

Minimal versus extensive pathology. In a report on microscopic examination of tumors remote from the treatment site (31), it was reported that lymphomas and pulmonary adenomas were probably spontaneous. The significance of other tumors, including tumors of the liver, was considered uncertain. To extend these findings, pathological data were evaluated from approximately 130 dermal carcinogenesis studies, which included more than 6,000 mice. There was no consistent evidence of treatment-induced nonmetastatic visceral tumors (32). Thus, having at one time conducted exhaustive histopathology, we now do not normally recommend microscopic examination of visceral organs. We have continued to conduct microscopic examination of skin tumors and sections of skin from treatment sites. But visceral organs are only examined microscopically if lesions are grossly evident at necropsy.

Statistical Analysis of Data

Initial attempts to evaluate dermal carcinogenesis data were published by Standard Oil of New Jersey in 1951 (33). In that publication, it was noted that comparison of animal test data was often desirable but difficult unless biological activity could be expressed as a single value, i.e., tumorigenic potency. It was also noted that a number of methods of data analysis were available and ranged from arbitrary assignments to fairly sophisticated statistical treatments. Blanding and coworkers (33) opted for an intermediate method, believing that the arbitrary methods were too qualitative but that the sophisticated statistical methods were based on assumptions that were impossible to test (i.e., that animals without tumors when they died would have developed tumors in the same proportion as survivors). Although Exxon has modified the methods of data treatment since 1951, we believe that the opinions of Blanding et al. (33) remain scientifically sound.

Assumptions of the Weibull method. One convenient method of data treatment is to estimate median latency by Weibull statistics. The utility of this method for evaluating dermal carcinogenesis data has been well described elsewhere (28,29,34). It has been suggested that if certain assumptions are made about the parallelism of dose-response curves and reproducibility of data, the Weibull statistic can be used as a means of comparing the tumorigenic potency of materials tested at different times and in different laboratories. In our view, comparisons should be approached cautiously, as those assumptions may not be well supported.

To test the reproducibility of dermal carcinogenesis bioassays, tumor-response data from 13 Exxon-sponsored bioassays of CCO were analyzed. These data were taken from three study series, initiated in 1975, 1978, and 1979 and containing four, four, and five study groups, respectively. The first of these studies used 40 animals per test group, and the remainder of the studies used 50. Otherwise, the studies were conducted under identical protocols in the same laboratory by the same personnel and with the same batch of test material.

Dose response curves were obtained for each study series with the median latencies (expressed in logarithms) plotted against the dose in mg/week (also expressed in logarithms) (Fig. 1). A test for equality of slopes of the dose-response curves was performed using a general linear model with the experimental study series as the nominal levels of the dependent variable and the dose as a covariate. The interaction term for the nominal-level variable and the covariate was statistically significant at the .01 level ($F=9.98$, $df=2.7$), indicating that the three dose-response curves did not have equal slopes. This does not seem to be merely a statistical difference without biological significance, as the variability within individual experiments (mean square error$=0.007$, $df=7$) was significantly

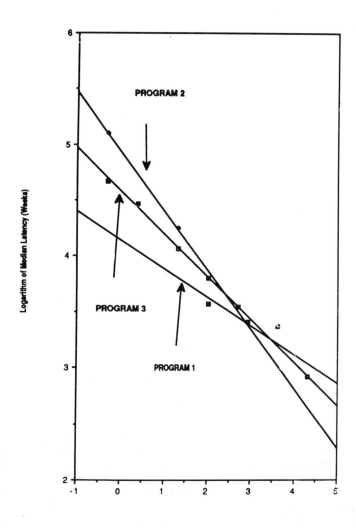

Figure 1. Comparison of the dose responsiveness of catalytically cracked clarified oil (CCO) as measured in three programs. Program 1 was initiated in 1975, program 2 in 1978, and program 3 in 1979. Median latencies were estimated by the Weibull method. Dose was the amount of material applied per week. The slopes are significantly different at the .01 level (F=9.98, df=2.7).

smaller than the variability that resulted when all studies of a single test material were combined (mean square error=0.024, df=11). This analysis indicated that there were sources of variation between experiments that were not present within experiments (35). Thus, this analysis demonstrated that dermal carcinogenesis studies, even if conducted in as similar a manner as possible, were not quantitatively reproducible.

Other Sources of Variability

Interlaboratory variability. When results from different laboratories were compared, the results were even more disparate. Table 3 summarizes a comparison study sponsored by Exxon and conducted in two laboratories. Qualitatively similar data were obtained; however, in some cases large differences in both tumor incidence and median latency were observed. Some differences in latency might be expected, inasmuch as the data were based on subjective judgments by different individuals and depended to some extent on the frequency of animal examination. However, tumor frequency data were based on microscopic examination of the treated sites and might have been expected to show greater similarity.

Table 3. Comparison of Dermal Carcinogenic Response Data in Studies from More Than One Laboratory*

	Laboratory 1		Laboratory 2	
Test material	Fraction of tumor-bearing animals†	Median latency (weeks)‡	Fraction of tumor-bearing animals	Median latency (weeks)
Solvent-refined naphthenic base oil	0%	—	0%	—
Aromatic extract of naphthenic distillate	32%	86	10%	122
Aromatic extract of paraffinic distillate	62%	76	15%	113
Middle distillate fuel containing cracked stocks	2%	—	10%	124
Distillate from catalytic cracking unit (338–370°C)	40%	84	50%	90
Heavy clarified oil, 10% solution in mineral oil	92%	44	100%	28
Heavy clarified oil, 2% solution in mineral oil	30%	107	96%	64

*Unpublished Exxon data.
†Number of tumor-bearing animals divided by the number initially tested (usually 50).
‡Median latency estimated by the Weibull method.

Table 4. Summary of Tumor and Survival Data from Mice Treated with Benzo[a]pyrene and Housed Under Differing Conditions *

	Plastic shoebox cage groups				Metal cage groups			
	1	2	3	4	1	2	3	4
Concentration (%)	0.25	0.05	0.01	0	0.25	0.05	0.01	0
Dose (µg/ application)†	50	10	2	0	50	10	2	0
Median survival time (days)	250‡	300‡	559	528	286	346	530	509
Animals with papillomas only	1	1	2	0	0	0	1	0
Animals with carcinomas	36	33	25	0	37	31	13	0
Animals with papillomas or carcinomas	37‡	34‡	27	0	37	31	14	0
Median time to tumor (weeks)	23	34	71	—	34	42	85	—

*Reproduced from DePass et al., Fundam Appl Toxicol 7:601-608, 1986, with permission.
†Total application volume was held constant at 25 µl.
‡Differences between groups that received the same dose of BaP under different housing conditions were statistically significant according to both the Breslow statistic and the Mantel-Cox statistic. $P < .001$.

Table 5. Effect of Vehicle on Tumorigenic Response*

	Mineral oil		Toluene	
Test material	Fraction of tumor-bearing animals†	Median latency (weeks)	Fraction of tumor-bearing animals	Median latency (weeks)
0.01% BaP	0%	—	30%	100
0.25% BaP	6%	139	80%	68
0.50% BaP	14%	110	94%	52
3.30% CCO	78%	65	88%	65

*Unpublished Exxon data.
†All studies utilized 50 animals per group.

Effect of housing. Relatively minor protocol differences can lead to quite substantial differences in tumor outcome. An experiment was conducted to assess the effects of animal housing on tumor response. Groups of mice housed in either polycarbonate shoebox cages or wire mesh cages were treated with graded doses of benzo[a]pyrene (BaP). Other than the caging conditions, the protocols were identical. It is apparent (Table 4) that the mice housed in polycarbonate cages developed more tumors in a shorter period of time than did the mice in the metal cages (36).

Effect of vehicle. Another study compared toluene and mineral oil as vehicles for BaP and CCO. The tumorigenic activity of BaP applied in toluene was significantly greater than equivalent amounts applied in mineral oil. In contrast, there was no discernible difference in the CCO study (Table 5). Thus, depending on the test material, choice of application vehicle may profoundly affect study outcome.

Qualitative versus quantitative studies. From the discussion provided above, it is evident that the mouse dermal carcinogenesis assay is not quantitatively reproducible. However, the assay is useful for hazard identification and for other purposes for which a qualitative comparison is adequate. As one example, four groups of investigators recently published studies of the dermal carcinogenic potential of lubricating base oils (21,23,37,38). These studies were conducted under similar but not identical protocols in four separate laboratories and utilized three different strains of mice. Nevertheless, each of these studies reached similar conclusions—that unrefined lubricating oils are carcinogenic and that carcinogenic potential may be reduced or eliminated by various refining practices. In particular, in each of the studies, it was found that solvent-extracted lubricating oils were not carcinogenic. Thus, data from the mouse dermal carcinogenesis assay provide a basis for qualitative comparisons of various materials but may not be appropriate for purposes requiring a high degree of precision.

Section Summary

The dermal carcinogenesis assay was developed as a qualitative test. When used for that purpose, a limited protocol (i.e., utilization of a single sex, species, and dose level as well as limited pathological examination) is appropriate. It is also evident that the assay is not quantitatively reproducible; seemingly minor differences in protocol can significantly affect tumor response. Thus the utility of dermal carcinogenesis data for purposes requiring a high degree of precision (e.g., risk assessment) may not be justified.

SYNOPSIS OF EXXON'S EXPERIENCE

Results of Studies and Utilization of Data

The first of Exxon's experimental studies demonstrated that catalytically cracked oils boiling above 370°C were highly carcinogenic (Table 6). As a result,

Table 6. Effect of Boiling Range on Carcinogenic Potency of Catalytically Cracked Oils*

Boiling range (°F)	Fraction of tumor-bearing animals 300 days after study initiation†
600–650	0
650–700	0
700–750	30
750–800	29
800–900	36
900–930	50
930–950	43
950–965	64
965–980	60
980–1010	46
1010+	15

*From Smith et al. Arch Ind Hyg Occup Med 4:229-314, 1951. Reprinted with permission of the Helen Dwight Reid Educational Foundation. Published by Heldref Publications, Washington, DC. Copyright © 1951.
†The number of tumor-bearing animals divided by the number of animals in the test.

Table 7. Fractionation of Raw Petroleum Distillates*†

Sample	Number of tumor-bearing animals‡	Median latency (weeks)
Raw petroleum distillate	23/40	69
Aromatic fraction of raw distillate§	36/40	51
Paraffinic fraction of raw distillate§	0/40	—
Aromatic fraction of raw distillate¶	37/40	45
Paraffinic fraction of raw distillate¶	0/40	—

*Unpublished Exxon data.
†The solvent-extractable fraction (i.e., the aromatic fraction) is similar to the liquid components removed from the distillate by mechanical force.
‡Numbers shown are the number of tumor-bearing animals and the number of mice initially in the test.
§The extraction solvent was phenol.
¶The extraction solvent was N-methyl pyrrolidone.

an industrial hygiene program was initiated to obviate the skin cancer hazard in refinery workers (39).

Another of the early Exxon-sponsored programs was initiated because an excess in scrotal cancer was observed among wax pressmen in one of the refineries. In that process, since discontinued, a raw vacuum distillate, i.e., a fraction of unrefined petroleum oil boiling between approximately 370 and 540°C, was passed through multiple cloth filter presses. The wax held up on the presses, and the liquid components were removed for further treatment. The pressmen were exposed to oil when they leaned over the plate and frame press to separate the frames and remove the wax. In addition, the workers tended not to use protective clothing, did not shower often, and tended not to change their clothes. Thus exposures were both heavy and prolonged.

The results of an experiment to assess the carcinogenic potential of the paraffinic and aromatic constituents of a vacuum distillate are shown in Table 7. The data shown were taken from a study to assess the efficacy of solvent refining, but they illustrate the principle that unrefined petroleum distillates boiling above 370°C contain carcinogenic components. The study also showed that the carcinogenic constituents are found in the aromatic (i.e., solvent-extractable) fraction of the oils. Thus the dermal carcinogenesis studies in mice supported the numerous epidemiological studies that have demonstrated that uncontrolled human exposure to raw vacuum distillates, aromatic extracts, and products derived from these materials can lead to occupational skin cancer (see refs. 3,40 for reviews).

Once it was learned that the liquid fraction from the wax presses contained constituents that could induce skin cancer, an industrial hygiene program was developed to provide greater protection during wax pressing operations (41). However, the efficacy of the industrial hygiene program was never tested because the wax pressing process was discontinued.

Contemporary Programs

The studies listed above illustrate the use of the dermal carcinogenesis assay as a means of identifying process streams that are unusually hazardous or may require particularly rigorous industrial hygiene procedures or engineering controls. This particular use of the assay continues. Contemporary studies, for example, assessed the carcinogenic potential of process streams associated with the production of liquid fuels from tar sands (42) or heavy oils (43). These recent studies demonstrated that the process streams were similar in carcinogenic potential to petroleum-derived materials of equivalent boiling range and process history. Thus these streams seemed likely to pose similar occupational hazards.

Similar studies led to the realization that the carcinogenic components in raw distillates could be reduced or eliminated by several processes, including solvent refining or catalytic hydrogen treatment. Recent publications have provided data demonstrating that N-methyl pyrrolidone (NMP) and phenol have similar extraction efficiencies and that vacuum distillates that have been extracted to meet modern industrial standards are not carcinogenic to mouse skin. Additionally, these reports have provided comparisons of solvent refining and catalytic hydrogen treatment as strategies for PAH mitigation (21,23,37,38).

Utilization of Single-Concentration Studies for Qualitative Purposes

The protocols used for the more modern studies did not differ substantially from those described in 1951. One feature that has been preserved is the use of single concentrations of test material. The reason is that the petroleum industry has used the mouse skin assay largely for qualitative purposes. In many situations, the experimental question, whether the test material is a dermal carcinogen, requires only a qualitative answer. The previously described studies of raw vacuum distillates, paraffinates (i.e., the material remaining after extraction), and aromatic extracts demonstrated that single-concentration investigations were clearly adequate to address that specific experimental question.

Even when more quantitative data are needed, single-concentration studies may still be adequate. In some cases, the experimental question is often semiquantitative—e.g., whether the test material is a more potent dermal carcinogen than some reference material. The materials could be ranked by median latencies as long as the limitations of the method were clearly recognized. However, it is important to note that, as the data are intended to provide guidance for engineering controls or industrial hygiene measures, small differences in carcinogenic potency, even if statistically significant, may ultimately have little relevance for worker protection.

Section Summary

As demonstrated by the various examples presented, the mouse dermal carcinogenesis bioassay is an adequate and efficient means of detecting potential dermal carcinogens. The information obtained from these studies can then be used for a number of purposes that do not require precise quantitative data. These include the identification of potentially carcinogenic products and process streams and the evaluation of engineering controls and industrial hygiene guidelines.

CURRENT STATUS OF BIOASSAY AND RESEARCH NEEDS

The mouse dermal carcinogenesis assay, as currently performed, is a sensitive and reliable method of assessing the dermal carcinogenic properties of PAHs and complex mixtures containing these molecules. However, it should be noted that the industry experience has tended to focus on liquids containing relatively high levels of PAHs, particularly certain refinery streams and synthetic fuels. Attempts to assess the dermal carcinogenic hazards of liquids low in PAHs, or other types of materials, have occasionally produced unexpected results. As one example, consider the results of a series of studies on a sample of lightly refined paraffinic oil (LRPO), a product that, because of its boiling range and process history, contains very low levels of PAHs (44). Repeated dermal application of this material produced a statistically significant increase in the yield of tumors in mouse skin. The tumor frequencies were low, and the median latencies were long in both studies, indicating low carcinogenic potency. However, the tumor frequencies seem clearly greater than the spontaneous incidence of skin tumors found in our recent studies (3 spontaneous, benign tumors in approximately 1,000 mice, unpublished Exxon data).

In other studies, LRPO was without activity in *Salmonella* assays and did not initiate tumors when evaluated in a two-stage assay in CD-1 mice (unpublished Exxon data). There was some evidence, however, that LRPO was a promoter of DMBA-initiated mouse skin (44). The promoting activity was weak; repeated application of relatively high levels of LRPO were required, and promoting activity was not detected within the first 6 months of study. The largest effect was associated with tumor progression; LRPO-promoted animals developed squamous cell carcinomas, whereas papillomas were found on the phorbol myristate-treated animals. Thus, LRPO behaved as if it were a second-stage promoter. Experiments to demonstrate this directly have not been conducted.

Research Efforts

The promoting effects of wound healing have been known for many years, and the relationship of skin irritation to tumor promotion has long been a subject of active investigation (45). Recent studies have focused on the role of irritation-induced hyperplasia in the carcinogenic process (46-49). Accordingly, a study was conducted to examine the effects of repeated application of LRPO on mouse skin. A gross examination indicated that from approximately week 4 to study termination (week 13), there was a relatively constant and high level of irritation and injury. Effects observed included eschar, cracking and fissuring, slight to moderate erythema, edema, atonia, desquamation, and recurrent exfoliation. Similarly, microscopic examination of treated tissue identified moderate inflammatory proliferative changes.

Thus, the data obtained to date are consistent with the hypothesis that the carcinogenic effects of LRPO may be the result of a promotional process. However, it is not yet known whether the promotional effects are a direct chemical effect or a secondary response related to skin irritation. Similar studies in other laboratories (see ref. 50) suggest that weak promotional effects are a general property of liquids in this boiling range.

Section Summary

The mouse dermal carcinogenesis model as currently used by the petroleum industry is a well-validated method of assessing the carcinogenic potential of complex PAH-containing materials. However, even within the range of petroleum products, assay interpretation is sometimes uncertain. It is particularly difficult to assess the potential clinical significance of materials that produce skin tumors only at treatment levels that also produce skin injury. Thus, when these assays are conducted, the limitations must be recognized, particularly when samples are tested that go beyond the range of materials for which the assay has been validated.

CONCLUSIONS

The petroleum industry primarily uses dermal carcinogenesis assays as qualitative indicators of potentially carcinogenic materials. For this specific application, the use of abbreviated protocols is a well-justified and widely accepted practice. However, the assay does have its limitations. First, it has been validated for only a few types of materials, and, second, dermal carcinogenesis data may be unsuitable for quantitative purposes.

To elaborate further on the limitations listed above, the assay was validated through studies of a number of PAH-containing, complex materials that were human carcinogens, and it is still a particularly good method of assessing the carcinogenic potential of materials of that type. However, even within the petroleum industry, there are materials that contain low levels of PAHs but still produce evidence of weak carcinogenic activity. The mechanism of tumor induction associated with these materials is unknown but may be related to repeated skin irritation and injury. Regardless of mechanism, the clinical significance of these findings is unknown. Clearly, the assessment of materials that fall outside the limits of assay validation should be regarded cautiously.

It is also important to understand that dermal carcinogenesis data do not appear to be quantitatively reproducible. Qualitative data are useful for a number of purposes, such as identifying potentially carcinogenic products and process streams. However, despite the availability of relatively sophisticated methods of statistical analysis, the data are not adequate for human risk assessment or other quantitative purposes.

To summarize the petroleum industry experience, it is common practice to utilize limited protocols to answer qualitative questions. Considering the types of materials that are tested and the purposes for which the data are intended, this approach is both efficient and well validated. However, the available evidence provides no assurance that studies conducted by more sophisticated protocols would yield substantially more information, particularly data that would be suitable for human risk assessment.

REFERENCES

1. Yamagawa K, Ichikawa D. Experimentelle studie uber die pathogenese der epithelialgeschwulste. Mitt Med Fak Tokyo 15:295-344, 1915.
2. Tsutsui H. Uber das kunstlich erzeugte cancroid bei der maus. Gann 12:17-21, 1918.
3. Eckardt RE. Industrial Carcinogens. New York: Grune and Stratton, 1959.
4. Kennaway EL. Experiments on cancer producing substances. Br Med J 2:1-4, 1925.
5. Cook JW, Heiger I, Kennaway EL, Mayneard WV. The production of cancer by pure hydrocarbons. Part I. Proc R Soc Lond 111:455-496, 1932.
6. Cook JW, Hewitt CL, Heiger I. The isolation of a cancer-producing hydrocarbon from coal tar. Parts I, II, and III. Journal of the Chemical Society, Transactions 1:395-405, 1933.
7. Leitch A. Mule spinners cancer and mineral oils. Br Med J 11:941-943, 1924.

8. Cruickshank CND, Squire JR. Skin cancer in the engineering industry from the use of mineral oil. Br J Ind Med 7:1-11, 1950.

9. Mastromatteo E. Cutting oils and squamous-cell carcinoma. I. Incidence in a plant with a report of six cases. Br J Ind Med 12:240-243, 1955.

10. Taylor WB, Dickes RE. The carcinogenic properties of cutting oils. Ind Med Surg 24:309-312, 1955.

11. Twort CC, Fulton JD. Experiments on the nature of the carcinogenic agents in mineral oils. J Pathol Bacteriol 32:149-161, 1929.

12. Twort CC, Twort JM. The relative potency of carcinogenic tars and oils. J Hyg (Lond) 29:373, 1930.

13. Twort CC, Twort JM. The carcinogenic potency of mineral oils. J Ind Hyg 13:204-226, 1931.

14. Twort CC, Twort JM. Suggested methods for the standardization of the carcinogenic activity of different agents for the skin of mice. American Journal of Cancer 17:293-320, 1933.

15. Twort JM, Lyth R. The concentration of carcinogenic materials in mineral oils by distillation processes. J Hyg (Lond) 39:161-169, 1939.

16. Gilman JPW, Vesselinovitch SD. Cutting oils and squamous-cell carcinoma. Part II. An experimental study of the carcinogenicity of two types of cutting oils. Br J Ind Med 12:244-248, 1955.

17. Sugiura K, Smith WE, Sunderland DA. Experimental production of carcinoma in Rhesus monkeys. Cancer Res 10:951-955, 1956.

18. Berenblum I. The carcinogenic activity of 9,10-dimethyl-1,2-benzanthracene on the skin and subcutaneous tissues of the mouse, rabbit, rat, and guinea pig. JNCI 10:167-174, 1949.

19. Smith WE, Sunderland DA, Sugiura K. Experimental analysis of the carcinogenic activity of certain petroleum products. Arch Ind Hyg Occup Med 4:229-314, 1951.

20. Horton AW, Denman DT. Carcinogenesis of the skin: A reexamination of the methods for the quantitative measurement of the potencies of complex materials. Cancer Res 15:701-709, 1955.

21. Halder CA, Warne TM, Little RQ, Garvin PJ. Carcinogenicity of petroleum lubricating oil distillates: Effects of solvent refining, hydroprocessing, and blending. Am J Ind Med 5:265-274, 1984.

22. Blackburn GR, Deitch RA, Schreiner CA, Mehlman MA, Mackerer CR. Estimation of the dermal carcinogenic activity of petroleum fractions using a modified Ames test. Cell Biol Toxicol 1:40-48, 1984.

23. Kane ML, LaDov EN, Holdsworth CE, Weaver NK. Toxicological characteristics of refinery streams used to manufacture lubricating oils. Am J Ind Med 5:183-200, 1984.

24. Holland JM, Rahn RO, Smith LH, Clark BR, Chang SS, Stephens TJ. Skin carcinogenicity of synthetic and natural petroleums. J Occup Med 21:614-618, 1979.

25. Renne RA, Wright CW, Smith LG, Buschbom RC. Epidermal carcinogenesis studies of fossil fuel material in mice. Toxicology 40:311-315, 1986.

26. Witschi HP, Smith LH, Frome EL, Pequet-Goad ME, Griest WH, Ho C-H, Guerin MR. Skin tumorigenic potential of crude and refined coal liquids and analogous petroleum products. Fundam Appl Toxicol 9:297-303, 1987.

27. Wilson JS, Holland LM. The effect of application frequency on epidermal carcinogenesis assays. Toxicology 24:45-53, 1982.

28. Holland JM, Wolf DA, Clark BR. Relative potency estimation for synthetic

petroleum skin carcinogenesis. Environ Health Perspect 38:149-155, 1981.

29. Holland JM, Frome EL. Statistical evaluation in the carcinogenesis bioassay of petroleum hydrocarbons. In Mehlman MA (ed): Advances in Modern Toxicology. New York: Halstead Press, 1984, pp. 151-166.

30. United States Department of Health, Education, and Welfare. Guide for the Care and Use of Laboratory Animals. DHEW publication number (NIH) 78-23, 1978.

31. Sunderland DA, Smith WE, Sugiura K. The pathology and growth behavior of experimental tumors induced by certain petroleum products. Cancer 4:1232-1245, 1951.

32. Freeman JJ, Lewis SC, McKee RH, Phillips RD. No systemic carcinogenic potential from skin application of petroleum hydrocarbons. The Toxicologist (in press) 1989.

33. Blanding FH, King WH, Priestly W, Rehner J. Properties of high-boiling petroleum products. Arch Ind Hyg Occup Med 4:335-345, 1951.

34. Whitmore A, Keller JB. Quantitative theories of carcinogenesis. SIAM Review 20:1-30, 1978.

35. Nicolich MJ, McKee RH, Simon GS, Lewis SC, Scala RA. Estimation of epidermal carcinogenic potency. Skin Cancer Symposium, Rouen, France, 1985.

36. DePass LR, Weil CS, Ballantyne B, Lewis SC, Losco PE, Reid JR, Simon GS. Influence of housing conditions for mice on the results of a dermal carcinogenesis bioassay. Fundam Appl Toxicol 7:601-608, 1986.

37. Doak SMA, Brown VKH, Hunt PF, Smith JD, Roe FJC. The carcinogenic potential of twelve refined mineral oils following long term topical application. Br J Cancer 48:429-436, 1983.

38. Gradiski D, Vinot J, Zissu D, Limasset JC, LaFontaine M. The carcinogenic effect of a series of petroleum-derived oils on the skin of mice. Environ Res 32:258-268, 1983.

39. Holt JP, Hendricks NV, Eckardt RE, Stanton CL, Page RC. A cancer control program for high-boiling catalytically cracked oils. Arch Ind Hyg Occup Med 4:325-334, 1951.

40. Bingham E, Trosset RP, Warshawsky D. Carcinogenic potential of petroleum hydrocarbons: A critical review of the literature. J Environ Pathol Toxicol 3:483-563, 1979.

41. Eckardt RE. Cancer prevention in the petroleum industry. Int J Cancer 2:656-661, 1967.

42. McKee RH, Stubblefield WA, Lewis SC, Scala RA, Simon GS, DePass LR. Evaluation of the dermal carcinogenic potential of tar sands bitumen-derived liquids. Fundam Appl Toxicol 7:228-235, 1986.

43. McKee RH, Lewis SC. Evaluation of the dermal carcinogenic potential of liquids produced from the Cold Lake heavy oil deposits of Northeast Alberta. Can J Physiol Pharmacol 65:1793-1797, 1987.

44. McKee RH, Plutnick RT, Pryzgoda RT. The carcinogenic initiating and promoting properties of a lightly refined paraffinic oil. Fundam Appl Toxicol (in press) 1989.

45. Mottram JC. A developing factor in experimental blastogenesis. Bacteriology 56:181-187, 1944.

46. Argyris TS, Slaga TJ. Promotion of carcinomas by repeated abrasion in initiated skin of mice. Cancer Res 41:5193-5195, 1981.

47. Clark LI, Murray AW. Tumor production and the induction of ornithine decarboxylase activity in mechanically stimulated mouse skin. Cancer Res 38:494-497, 1978.

48. Raick AN, Bardzy K. Ultrastructural and biochemical changes induced in mouse epidermis by a hyperplastic agent, ethylphenylpropiolate. Cancer Res 2:2221-2230, 1973.
49. Slaga TJ, Bowden GT, Boutwell RK. Acetic acid, a potent stimulator of mouse epidermal macromolecular synthesis and hyperplasia but with weak tumor-promoting activity. JNCI 55:983-987, 1975.
50. Gerhart JM, Halder CA, Hatoum NS, Warne TM, Garvin PJ. Tumor initiation and promotion effects of petroleum fractions in mouse skin. The Toxicologist 5:18, 1985.

Skin Carcinogenesis: Mechanisms and Human Relevance, pages 381–391
© 1989 Alan R. Liss, Inc.

Skin Carcinogenicity Bioassays of Petroleum Refinery Streams: Issues of Interpretation

Peter H. Craig

Mobil Oil Corporation, Princeton, New Jersey 08540

It has been recognized for many years that the presence of polynuclear aromatic hydrocarbons (PAHs) in coal and petroleum is associated with carcinogenic properties. Indeed, one or another member of this class of chemical, particularly benzo[a]pyrene (BaP), is the agonistic substance in most of the classic experimental models of carcinogenesis described in this book. In their monograph on petroleum in 1979, Bingham et al. (1) concluded as follows:

> The carcinogenic potential of petroleum and other fossil fuel materials to experimental animals appears to be associated with the presence of polycyclic aromatic hydrocarbons (PAH). High-boiling refinery streams from solvent extraction and from catalytic cracking processes should receive particular attention as possible sources of these compounds. Chemical analysis for one of the PAH, benzo[a]pyrene (BaP), shows that the BaP content of some samples may be correlated with their carcinogenic potency. However, samples free of BaP may also be carcinogenic. Although BaP has commonly been measured, it may not be the most important, prevalent, or significant of the PAH with carcinogenic potential in petroleum. Further chemical analyses of a variety of petroleum samples for PAH are needed. It is possible that correlation of such data with the results of bioassays of the same samples will reveal some compounds other than BaP as better indicators of carcinogenic potency.

In fact, far better indicators have now been identified, but we still have much to learn about the carcinogenic properties and related biological activities of petroleum and its many derivatives, which are commonly called refinery streams. The following is intended as a review of recent information concerning the dermal carcinogenicity of petroleum refinery streams.

A highly simplified schematic diagram of a modern petroleum refinery is shown in Figure 1—in this case, one producing lubricants. The first two major steps in refining are distillation of crude oil at atmospheric pressure and redistillation of the atmospheric still "bottoms" under reduced pressure. Other

A Typical Lube Refinery

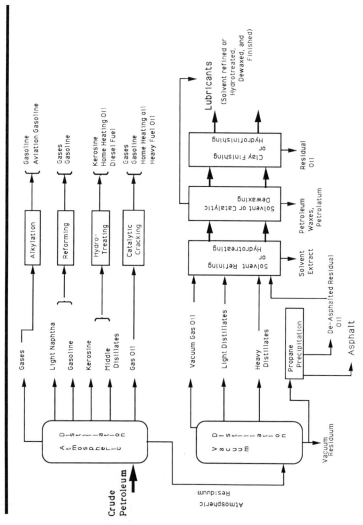

Figure 1. With an appropriate slate of crude petroleum, a refinery can produce lubricants, most of which boil between 500 and 1000°F. With a different crude slate, the outputs from the vacuum distillation tower are used mainly for the production of fuels.

important processes for refining streams effluent from the atmospheric tower are alkylation (assembly of two to four carbon gases into a C7-C9 mixture of paraffins), reforming (cyclization of naphtha to produce aromatics), hydrogenation (a variety of purposes and effects, depending upon feedstock and severity of treatment), and catalytic cracking. In the latter, larger molecules of limited utility are broken down by heat and catalysis into smaller moieties, most of which are useful as fuels. The resistant remnant from catalytic cracking (clarified oil) often has carcinogenic properties and may be incorporated in heavy fuels as a minor blending component (< 0.5% of the final product).

The lower half of the diagram in Figure 1 deals with the production of lubricant stocks and asphalt by vacuum distillation. Downstream processes for lubricants include solvent refining (extraction of PAHs with a suitable solvent, usually furfural), and dewaxing (usually with methylethyl ketone or toluene). Asphaltenes, very large and complex molecular structures, are collected from the residue of the vacuum tower by extraction/precipitation with liquid propane.

In those refineries that do not produce lubricants, streams effluent from the vacuum distillation process are mainly used for fuels and as feedstocks for the catalytic cracker. Some refineries have a coker, not shown in Figure 1. In the coking process, heavy, complex materials are reduced by pyrolysis to gases, lighter hydrocarbons, and a solid, highly carbonaceous remnant, petroleum coke.

The many intermediate and product streams in the petroleum refinery have been codified in the TOSCA inventory. This list also supplies generic descriptions of the streams, but the latter reveal little or nothing of the molecular composition of the streams, which are usually highly complex mixtures of hydrocarbon molecules.

Basically, petroleum refining is a series of processes that separate the crude oil into simpler mixtures of limited boiling range and useful viscosity. Both of these properties are, of course, a function of average molecular size. Figure 2 shows typical boiling ranges and hydrocarbon constituencies of the major products of refining. Although there is overlap, lighter materials have lower boiling ranges and lower average molecular weights. As you would expect, viscosity increases as a function of molecular weight.

Heavy streams such as clarified oil, which boil in the region of 600–950°F, often contain substantial percentages of three- to seven-ring PAHs, heterocyclics such as carbazoles and nitroaromatics, and small quantities of metals. Such streams are highly complex and very difficult to characterize fully by chemical analysis.

Vacuum residuum, the remnant from vacuum distillation, has an initial boiling point of approximately 900°F and contains molecules that are mostly larger than those of the other streams shown in Figure 2. This is of interest because vacuum residua are generally not carcinogenic, ostensibly because their PAHs and other constituents are too large and stable to be absorbed and metabolized in biological systems.

Tables 1–3 summarize preliminary results of systematic dermal carcinogenicity testing by the American Petroleum Institute in a series that ranges over the light to the heavy process streams. Several generalities emerge from this

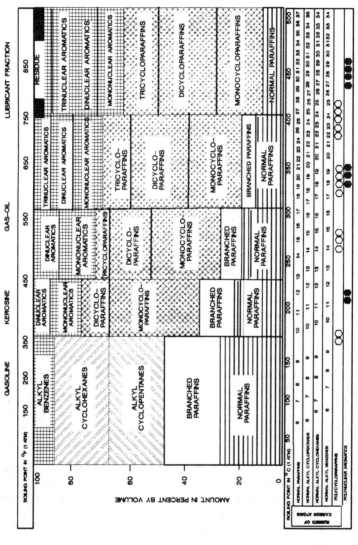

Figure 2. The sizes and proportions of molecular constituents in the distillation fractions of petroleum vary according to boiling range. This classification is useful for illustrative purposes only; in practice, the separations are not sharply defined. For example, pentanuclear and larger aromatics can be found throughout the 500 to 1000°F range.

Table 1. The Carcinogenic Potential of Naphtha Refinery Streams

Stream	API identifier	Boiling range (°F)	Dermal carcinogenicity
Light naphtha streams			
Light alkylate naphtha	83-19	103–331	–
Sweetened naphtha	81-08	98–262	–
Light cat-cracked naphtha	81-03	94–358	–
Heavy naphtha streams			
Heavy cat-reformed naphtha	83-06	248–365	–
Heavy cat-cracked naphtha	83-18	250–467	+
Heavy thermal-cracked naphtha	84-02	230–406	+

Table 2. The Carcinogenic Potential of Middle Distillate Streams

Stream	API identifier	Boiling range (°F)	Dermal carcinogenicity
Straight-run kerosene	83-09	238–520	++
Hydrodesulfurized kerosene	81-07	362–535	++
Light cat-cracked distillate	83-07	464–701	+++
Middle distillate (10% cracked)	83-01	356–589	+/–
Middle distillate (30% cracked)	83-02	358–606	+
Middle distillate (50% cracked)	83-03	358–620	++
Hydrodesulfurized middle distillate	81-09	502–574	++
Hydrodesulfurized middle distillate	81-10	342–651	+++

Table 3. The Carcinogenic Potential of Heavy Refinery Streams

Stream	API identifier	Boiling range (°F)	Dermal carcinogenicity
Lubricant stocks and related streams			
Light paraffinic distillate	84-01	579–803	++++
Furfural extract of light paraffinic distillate	83-16	NA	++++
Hydrotreated light naphthenic distillate	83-12	464–796	+
Paraffinic base stocks	78-09, 78-10	541–909	–
(solvent-refined)	79-03, 79-04	572–1016	–
	79–05	515–989	–
Napthenic base stocks	78-05, 79-01	470–1017	+/–
Residual stocks			
Cat-cracked slurry oil	81-15	E650–1000+	++++
Vacuum residuum	81-13	E925–1000+	–
	81-14	E925–1000+	–

series, but it must be recognized that individual samples may depart from the norm, depending upon crude oil source and other factors. This series of tests was conducted over a period of years, using standard protocols and the C3H mouse, under the auspices of the American Petroleum Institute (2).

In Table 1, we consider the naphtha streams, light and heavy. The naphtha streams are blended to produce gasoline and may be further refined in order to produce solvents. The polynuclear aromatic content of these streams is very low, in the ppm range if any are found at all. Characteristically, the lightest streams are not carcinogenic, but the heavier naphthas may be slightly active in mouse bioassays.

Rather greater levels of carcinogenic activity are often encountered with the middle distillates (Table 2), with most of the samples having boiling ranges between 350 and 600°F. These streams are the source of kerosenes, aviation jet fuels, diesel fuels, and home heating oils. Many of the middle distillate streams are irritants to the skin as well, although this feature is highly variable in mouse skin painted over a lifetime.

Table 3 lists some of the heavier, higher-boiling streams, in which substantial quantities of PAHs are likely to exist. An example is seen in the pair of samples, light paraffinic distillate and its LPD extract. The distillate was highly carcinogenic, and that biologic activity was transferred to the solvent during the process of extraction. Furfural is the solvent in most common use for refining lubricant stocks, and one of its most important effects is the removal of PAHs. In Table 3, the three solvent-refined paraffinic stocks are not carcinogenic, the PAH content having been reduced to very low levels by solvent extraction. These processing effects have been documented in detail by Kane et al. (3).

The development of a modification of the Ames test (Figure 3) has been of great help in codifying and understanding the carcinogenic properties of petroleum and its derivatives (4). In this modification, a dimethyl sulfoxide extract of the sample in question is tested in a system containing additional quantities of S9 liver fraction and NADP cofactor. The correlation between the mutagenicity index from the modified Ames test and dermal carcinogenicity bioassay results is shown in Figure 4. A 2 x 2 contingency array showing the predictivity of the index is in Table 4.

The excellent correlations are based primarily upon the fact that both the modified Ames procedure and the dermal carcinogenicity bioassay in the mouse are responsive to a particular size range of polynuclear aromatics. The great majority of biologically active PAHs appear to have from three to seven rings. In Figure 5, oils with known carcinogenicity profiles and originating from several sources were analyzed for their three- to seven-ring PAH content (5). The plot depicts the correlation between the mutagenicity index (MI) and the PAH content for the same 39 samples shown in Figure 4 and Table 4.

Table 5 gives multiple correlation coefficients, normal and weighted, for the 39 oil samples (for further details, see ref. 5). There is no doubt that, within the framework defined by samples boiling in this range (~500 to 1000°F), the modified Ames test and the bioassay are responding to the same kind of agents and that those agents can be found in the PAH class.

MODIFIED AMES TEST

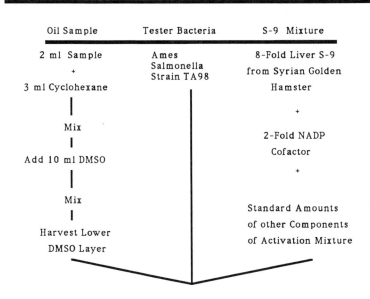

Oil Sample	Tester Bacteria	S-9 Mixture
2 ml Sample + 3 ml Cyclohexane	Ames Salmonella Strain TA98	8-Fold Liver S-9 from Syrian Golden Hamster
Mix		+
Add 10 ml DMSO		2-Fold NADP Cofactor
Mix		+
Harvest Lower DMSO Layer		Standard Amounts of other Components of Activation Mixture

Combine, Incubate and Pour Plates

Incubate 48 hr @ 37 C

Count Revertants

Figure 3. In the modified Ames test, mutagenicity is evaluated in strain TA98, with an augmented activation mixture. Generally, this system is responsive to the presence of three- to seven-ring polynuclear aromatic hydrocarbons.

Table 4. The Predictivity of the Modified Ames Test for Carcinogenic Potential

	Mutagenicity index	
Carcinogenicity index*	1 or less	More than 1
5 or less	16	1
More than 5	0	22

*(Percent tumors/latent period) x 100 (see ref. 5).

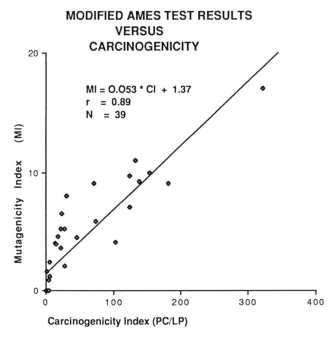

**MODIFIED AMES TEST RESULTS
VERSUS
CARCINOGENICITY**

MI = 0.053 * CI + 1.37
r = 0.89
N = 39

Mutagenicity Index (MI)

Carcinogenicity Index (PC/LP)

Figure 4. There is a highly significant linear correlation between the mutagenicity index and the carcinogenicity of 39 samples, as evaluated in the standard dermal mouse bioassay. The samples had boiling points in the 500–1000°F range.

It is important to recognize, however, that lighter materials such as naphtha and light distillates (kerosene, jet fuels) may have a very low PAH content and very low mutagenicity indices in the modified Ames test yet often elicit tumorigenic responses in the mouse skin bioassay. At this time, we are uncertain of either the causal constituents or mechanistic basis for such responses when the PAH content is minimal. Perhaps there are significant concentrations of compounds not yet recognized as carcinogenic. More likely, the lighter materials enhance the rate of appearance of skin tumors by some indirect means.

Because this book has risk assessment as its central focus, it is appropriate to consider the foregoing as a potential basis for the prediction of risk in man. Although many refinery streams exist only in closed systems, there is potentially extensive human contact with fuels, lubricants, solvents, and other petroleum derivatives. What would qualify a test system as a scientifically reasonable basis for the quantitative extrapolation of risk from one species to the other? I propose the following: (1) A test system in which the biologically active substances that produce the carcinogenic response have been identified, and at least preliminary information exists on how that response is produced. For pure substances, the

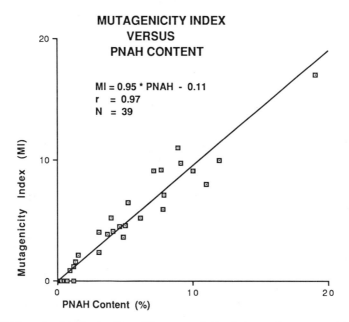

Figure 5. There is a highly significant linear correlation between the mutagenicity index and the content of three- to seven-ring polynuclear aromatics. These are the same samples depicted in Figure 4.

identity of the active metabolites is important. For mixtures, the identity of the biologically active classes of chemicals and their metabolism are of analogous utility. (2) Adequate data and a mathematical model to relate the dose and response in the test system and to scale the relationship between the test species and man. (3) A measure of the comparative sensitivity of human populations and the bioassay species. Other chapters in this book emphasize the importance of human genetic subpopulations, a concept that probably applies in full measure to skin carcinogenesis. (4) A method for defining the limit of applicability of a test system.

In relation to those criteria, the mouse skin bioassay of petroleum deriva- tives containing three- to seven-ring PAHs appears to be an excellent candidate for development as a basis for human quantitative risk assessment. Chemical identities and mechanisms have been studied as much as those of any carcinogen class. It has been established that humans develop tumors as the result of extensive exposure to PAH-containing oils. Dose-response relationships have been developed in experimental systems for many PAHs. Establishing a com- parative measure of sensitivity and defining the limit of applicability of the test system are related problems and, of course, these have yet to be accomplished.

Table 5. Multiple Regression of Variables from 39 Oil Samples

Variable 1	Variable 2	Correlation coefficient
1/LP	MI	0.84
1/LP	PAC	0.78
1/LP	(MI x dose)	0.77
1/LP	(PAC x dose)	0.76
1/LP	Dose	0.53
1/LP	SXST	0.40
% T	MI	0.87
% T	PAC	0.86
% T	(MI x dose)	0.66
% T	(PAC x dose)	0.65
% T	Dose	0.08
% T	SXST	0.01
% T/LP	MI	0.88
% T/LP	PAC	0.87
% T/LP	(MI x dose)	0.79
% T/LP	(PAC x dose)	0.76
% T/LP	Dose	0.13
% T/LP	SXST	0.03

Abbreviations: MI, mutagenicity index, modified Ames test; % T, percentage of tumor-bearing animals, carcinogenesis bioassay; 1/LP, reciprocal of latent period in weeks; % T/LP, carcinogenicity index: (% T) x (1/LP); PAC, polynuclear aromatic content, 3–7 rings, percentage; SXST, categorization by sex and strain.

As to the tumorigenic responses produced by petroleum derivatives containing little or no PAH, the basis for this biological activity is not understood. Indeed, none of the criteria of a test system adequate for quantitative risk assessment can be fulfilled. For many years, such results have been used in the petroleum industry as a trigger for labels and warnings and as an indicator of the need for protective handling practices. This is a prudent and appropriate approach to the need for protection of those involved in manufacture, transport, use, and disposal of petroleum products. A mathematical prediction of human risk, however, should await the development of more information than is available now.

REFERENCES

1. Bingham E, Trosset R, Warshawsky D. Carcinogenic potential of petroleum hydrocarbons. J Environ Pathol Toxicol 3:483-563, 1979.
2. American Petroleum Institute. Reports 30-32847, 33-31451, 34-32865, and relevant preliminaries. Washington, DC.
3. Kane M, Ladov E, Holdsworth C, Weaver N. Toxicological characteristics of refinery streams used to manufacture lubricating oils. Am J Ind Med 5:183-200, 1984.

4.   Blackburn G, Deitch R, Schreiner C, Mackerer C. Predicting carcinogenicity of petroleum distillation fractions using a modified *Salmonella* mutagenicity assay. Cell Biology and Toxicology 2:63-84, 1986.
5.   Roy T, Johnson S, Blackburn G, Mackerer C. Correlation of mutagenic and dermal carcinogenic activities of mineral oils with polycyclic aromatic compound content. Fundam Appl Toxicol 10:466-476, 1988.

Skin Carcinogenesis: Mechanisms and Human Relevance, pages 393–399
© 1989 Alan R. Liss, Inc.

Application of Short-Term Assays by the Petroleum Industry to Identify Skin Carcinogens

F. B. Thomas and B. J. Simpson

*Shell Oil Company, Houston, Texas (F. B. T.) and
Shell Internationale Petroleum Mij. B.V. (B. J. S.)*

If you take pollen from a plant and heat it for a few days under pressure, a liquid that is remarkably similar to crude oil will be produced. This should not be surprising because this process simulates the geothermal conditions by which crude oil is formed in nature. However, if you start with pollen or leaves from a different type of plant, the liquid you derive has a qualitatively and quantitatively different chemical composition from our first sample. The crude oils found in nature also show significant differences in their chemical and physical properties. For example, crude oils range from a liquid with about the viscosity of kerosine to "heavy" oils that are essentially solid at atmospheric temperatures. They are termed sweet or sour, depending on their sulfur content.

The petroleum industry further characterizes crude oils on the basis of their relative content of paraffinic (i.e., aliphatic), naphthenic (i.e., cycloaliphatic), olefinic, and aromatic compounds. Different combinations and sequences of petroleum processing complicate the situation even more, producing literally hundreds of highly diverse refinery streams. These may be further blended, combined with complex additive mixtures, packaged, and sold for various uses. It is important to recognize that petroleum products are generally defined by performance specification rather than chemical analysis. For example, the types and quantities of refinery streams that are blended together to form automotive gasoline are different for gasoline sold in winter compared with that sold in the summer, and that sold on the Gulf Coast differs from that sold in the mountains of Colorado.

The industry has sought to characterize the toxicological characteristics of the materials it uses and the products it sells. Research sponsored by the American Petroleum Institute (API) beginning in the 1960s led to the understanding that the tumorigenic potential of petroleum oils is due primarily to the presence of certain polycyclic aromatic hydrocarbons and heterocyclic compounds (hereafter referred to collectively as PAHs). API-sponsored research also demonstrated that simply washing PAH-contaminated skin with soap and water reduced the risk of skin tumor development (1). Indeed, this remains the standard workplace recommendation for PAH-containing materials—that is, minimize getting the material on your skin, but if you do, wash the affected area with soap and water (detergents are not as effective). This recommendation is applied to the workplace handling of all oil products. For that reason, the finding that a particular material was tumorigenic in a mouse skin-painting study, while it would emphasize the need for extra care, would not change the basic workplace handling procedures already in place.

Why then does the industry continue to characterize the tumorigenic potential of its products? Part of the answer is that the industry recognizes its obligation to understand the properties of its products and to assure that they are used safely. In addition, a number of recent worker and community right-to-know regulations require the manufacturers/users of materials to inform people of the hazardous properties of the chemicals to which they are exposed.

The tumorigenic potential of a particular class of refinery stream can be described in a general way, but the chemical and physical properties of the stream produced by each particular plant vary to some extent because of the specifics of refinery processing (e.g., crude source, temperature, hydrogen pressure and residence time in the hydrotreater, type and age of the catalyst used, and degree of solvent extraction). It is assumed that because the chemical and physical properties of the product stream differ, so might the biological activity of that stream. As it is impractical to test every refinery stream and all of the various blends in a lifetime cancer bioassay, the industry has sought short-term predictors of tumorigenic potential for use with its refinery streams and products.

This chapter presents a brief overview of some of the research programs that have been mounted by petroleum companies during the past 20 or so years.

SHELL PROGRAM

In the early 1970s, Shell began a long-term program examining the relationship between specific refinery processes and the tumorigenic potential of lubricant base oils. Mouse skin-painting studies were conducted on 21 lubricant base stocks at the Shell Toxicology Laboratory at the Sittingbourne Research Centre. The technical details of these studies have been described by Doak et al. (2,3), but in general, female CF-1 mice were treated with the test material twice weekly for 18 months. At the end of this period, histopathological evaluation of the skin and major viscera was performed. Using the percentage of animals that develop skin tumors and the mean latency period to first tumor development, it was possible to rank these oils according to potency.

These test materials were also subjected to a variety of analytical procedures in an effort to identify a simple indicator of tumorigenic potential. It was hoped that such an index could be used by any Shell location worldwide as a quick method of characterizing the degree of biomedical concern to be associated with a lubricant base stock, regardless of its processing history. In identifying potential indices, chemists at the Shell Oil Company suggested methods involving the measurement of the absorbance at specific wavelengths of ultraviolet (UV) light that are related to the ring size of PAHs. Shell Internationale's chemists favored a method involving the extraction of the test material into dimethyl sulfoxide (DMSO), followed by determination of the gravimetric weight of material extracted, as well as the refractive index of the extract. DMSO selectively favors the extraction of three- to seven-ring PAHs, along with certain heterocyclic compounds suspected to have carcinogenic potential. This procedure was subsequently adopted by the Institute of Petroleum in the U.K. as Method IP-346/80 for use with lubricant-range base stocks (4).

The results from each proposed method showed a clear relationship with the tumorigenicity data determined by Shell's Sittingbourne Research Centre, but the amount of substance extractable with DMSO, as determined by IP-346/80, was found to distinguish tumorigenic and nontumorigenic oil base stocks most clearly. It was possible to utilize these data to establish a content of 3% (wt) of DMSO-extracted material as the criterion below which a material could be considered to be without significant tumorigenic potential. It should be noted here that Shell's focus has been on lubricant base stocks and that IP-346/80 is inappropriate for formulated oils because various additives may also be extracted by DMSO, leading to uninterpretable results.

MOBIL PROGRAM

The hydrocarbons found in lubricant-range oil samples are poorly soluble in the aqueous media used in most in vitro bioassays, limiting the usefulness of the common mutagenicity assays (5). Several industrial research groups have therefore examined the mutagenic potential of DMSO extracts of lubricant base stocks in assays utilizing *Salmonella typhimurium* (6-9). As mentioned above, DMSO extracts PAHs with some preference for compounds with three to seven rings. It is these ring structures that are commonly considered to be the major mutagenic and tumorigenic compounds in petroleum oils, although this relationship is apparently complex (see ref. 10).

Perhaps the most influential of the mutagenicity studies has been that conducted by the Mobil Environmental and Health Science Laboratory, which has utilized an assay system incorporating increased quantities of S-9 and cofactors to achieve an optimization of mutagenic activation (11,12). Using oil samples that have been tested in mouse skin-painting studies not only by Mobil but also by API, Shell, and other companies, the Mobil investigators have found a striking correlation between carcinogenic activity and the mutagenic activity of DMSO extracts in this modified *Salmonella* assay system as determined by a nonlinear regression analysis of the data (13). Correlation is also seen with the weight percentage of three- to seven-ring PAHs as determined by Mobil's GC/FID and GC/MS method (14). Indeed, the data of Roy et al. (13) indicate that the combination of mutagenic activity and PAH analysis improves their ability to distinguish tumorigenic and nontumorigenic oils.

PENNZOIL PROGRAM

Skisak et al. (15) have utilized the modified Ames assay described by Mobil but have defined mutagenic potency by a method involving linear regression analysis of the data derived on 26 lubricating oil base stocks. These investigators have found a good correlation of their mutagenic potency index with tumorigenic potential as determined in mouse skin-painting studies. The Pennzoil investigators have examined the effects of various refining processes and conditions on the mutagenic potency index (16).

SUN PROGRAM

Recently, Haas et al. (17) of Sun Refining and Marketing Company reported on their use of the spectrophotometric method specified by the United States Food and Drug Administration for determining the purity of white oil for use as an indirect food additive [21 CFR 178.3620(b)]. This method measures the UV absorbance of a DMSO extract of petroleum at selected wavelengths in the range of 260 to 350 nm, but the Sun investigators indicate that the absorption maximum, measured in the range of 280 to 289 nm, gave the best correlation (r = 0.91) with the mutagenicity index [as determined by the method of Blackburn et al. (11,12)] in a series of 23 oils. A somewhat poorer correlation (r = 0.77) was seen with the tumorigenic potency (as defined by the percentage of mice with tumors) for the Sun oils. The Sun investigators suggest that the predictability of their method improves with the inclusion of a viscosity correction factor, which was defined for a series of oils found to have a maximum absorbance of about 700 units (presumably, within the wavelength range of 280 to 289 nm). Although the Sun paper lacks technical detail, it provides a perspective on a different approach to developing a short-term index of tumorigenic potential.

OTHER SHORT-TERM INDICES

Work on other types of short-term indices is ongoing. Dr. Grasso discusses his program at British Petroleum examining the value of the nuclear enlargment assay in chapter 13 (see also ref. 18). Other biological end points being evaluated include the sebaceous gland suppression assay, in vitro cell transformation with C3H/10T1/2, aneuploidy, unscheduled DNA synthesis, adduct formation with various macromolecules, dermal hyperplasia, and dermal irritation.

It is clear that the carcinogenic process as seen in the skin of mice reflects a series of complex phenomena. Recent findings by the American Petroleum Institute that skin tumors can be reproducibly induced by certain fuel-range materials containing essentially no PAHs has led to an increased appreciation of this complexity within the industry. It has been noted that the repeated application of such materials to the skin likely results in some degree of chronic defatting and/or irritation of the skin, which may play a role in tumor development. We are now examining histological measures of skin irritation and the role of the resulting cell division in the expression of tumors in the skin of treated mice. We are also examining the implications to our industry of the explosion of information on carcinogenic initiation and promotion, gene-mapping technology, and oncogene expression. Thus, although industry-sponsored research programs are commonly justified on the basis of practical benefit and regulatory requirements, they are now focusing also on basic mechanistic understanding—a biological understanding required by the need to make sound policy judgments on the most effective way of protecting the health of refinery workers and customers.

OPEN FORUM

Dr. J. Smith: I think, as supported by this presentation by the petroleum industry, that when the information suggests that you have a good causal relationship as opposed to just correlation, you can develop a short-term assay that is probably very predictable. Is there any epidemiology to indicate which kerosene streams are or are not carcinogenic to man? Could you expand on that particular work, the predictivity of that, and extrapolating that to man?

Dr. F. B. Thomas: I am not aware of any suggestion of an increase in human skin cancer from kerosene.

Dr. Donald Stevenson: There are several epidemiology studies on refinery workers and distribution workers. There is no general pattern in these studies, other than that the level of tumors fits in with the general background or the healthy worker effect. There are occasions when you get a specific cluster of tumors. For instance, we had a cluster of leukemias in a refinery that has been reported. But I cannot recall any positive information for dermal carcinogenesis.

Dr. Thomas: What I am really asking is: Is the positive in that study false or true?

Dr. Stevenson: The answer to that lies in the exposure data, which indicate that people are not normally chronically exposed to kerosene. However, there are some misuse situations under which you might get considerable dermal exposure.

Dr. Thomas: In the 1960s, when the American Petroleum Institute did its study at Kettering and determined that the polynuclear hydrocarbons seemed to concentrate in materials that were boiling at 500°F or higher, they also did a study that looked at the ability of various treatments to reduce tumor incidence once exposure had occurred. The result was that washing with soap and water seemed to reduce the tumor response of the animals painted with PAHs. That has formed the basis of our worker protection strategy, which is to maintain education of our employees, minimize exposure to all kinds of materials, and advise workers to wash with soap and water if they get anything on their skin. As Dr. Stevenson says, we don't see people who abuse kerosene, certainly not to the point where it ulcerates their skin, so that has colored our epidemiology studies.

REFERENCES

1. Bingham E, Horton AW, Tye R. The carcinogenic potency of certain oils. Arch Environ Health 10:449-451, 1965.
2. Doak SMA, Brown VKH, Hunt PF, Smith JD, Roe FJC. The carcinogenic potential of twelve refined mineral oils following long-term topical application. Br J Cancer 48:429-436, 1983.
3. Doak SMA, Hend RW, Vanderweil A, Hunt PF. Carcinogenic potential of hydro-treated petroleum aromatic extracts. Br J Indust Med 42:380-388, 1985.
4. Institute of Petroleum. Method IP-346/80: Polycyclic aromatics in petroleum fractions by dimethyl sulphoxide-refractive index method. London: Institute of Petroleum, 1986.
5. Cragg ST, Conaway CC, MacGregor JA. Lack of concordance of the Salmonella/ microsome assay with the mouse dermal carcinogenesis bioassay for complex petroleum hydrocarbon mixtures. Fundam Appl Toxicol 5:382-390, 1985.
6. Hermann M, Durand JP, Charpentier JM, Chaudé O, Hofnung M, Petroff N, Vandecasteele J-P, Weill N. Correlation of mutagenic activity with polynuclear aromatic hydrocarbon content of various mineral oils. In Bjorseth A, Dennis AJ (eds): Polynuclear Aromatic Hydrocarbons: Chemistry and Biological Effects. Columbus, Ohio: Battelle Press, 1980, pp 899-916.
7. Hermann M, Chaudé O, Weill N, Bedouelle H, Hofnung M. Adaptation of the salmonella/mammalian microsome test to the determination of the mutagenic properties of mineral oils. Mutat Res 77:327-339, 1980.
8. Carver JH, MacGregor JA. Two aromatic subfractions of high boiling (700-1070 F) petroleum distillates tested in the Salmonella microsome assay (abstract). Environ Mutagen 5:445, 1983.
9. Carver JH, Machado ML, MacGregor JA. Petroleum distillates suppress in vitro metabolic activation: Higher [S-9] required in the Salmonella/microsome mutagenicity assay. Environ Mutagen 7:369-379, 1985.
10. Watson WP, Brooks TM, Gonzalez LP, Wright AS. Genotoxicity studies with mineral oils: Effects of oils on the microbial mutagenicity of precursor mutagens and genotoxic metabolites. Mutat Res 149:159-170, 1985.
11. Blackburn GR, Deitch RA, Schreiner CA, Mackerer CR. Predicting carcinogenicity of petroleum distillation fractions using a modified Salmonella mutagenicity assay. Cell Biology and Toxicology 2:63-84, 1986.
12. Blackburn GR, Deitch RA, Schreiner CA, Mehlman MA, Mackerer CR. Estimation of the dermal carcinogenic activity of petroleum fractions using a modified Ames assay. Cell Biology and Toxicology 1:40-48, 1984.
13. Roy TA, Johnson SW, Blackburn GR, Mackerer CR. Correlation of mutagenic and dermal carcinogenic activities of mineral oils with polycyclic aromatic compound content. Fundam Appl Toxicol 10:466-476, 1988.
14. Roy TA, Johnson SW, Blackburn GR, Deitch RA, Schreiner CA, Mackerer CR. Estimation of mutagenic activity and dermal carcinogenic activity of petroleum fractions based on polynuclear aromatic hydrocarbon content. In Cooke M (ed): Polynuclear Aromatic Hydrocarbons: A Decade of Progress. Columbus, Ohio: Battelle Press, 1986, pp 809-824.
15. Skisak CM, Venier CG, Baker DO. Ames test of lubricating oil products: The mutagenic potency index. In Vitro Toxicology 1:263-276, 1987.
16. Venier CG, Skisak CM, Bell DA. Ames test of lubricating oil products: The effect of processing variables. In Vitro Toxicology 1:253-261, 1987.

17. Haas JM, Dimeler GR, Basil EW, Wilkins GW, Nutter JS. A simple analytical test and a formula to predict the potential for dermal carcinogenicity from petroleum oils. Am Ind Hyg Assoc J 48:935-940, 1987.
18. Ingram AJ, Grasso P. Nuclear enlargement produced in mouse skin by carcinogenic mineral oils. J Appl Toxicol 7:289-295, 1987.

Viewpoints and Critical Issues

The exchange that follows took place at the December 1987 symposium Dermal Carcinogenesis: Research Directions for Human Relevance. In fact this book is based on and summarizes the critical viewpoints and issues that were discussed there.

Dr. Michael Fry: Most sponsors of this meeting are interested not only in the mechanisms of carcinogenicity but also in risk assessment. One key question is whether animal data can be extrapolated to humans. Perhaps the panelists would like to comment on whether animal data can be used for human risk assessment and, if not, what information is needed.

Dr. John DiGiovanni: Our approach is to try to develop quantitative predictors based on biochemical responses. The problem is having a biological end point to relate that to. I do not think there is currently any good way to measure how the level of a particular adduct leads to some type of change in a mouse versus a human epidermal cell that can be called cancer. We need to develop model systems in which we can take human cells and make that quantitative type of assessment. Dr. Rheinwald described a mutagenesis system with human cells that may begin to approach this goal.

Dr. Ronald Ostrow: As far as papillomaviruses are concerned, I think it would be difficult to develop risk assessments for humans based on animal models. However, I think the important thing is showing the biological activity of the agents and how this activity relates to tumorigenesis. In the papillomavirus model systems, different papillomaviruses have different oncogenic potentials. But it is becoming evident that the process of malignant transformation is the same in each case. Thus, animal systems are useful for mechanistic studies, but epidemiological studies must be conducted to directly assess the risk in humans.

Dr. Kenneth Kraemer: The human population is not homogeneous. Some of the laws require protection of all exposed humans. The most sensitive individuals in the population must be identified, and regulations must be based on that sensitivity. For certain substances, patients with the diseases I discussed may comprise the most sensitive population. Cells from those patients can be readily studied.

Comment: With continuous or complete carcinogenesis studies using relatively low dose rates of benzo[a]pyrene repeatedly, I have observed that if the lesions are excised at the point of inception, when their total volume is 1 mm or less, and examined histologically, they are uniform in their morphological characteristics, and there are approximately equal numbers of carcinomas and papillomas. I have concluded that a tumor does not need to go through a papilloma stage to become a carcinoma. I believe (1) that either cells can make this transition rapidly under the appropriate stimulus without having to exist in or develop into a so-called benign state for any length of time, and (2) that carcinomas can arise de novo as well under the appropriate stimulus.

Dr. Henry Hennings: That is definitely a possibility with carcinogens that are applied repeatedly. All the studies I was talking about were initiation-promotion, and there I think it is clear that you need a papilloma stage. Irradiation may produce carcinomas without a papilloma precursor stage, however.

Dr. Fredric J. Burns: I agree that after repeated applications of a carcinogen without a promoter, de novo cancers without antecedent papillomas will arise frequently—roughly 50% of the cancers arise without an obvious precursor papilloma.

Comment: I thought there was some consensus on this point. Are we really looking at comparable phenomena? Is carcinogenesis per se really a phenomenon apart from initiation and promotion? In other words, is there a qualitatively different kind of promotion operating in complete carcinogenesis that results in these much greater probabilities of de novo malignant conversion than operates in the case of the traditional two-stage mouse model?

Dr. Burns: I don't think we can eliminate the possibility that we are looking at two very separate phenomena. My feeling is that the kinds of genetic alterations we are dealing with are the starting points of carcinogenic progression—that we might expect some connection between these two groups. I presented possible explanations of how similar basic genetic alterations could lead to quite different dose and time responses. I certainly agree that there are other possible explanations.

Dr. Hiroshi Yamasaki: One issue that was not really discussed is the possible effects of carcinogens on future generations. Dr. Burns showed transplacental carcinogenesis in offspring, and there is clear evidence from initiation-promotion skin carcinogenesis that there are effects in both F_1 and F_2 generations. If this effect also occurs in humans, it would be very important from a public health standpoint. This could be a future research area. Dr. Burns, do you have any data concerning multigenerational effects?

Dr. Byron Butterworth: Are you talking about germ cell mutagenesis?

Dr. Yamasaki: Yes. Through transplacental initiation, you may be damaging some germ cell genes.

Dr. Burns: I cannot really comment on the possibility that there could be damage to the germ cells that would be transmitted to offspring. These embryonic exposures were somatic; in other words, the embryo was in the process of development. We have not studied further generations of those animals.

Dr. Butterworth: It is a very interesting issue. Does skin exposure lead to risk of genetic damage or cancer within other internal organs?

Dr. Donald Stevenson: We tend to home in on the chemical hazard aspect, but it is also important to focus on the other risk components, such as exposure. An important question raised was the question of the duration and time of exposure. That must be looked at in greater detail. In many cases, we may be exposed to a carcinogen for only a short period of time. Clearly, route is important, although we are focusing here on skin. One compound on the slide of Dr. Slaga's data was hydrogen peroxide. Some recent information shows that hydrogen peroxide given orally to mice produced reasonably large numbers of stomach tumors. So something that we regard as potentially noncarcinogenic via the skin may, in fact, turn out to be carcinogenic via other routes.

Dr. Butterworth: Dr. Argyris, do you think that studies that involve continually painting the substance on the back of the mouse apply to the human situation?

Dr. Thomas Argyris: We don't have enough information to answer that question. I wonder about its importance in terms of risk assessment. I have a gut feeling that whether a company gets sued or not will be based not just on the quality of the science it is doing but also on how society views what they have done. The reality is, if I got a result showing that a substance produced cancer in a mouse with a probability of 1 in 1,000, that result probably would not seem important. Yet this would be considered a significant probability if it applied to humans.

Dr. Butterworth: I think that in dealing with the problem of skin cancer, industry and the regulators should pay attention to the duration and extent of human exposure. It makes quite a difference whether someone is exposed to a substance every day or once a year, particularly for promoters.

Dr. Stevenson: I agree. I think there is a groundswell of opinion that our approach using risk assessment is not going to solve the problem. In other words, we can chip away at all these small risks, but there is still a 1 in 4 risk of getting cancer, and that is what we should be addressing—not the 1 in a million risk. I think we should consider all the factors that can reduce the overall risk of skin cancer, not just the chemical factors.

Dr. Argyris: We have enough information on smoking alone that if it were discontinued, a major cause of cancer would be removed. Yet the population as a whole doesn't see it that way. So I am not sure that addressing the large factors is the right approach; people aren't changing their behavior.

Dr. Butterworth: It seems to me that a very good public education campaign on the national news and in national magazines would be very effective. As the scientific group that knows the most about skin cancer, if you all believe that exposure to sunlight is the most important factor, maybe we should be pushing our government agencies to do more of those practical things.

Dr. G. Tim Bowden: I think public education is very important in preventing skin cancer. In Arizona we have rapid increases in melanoma and nonmelanoma skin cancers. A vigorous public education campaign starts in primary schools to make people aware of UV (ultraviolet) effects on the skin. Also, an index showing the erythemic dose of UV in terms of time is published in the Tucson newspaper.

Dr. Argyris: There is a downside to education. Today, information is publicized so rapidly that much of it changes, so there is a danger that scientists may lose credibility with the general public.

Dr. Butterworth: Perhaps the scientific community should take more responsibility for public cancer policy. The human suffering and economic burden caused by cigarette-induced cancer tends to make other problems pale into insignificance. Yet, for the layperson, the warning on a pack of cigarettes is not that much different from the warning on a packet of saccharin.

Dr. Andre J.P. Klein-Szanto: Although skin cancer accounts for fewer than 2% of deaths in the human population, I believe that the investigation of skin cancer in experimental models is extremely relevant to illuminating the mechanisms of cancer in general. In addition, the skin model is also important as a model for squamous cell carcinoma, which is one of the most important carcinomas in humans. Among our presentations was a good example of how a study on skin was relevant to lung carcinogenesis.

Dr. Andrew T. Huang: How do you define a human carcinogen?

Dr. Paul Grasso: One of the many sources of data on human carcinogenicity is epidemiology. Most of the examples I indicated were based on epidemiological studies. I did not include those compounds that are thought to be human carcinogens because they are animal carcinogens.

Comment: At the International Agency for Research on Cancer, only epidemiological data are used to determine whether a substance is a human carcinogen.

Dr. Butterworth: Dr. Burns pointed out that if you treat with a promoter, you can linearize the dose-response curve. How do you view the risk assessment process? What kind of model would you use with a promoter—one that was more linear or one that had a threshold?

Dr. Burns: I think the point is not to take the animal data in toto and apply it to humans unless you have alternative human data that might lend some validity to the animal results. There is another problem that has not been mentioned much here. It has to do with subpopulations that might be unusually sensitive to the carcinogenic effects of environmental agents.

In particular, there is an epidemiological study of patients who were x-irradiated at approximately 11 years of age for ringworm of the scalp. Thirty-five years later, approximately 10% of that population has developed skin cancers, and approximately 10% of those who have cancer, i.e., 1% of the total population, have developed multiple cancers. Some have developed up to nine cancers. In my mind, these individuals with multiple cancers represent an unusually sensitive subpopulation, which in this case would represent about 1% of the 2,000 individuals exposed. I don't know of any evidence for this kind of sensitive subpopulation in rats. In mouse skin, there is evidence of subpopulations of sensitive mice, especially in Swiss outbred mice. Sensitive subpopulations are an important area for future research.

Comment: In the UV system of mouse skin tumor induction, it has been shown that UV radiation itself induces an immunosuppression and this predisposes the mice to develop UV-induced tumors. There is a corollary in the human situation. People who have received renal transplants and are undergoing sustained immunosuppression have a very high incidence of skin tumor induction—40 times that of the normal population. So some subpopulations are known.

Dr. Butterworth: People who chew tobacco voluntarily expose themselves to mutagens on a daily basis on a localized area. Couldn't we do a better job in studying that population? Is the cellularity and morphology of the skin inside the lips sufficiently similar to that outside the lip to make some comparisons?

Comment: Although the oral mucosa in humans is different from mouse skin, I think mouse skin is still a reasonable assay for studying oral mucosa. The oral mucosa in humans is nonkeratinized. The top layers are nucleated, and they are more permeable than the epidermis.

Dr. Butterworth: We heard here about important biochemical techniques to detect markers such as activation or overexpression of oncogenes. If you could begin to identify those as significant, maybe you could take a few cells from individuals who are voluntarily exposing themselves to mutagens or carcinogens and see whether the same events are taking place in human beings.

Dr. Stevenson: I think models should fit the data and we shouldn't put artificial constraints on models—such as imposing a threshold or a nonthreshold situation or requiring the results to be positive. We are moving through a generation of models that are much more flexible, so the old battles are no longer relevant.

Dr. Jerry Smith: The carcinogenic/tumor-promoting potential of substances varies widely. If I want to do a promotion study with a new material, what treatment regimen do I use? What I learned here is that if I select the treatment regimen so as to obtain sustained hyperplasia, I probably can generate data that show some promotional activity. Dr. Grasso suggests that we need to concentrate on the maximum tolerated dose. What is the maximum tolerated dose for a tumor-promotion study? The Environmental Protection Agency has tremendous problems with new materials for which premanufacturing notices are required. It is now taking entire classes of chemicals for which there have been only a few carcinogenic responses in skin under promoting or irritating dose levels and labeling those classes carcinogenic. Yet when I look at the overall data base, I have to ask whether carcinogenicity of the skin isn't a nonproblem. Other than after irradiation and exposure to polycyclic hydrocarbons, I am not aware of it being a problem in humans. Even though the skin is an excellent model, we need to the address the questions of what an appropriate study is and how we interpret the results. It is not easy. But we need to determine what really does pose a human health risk. Can we define a set of criteria to indicate this?

Dr. Grasso: I don't think there is a consensus on what constitutes a maximum tolerated dose. It depends entirely on what question you are trying to answer. If you want to know whether a compound is a complete carcinogen, you should first do a toxicity test to identify the target organ and then find the dose that produces a minimal effect in the target organ—and I really mean minimal— for example, a threshold level of organ enlargement. This could be controlled during the experiment to look for an increase in pathological lesions. Then you may need to redefine the maximum tolerated dose. In my opinion, this is one way to define a carcinogen that is a hazard to man.

I was involved in a large nitrosamine study with about 16 dose levels. I noticed that at the highest dose levels, there was tissue damage in the liver, and tumors started to appear within about 6 months. They were all malignant and metastasized. At the lower end of the dose scale—approximately 100 ppm—we still had something like a 10% to 15% incidence of hepatocellular carcinomas. There was no histological, electron microscopical, or histochemical evidence that there was any change at all at the lower dose level. So I think it is important to conduct long-term carcinogenic studies at a level at which tissue damage is either minimal or absent. As far as skin is concerned, I think that you have to avoid producing the sort of hyperplasias that have been described for agents classified as promoters and the degree of ulceration I showed here. To my mind, the maximum tolerated dose on the skin is one that produces a minimal effect. If you find a strong effect and you can't dilute the compound, you must wait until the induced response ends, usually in a week or 10 days, and then start again.

Dr. Mark Naylor: To look at risk assessment realistically, you should try to determine the absolute risk, not given any possible exposure but rather based on the actual or estimated exposure levels in humans.

Dr. Butterworth: One problem is that the test animal population is much smaller than the potentially exposed human population so that one wants to look at as high a dose as is reasonable. The other side of the coin is that low doses may not produce effects that might occur at higher doses.

Dr. Stevenson: In the case of pesticides, you can determine the expected human dose from application rates and residue levels. This can be fed into the design of long-term studies, because clearly there must be a no-effect level that relates to that potential exposure. There must also be a series of doses above that baseline dose. You end up with a much wider range of doses than is classically used, for example, in a National Toxicology Program (NTP) study, which might have a maximum tolerated dose and one other dose. In my experience, you often need five or six doses over three or four orders of magnitude to come up with a realistic dose-response relationship.

Dr. Butterworth: I agree, and I think that is one of the positive suggestions we should make from this conference—that we should have a complete dose-response curve. I also suggest that more animals be added to the study to measure the degree of sustained hyperplasia with all doses, so that we can begin to correlate the hyperplastic and carcinogenic responses. That will help us scientifically and in risk assessment.

Dr. Stevenson: Unfortunately, the maximum dose to the skin is limited by how much of the substance will stay on the surface area of the skin. This is a problem with many low-grade carcinogens. With the skin, it is difficult to know precisely what the dose was, so the experiment becomes semiquantitative.

Dr. Argyris: Dr. Butterworth, suppose you could do what you just suggested for a particular chemical substance. How confident would you be in those results? Do you think the government would accept that approach in retrospect as being the best possible approach if, 10 years later, the chemical turned out to have some other human health effects? You are trying to get a risk assessment answer that I am not sure is available.

Dr. Butterworth: I think that we have to apply the best science and mechanistic information that we have. Do you really trust the current skin-painting studies so much that you would bet your life that those are distinguishing between chemicals with risks and those without?

Dr. Argyris: Absolutely not.

Comment: I think we will never know whether the results of single-stage, two-stage, or any animal test are valid for quantitative human risk assessment until we know what the disease burden is in humans and what the quantitative human exposure is that validates that test and draws the nexus between the results of animal tests and human risk. I submit that the answer to the question, Are these data relevant for quantitative risk assessment? is no. They never will be until we have done prospective epidemiology that tells us what the disease burden is and until we have done the prospective exposure assessment that allows us to make the connection.

Dr. Smith: To answer the question, How are we going to be held accountable for our risk assessments? look at how we are being held accountable today for exposure that happened in the 1940s. People are being held accountable for the results of those exposures even though the state of the art was practiced at the time. Unfortunately, we have created a societal type of insurance policy that is saying that those individuals with the deepest pockets will be held accountable and pay for the overall societal risks. I would encourage those people who don't have to make these decisions not to take the position that we really don't know, therefore, we can't make a decision. We have to make the best decision we can based on limited data and resources. I would encourage the development of a profile of or criteria to define chemicals that represent a hazard.

Comment: People have been looking into ecogenetics recently—that is the human variation in susceptibility to chemical agents or UV. Certainly, in pharmacology certain people metabolize drugs better than others, and therefore there may well be a substantial range in the human response to individual carcinogens.

Question: What significance do each of the panel members see for promotional studies for human carcinogenesis?

Dr. Peter Blumberg: Perhaps what we are seeing in tumor promotion in the mouse is really a subversion of normal physiological processes. For example, the phorbol esters look like they are activating a normal cellular signaling pathway—that of phosphatidylinositol turnover. The fact that the phorbol esters are unusual xenobiotics may therefore not be so relevant. The same sort of physiological perturbations leading to a cancer response could occur through several other initial events. For example, we know that half a dozen oncogenes elevate diacylglycerol levels and could thereby activate protein kinase C, so genetic mechanisms could go through the same pathway that we study with the phorbol esters. Likewise, other classes of chemical agents may affect protein kinase C. There have been some suggestions, for example, that the bile acids may be able to activate protein kinase C in colonic epithelia. Perhaps that is related to their promoting activity in the colon.

Dr. Thomas G. O'Brien: There is a danger in extrapolating too much from work based on phorbol esters to the human situation. There are undoubtedly other classes of human tumor promoters. I think we can use the data from TPA (12-O-tetradecanoylphorbol-13-acetate) in the mouse skin model to look at important targets of promoters in human tissue. We have suggested that the regulation of a gene, ornithine decarboxylase (ODC), that we think may be important for promotion in mouse skin might be altered in epidermal tumors. We then looked at human tumors. Though undoubtedly the tumors we studied were initiated by quite different agents than DMBA (7,12-dimethylbenz[a]anthracene) and promoted by quite different agents than TPA, we still saw in some tumors the same kinds of changes that we saw in the mouse epidermal tumors. That suggests that a set of fundamental genes is altered by different mechanisms and promoters create selective conditions. So those genes can force the clonal expansion of initiated cell populations if they are expressed after promoter treatment.

The fundamental point that most of us agree on is that promoters somehow cause the evolution of populations in a tissue that would not normally occur. An assay for this property of promoters is difficult to develop. Dr. Yamasaki has one assay. I would like to see other assays using epithelial model systems. There are many kidney and intestinal cell lines now in culture that are polar epithelial lines. There are tight junctions between these cells that restrict the flow of molecules between two compartments—blood and lumen in the intestine and kidney, for instance. In the kidney epithelial system, promoters appear to open these junctions, allowing the passage of molecules that normally would not pass. Jim Mullen at the Lankenau Medical Research Center in Philadelphia is looking at the flux of such growth factors as EGF (epidermal growth factor) in this kidney model system. Normally, EGF cannot flow from one compartment through the epithelial junctions to the other compartment. In the presence of promoters, the junctions open up wide and growth factors can cross to the other side. That may constitute a profound disturbance in homeostasis in that tissue. These lines of research must be developed to a point that we can look at a wide class of promoters.

Dr. Thomas J. Slaga: I believe we are still far from the point where we can regulate tumor promoters. We cannot even regulate carcinogens. We are not always convinced what a carcinogen is. Because carcinogenesis involves many natural physiological processes, these are difficult issues. Do we know of a biochemical event that relates to promotion, at least in the experimental animal? If so, is there a possibility that that might extrapolate to humans? What type of biochemical event best correlates?

Dr. Susan Fischer: I was impressed with Dr. Argyris' work with physical wounding and similarities with chemical wounding. In some respects, it seems as if a pathological approach may be a good one.

Dr. Slaga: I agree that hyperplastic response correlates very well. Is there an even simpler biochemical event? Under the right conditions, could you be pretty certain you would pick up all promoters by measuring ODC?

Dr. O'Brien: I would not recommend ODC as an assay. We certainly know many physiological agents that induce the enzyme. For example, we have found that one of the best inducers of ODC in culture is distilled water. I think disturbances in the control of the enzyme might be important if we had an easy assay for that. So I don't think we can design a simple test at this point.

Dr. Carl Mackerer: As a pathologist looking at the human literature and thinking about how the two-stage model relates to what we see clinically and how that might compare with what we see when we do complete carcinogenesis studies in animals, I wonder where the papillomas are. There seems to be a missing class of lesions in humans. If the initiation-promotion slow evolution multistage hypothesis is valid, if we really are as "initiated" as the researchers here indicate we are, and if we are subjected in our lifetime to the incredible variety of promoting stimuli that we appear to be exposed to (sunlight, wounding, etc.), then one would predict more benign lesions in the average human. My understanding is that we tend to see, in the normal, average human, malignant lesions—basal and squamous cell carcinoma—that occur singly. They do not tend to arise from preexisting benign papillomas that have been there for any period of time.

Comment: I think the papillomas in mice per se are not important but are the equivalent of the malignant lesions in humans, such as oral and genital leukoplakias and colonic polyps. We are saying that papillomas are not important as an entity but as premalignant precursors of cancer.

Dr. O'Brien: My dermatologist friends tell me there are premalignant lesions, such as Bowen's disease and actinic keratoses. The frequency of progression is usually quite different from the frequency that we see in the mouse. Bowen's disease is much rarer in the human population than basal cell carcinoma, but I think both lesions are considered premalignant lesions, and I think they should be studied for some of the properties that we are interested in.

Dr. Klein-Szanto: That is absolutely correct. These are premalignant lesions, and there are even basal cell carcinomas in situ. There are many more preneoplastic lesions than full-fledged tumors and, practically, solar keratosis is considered to be the premalignant state of the squamous cell carcinoma of the human skin. Solar keratosis is very common.

Dr. Kraemer: The dysplastic nevi are precursors of melanomas and they are not rare. There may be at least 12 million people in the United States that have at least one dysplastic nevus.

Dr. Slaga: Obviously, the typical papilloma-type lesion that we see in the mouse does not occur in humans. I think the important thing that was brought out is the preneoplastic condition.

Dr. R.K. Boutwell: The DMBA-TPA model was picked because in the laboratory we want to get benign tumors quickly. Other initiators with TPA do not cause such a high yield of benign tumors. We picked that model for research purposes.

Dr. Slaga: It gives us a way to look at the preneoplastic condition, even if it is artificial.

Dr. Thomas W. Kensler: I agree with the consensus of my colleagues that we do not appear to have any unifying mechanism for tumor promotion. But I do think there is a utility to some of these short-term biochemical end points, at least in the design of bioassays. I think they can be very useful for establishing dose, exposure frequency, and toxicity thresholds. I think that if investigators used some of these biochemical markers when they designed their bioassays, they would generate more consistent and informative experiments.

Dr. Slaga: In the skin, if you induce sustained hyperplasia, you get a good ODC response, and I think you have a better chance to bring about tumor promotion.

Dr. Boutwell: A battery of tests is indicative of potential promoting activity. No single test is adequate. False positives and false negatives are less frequent if several tests are used to make a judgment, whether one is using whole animal or in vitro test systems. We do not have to achieve the maximum tolerated dose in tests for promoting activity. We pick the dose and frequency based primarily on the degree of induction of ODC activity in the epidermis of the mouse that has been shown to be important to the mechanism of promotion. These changes include the induction of ODC activity, increases in the level of cyclooxygenase products, and an ear redness/inflammatory reaction test.

Dr. Yuspa: I think the general lack of negatives is the essence of the problem.

Dr. Slaga: In studies of complete carcinogenesis or initiation-promotion activity of an agent on the skin, I think acute studies are essential to see what is happening to the skin—to determine whether the reaction is hyperplastic or cytotoxic, for example. For promoters, it would be nice to have some additional data concerning ODC.

I would like to pose a different question. What do you do with data when it is very marginal and the experiment was not properly designed? Can we actually use that type of data?

Dr. Stephen Nesnow: That is a tough question. Someone mentioned earlier that a study that is not done properly opens up more questions than one that is done properly. In some cases, if there are insufficient numbers of animals, you can define bounds as to potential activity or inactivity. If the dose is insufficient, we can tell little about the activity of the chemical.

Dr. Smith: Would some of the pathologists here comment on what criteria they would like to see from a histological point of view for choosing initiating doses and promoting doses? I think this is going to be critical in interpreting the information that is going to come out of these studies.

Dr. Paul Grasso: I think that the initiating dose should be sufficient to produce a minimal amount of cell enlargement that can be seen histologically. Twenty micrograms should certainly produce this. One must avoid having either ulceration or hyperplasia by the carcinogen itself. Otherwise it would make the entire test quite uninterpretable.

Dr. J. Michael Holland: As a pathologist, I disagree with Dr. Grasso that nuclear enlargement is something that we should give a great deal of consideration to until we know much much more about what role these subtle cytological effects are playing. I would prefer using simple clinical criteria—that doses of either an initiator or promoter that evoke any sort of clinical inflammatory process should be avoided. Anything that results in frank, observable skin damage is unacceptable because of confounding influences of all killing and wound repair. Other more subtle effects should be allowed to participate in the evolution of whatever end point one obtains. Eventually, we may be able to sort out the relative contributions of these factors. Finally, I would like to point out that simple, serial photographs of animals are in many respects simpler, easier, and less expensive than diagrams.

Dr. Ben Thomas: It has been difficult for some time for industrial toxicologists to evaluate the role of irritation and what parameters should be used to judge irritation. In Europe, the suggestion was made that many of the tumors that we saw in some of our middle distillate skin-painting programs at the American Petroleum Institute might not be the result of carcinogenic potency per se but rather chronic irritation and prolonged hyperplasia. It was suggested that we might want to reduce the administered dose to nonirritating levels. I think the problem lies in the purpose of the experiment. In the initial screens by NTP and the industry and, in many cases, academia, the idea was to identify agents that caused a specific type of hazard. The problem we immediately saw was that, having designed a study and reduced the dose to reduce the degree of irritation, we were criticized that our lack of result in the bioassay was caused by the fact that we did not treat with enough material. That is something we need to keep in mind when we are considering the design aspects of the bioassay. I think it is very important to think in terms of whether we are trying to do this to identify hazard (i.e., a yes or no response) or whether it is a risk study.

Dr. Grasso: I did not mean that nuclear enlargement should be a criterion for the initiating dose. I meant that if you are using a high initiating dose, you must not go beyond that stage. There is no doubt that you can see this nuclear enlargement even after one or two applications. I agree that if you have a negative result, you may be accused of not putting enough on the backs of the animals. This is why we should carry appropriate positive controls using known carcinogenic oils if we are going to test an unknown oil.

Dr. Thomas: This issue has given us some degree of pause. In reviewing our data for real world samples in this highly artificial mouse skin-painting system, we found evidence of irritation for virtually everything that we tested that turned out to be tumorigenic. This irritation could be expressed as an increase in the thickness of the epithelial layer or as one of the other parameters I mentioned. If chronic irritation is in fact a confound, then repeated application of materials that defat the skin, make it more prone to infection, or cause direct irritation effects make it very difficult to evaluate our data.

Comment: We have seen a fair amount of irritation with treated samples that did not get tumors. So we question the concordance between chronic irritants and carcinogens.

Dr. John J. Reiners: I have attended several meetings like this in the past several years. I think the contribution of the immune system to the carcinogenic process is totally overlooked. For skin alone, there is a significant data base that implicates the immune system in UV carcinogenesis, hydrocarbon carcinogenesis, and melanoma metastases. I also think that modification of the immune system is relevant to the mechanism of tumor promotion. I don't think we can continue to overlook the immune system and its relevance to dermal carcinogenesis.

Dr. A.S. Wright: It is worth noting that Ehrenberg's rad-equivalence approach seeks to improve the extrapolation of experimentally determined cancer risk data to man by compensating for species differences in the operation of all systemic determinants of carcinogenesis (including the immune system) and general extrinsic factors (including general promotional pressure) that determine the relationships between exposure and the overt biological effect. A sound theoretical basis and substantive experimental data support this approach. However, it is important to recognize that the rad-equivalence approach is designed to estimate risks posed by low exposures to genotoxic carcinogens. The method cannot be applied in cases of high exposures that exert a significant promoting action, e.g., carcinogenic doses of mineral oils. There is an obvious need to develop approaches to evaluate the impact of experimentally determined promoting action on human carcinogenesis.

Dr. Thomas: I certainly agree that the role of the immune system has been underrepresented here. I am also disappointed that we have not talked more about the responses of receptors to growth factors. We are aware of data showing that partial hepatectomies have induced skin tumors in mice, presumably because the epidermal growth factor was induced. Likewise, data from the National Institutes of Health indicate Kaposi's sarcoma can be transformed or not tranformed simply by adding growth factors into the culture medium. These kinds of things also create difficulties in interpreting our bioassays. I agree that the process by which a cell evolves into a clone that has a particular competitive advantage in its tissue environment is complicated, and we should examine all the factors.

Dr. Smith: I think we need more studies of the validity of animal testing for extrapolation to man. We need prospective epidemiology studies that involve detailed data on skin examinations from periodic physical examinations in industry, which is a routine part of worker health surveillance. Although I think we do a pretty good job of monitoring employee health, we are not looking at a very high risk population because we have instituted industrial hygienic measures that really virtually prevent exposure. This is underscored by the fact that we know from tumor registry experiences that skin tumors are among the most underreported of all neoplasms. That is in part because they are generally not life threatening, and they are often treated by family practitioners or dermatologists on an outpatient basis. Data are not available for tumor registry and epidemiologic purposes. If we are truly going to estimate this, we will need an extremely aggressive commitment to gathering data.

Dr. Wright: One problem associated with epidemiological studies is in estimating exposures to ultimate genotoxic agents, particularly unanticipated and unexpected exposures that could confound the interpretation of the results. This problem has fueled the development of biomedical monitoring techniques based, for example, on the measurement of hemoglobin or DNA adducts. I believe that information from these studies and from the parallel analysis of health problems will prove useful in determining the causes of the health effects. Some of these monitoring techniques are already being applied in molecular epidemiological programs in the United States and Europe to identify the specific chemical initiators of human cancer. In the case of dermal carcinogenesis, it is worth noting the good correlation between dermal exposure to benzo[a]pyrene and covalent binding to skin DNA and to hemoglobin in the circulating erythrocytes. These findings suggest that hemoglobin may be a useful dose monitor for determining dermal exposures to polycyclic aromatic hydrocarbons. Rapid GC/MS (gas chromatography/mass spectroscopy) methods have been developed to distinguish hemoglobin adducts, ranging from methyl to polycyclic adducts. Furthermore, immunochemical methods have been developed to monitor polycyclic adducts at the level of white blood cell DNA, and class-specific antibodies aimed at recognizing whole classes of polycyclic adducts rather than individual adducts are being developed.

Index

A23187, and dark cell induction, 49
Abrasion, and tumor production, 51, 63–73
    epidermal cell enlargement in, 68–70
    epidermal cell number in, 70
    growth kinetics in, 68–73
    hair plucking in, 67, 73, 78
    relevance for humans, 77
    and ribosome accumulation in cells, 70, 72
    sandpaper use in, 67
    tape stripping in, 71, 79
Acetic acid
    epidermal response to, 74–76, 78
    hyperglasiogenic action of, 49
    and initiating potency of agents, 12
Acetone, as solvent in animal testing, 9
β-Actin genes, expression in tumors, 153–154
Age, and susceptibility to carcinogenesis, 5
Alcohol, as solvent in animal testing, 9
Alopecia from carcinogens and promoters, 51
Ames test, 8, 386
cAMP, inhibiting cell transformation, 270
Anhydrodebromoaplysiatoxin, as tumor promoter, 284, 286
Animal studies
    abrasion in, 63–73
    basal cell carcinoma in, 55–57
    chemical agents in, 54–59
        affecting mouse skin and human skin, 122
    cocarcinogenesis in, 12
    comparison of initiators in, 58–59
    dose-related effects in, 58, 59
    experimentally induced skin tumors, 54–57
    genotoxic metabolism in mouse skin, 319–322
    initiators and promoters in, 10–14
    keratoacanthoma in, 55

melanotic tumors in, 57
metabolism of phorbol esters by mouse skin, 183–189
mouse Harvey-*ras* gene mutations in, 137–142
    relevance to human cancer, 142
papilloma in, 54–55
papillomavirus DNA studies in, 38, 39
progression of papillomas to carcinoma, 81–91
rapid tests in, 8–9
relevance for man, 17–23
    dose-response relationship in, 19
    structure-activity relationships in, 19
    tests for genotoxicity in, 19–22
solvents in, 9–10, 13–14
species and strains in
    in dermal carcinogenesis bioassays, 364–365
    in initiation-promotion protocol, 10
    in response to TPA, 185
squamous cell carcinoma in, 55
in testing for initiation and promotion of neoplasms, 3–12
xenografts of human skin in, 114–115, 178
Anthralin, as tumor promoter, 186
Anthrones, as tumor promoters, 187–188
Antioxidants
    affecting oxygen radical metabolism, 235
    and hydrocarbon metabolism by mouse skin, 171
Aplysiatoxin
    and superoxide production, 235
    as tumor promoter, 186, 284, 286
Apocrine glands, 47
Arachidonic acid metabolism
    studies in skin, 256–260
    and tumor promotion, 252–256
    in two stocks of mice, 257–259
Asbestos workers, lung cancer in, 333

415